from here to
nirvana

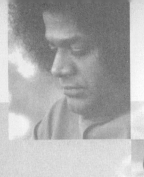

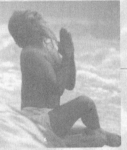

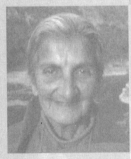

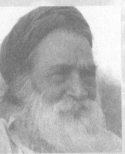

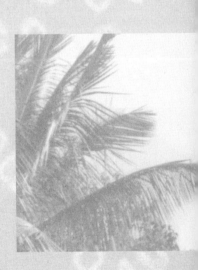

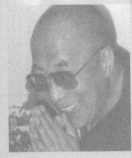

RIVERHEAD BOOKS

New York

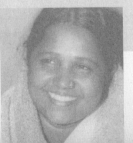

from here to nirvana

the *yoga journal* guide to spiritual india

anne cushman and jerry jones

RIVERHEAD BOOKS
Published by The Berkley Publishing Group
A member of Penguin Putnam Inc.
375 Hudson Street
New York, New York 10014

Copyright © 1998 by Anne Cushman and Jerry Jones
Book design by Deborah Kerner
Map by Jeffrey L. Ward
Photograph of His Holiness the Dalai Lama courtesy of James Gilbaugh
Photograph of B.K.S. Iyengar courtesy of Pablo Bartholomew
All other photographs courtesy Jerry Jones
Cover design copyright © 1998 by Tom McKeveny
Cover photograph copyright © 1998 by Sipa Image/Leo de Wys, Inc.

First Riverhead hardcover edition: April 1998
First Riverhead trade paperback edition: January 1999
Riverhead trade paperback ISBN: 1-57322-715-3

The Penguin Putnam Inc. World Wide Web site address is
http://www.penguinputnam.com

The Library of Congress has catalogued the Riverhead hardcover edition as follows:

Cushman, Anne.
    From here to nirvana : the Yoga Journal guide to spiritual
India / by Anne Cushman and Jerry Jones.
        p.   cm.
    ISBN 1-57322-086-8
    1. India—Religion—Guidebooks.   2. Ashrams—India—
Guidebooks.   3. Religious institutions—India—Guidebooks.
I. Jones, Jerry, date.   II. Yoga journal.   III. Title.
BL2003.C97   1998   97-46026 CIP
200'.954—dc21

Printed in the United States of America

10 9 8 7 6 5 4 3

acknowledgments

Prostrations at the feet of: *Yoga Journal* editor-in-chief Rick Fields, for helping dream up this crazy idea. The whole *YJ* staff, especially Linda Sparrowe and Jennifer Barrett, for getting the magazine out while I wandered around India. My coauthor, Jerry Jones, for visiting more ashrams than I would have thought possible in a single lifetime. All the friends and fellow travelers who offered advice and support in India, especially Shantum and Gitanjali Seth, for giving me a home in Delhi. Lou Hawthorne, for joining me on the road and blasting through my writer's block. Jeff Greenwald, for inspiring the letter that became the introduction. And all my friends at home, especially Jill Edwards, whose friendship, Jacuzzi, and home-cooked dinners kept me sane while I wrote.

—ANNE CUSHMAN

In the ten years I traveled in India seeking out evolved beings, looking for ashrams, and working on this book, many people assisted me with suggestions, advice, and direction. If I could recall them all, the list would be very long indeed and no doubt incomplete. So I give thanks to all the friends and fellow travelers who wrote a name on a scrap of paper or otherwise provided information and assistance.

Special thanks to Gunther Leising, for his original list of names that got me started, and to Alex Merrin and Shannon Jones for their contributions and encouragement of this project early on. To Teresa Kirsch, Deanna Berg, and Linda Kasbohm for research, organizational, and secretarial assistance. To Murray Feldman, David Godman, Catherine Ingram, and John Nance for their review of the manuscripts, valuable input, and friendship. To my wife, Kristayani, for her unflagging encouragement, love, and support.

And lastly to my coauthor, Anne, for her honesty, skill, and tact in editing, adding to, and revising my original drafts and for her research, writing, and the coordination of the overall project.

I would like to dedicate this book to Poonjaji, for showing what is possible.

—JERRY JONES

Guidebook correspondents include:

LEA TERHUNE, a journalist based in New Delhi, India, and the coauthor (with the 12th Tai Situpa) of two books on Tibetan Buddhism: *Relative World, Ultimate Mind* and *Awakening the Sleeping Buddha*.

SITA SHARAN, a Vaishnav sadhu, writer, and teacher of Hindu rituals who divides her time between Boulder, Colorado, and India.

LORILIAI BIERNACKI, a graduate student in East Asian Studies at the University of Pennsylvania.

ELIZABETH USHA HARDING, the author of *Kali: The Black Goddess of Dakshineshwar* (Samuel Weiser) and founder of Kali Mandir, a non-profit organization dedicated to facilitating Kali worship in the West.

contents

from here to
nirvana

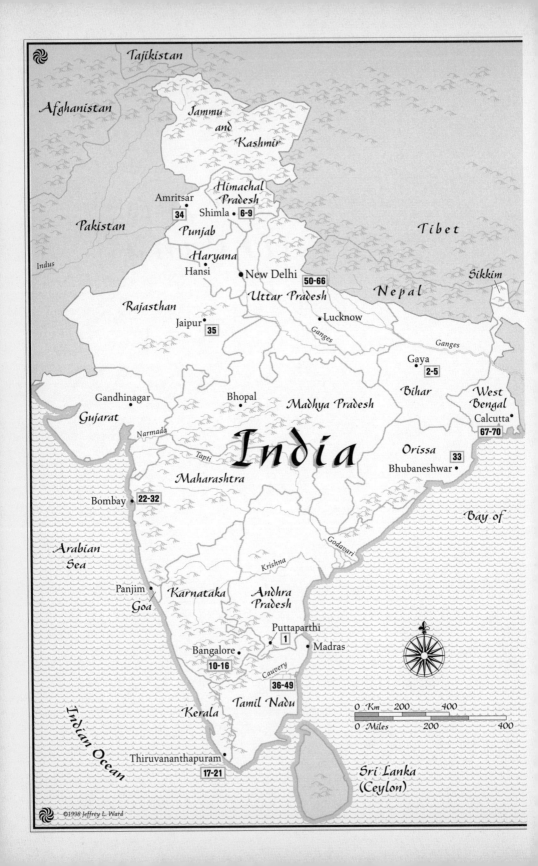

Tajikistan

Afghanistan

Pakistan

Indus

Jammu
and
Kashmir

Himachal
Pradesh

Amritsar •
Shimla • 6-9
34

Punjab

Haryana
Hansi •

• New Delhi
50-66

Rajasthan

Jaipur •
35

Uttar Pradesh

• Lucknow

Ganges

Tibet

Nepal

Sikkim

Ganges

Gaya •
2-5

Bihar

West
Bengal
Calcutta •
67-70

Gandhinagar •

Gujarat

Narmada

Tapti

Bhopal •

Madhya Pradesh

India

Orissa

Bhubaneshwar •
33

Maharashtra

Bombay • 22-32

Arabian
Sea

Godavari

Krishna

Bay of

Panjim •
Goa

Karnataka

Andhra
Pradesh

Bangalore •
10-16

Puttaparthi •
1

• Madras

Cauvery

36-49

Indian Ocean

Kerala

Tamil Nadu

Thiruvananthapuram •
17-21

| 0 Km | 200 | 400 |
| 0 Miles | 200 | 400 |

Sri Lanka
(Ceylon)

©1998 Jeffrey L. Ward

Andhra Pradesh
1 Prasanthi Nilayam Ashram

Bihar
2 International Meditation Centre
3 Root Institute for Wisdom Culture
4 Wat Thai Bodh Gaya
5 Bihar School of Yoga

Himachal Pradesh
6 Library of Tibetan Works and
  Archives
7 Tushita Meditation Centre
8 Chinmaya Mission
9 International Meditation Institute

Karnataka
10 Sri Kailash Ashram
11 Sri Mathrudevi Vishnas Shanti
   Ashrams
12 Shri Shivabalayogi Maharaj Trust
13 Vivekananda Kendra Yoga
   Research Foundation
14 Art of Living Foundation
15 Ashtanga Yoga Research Institute
16 Ganapathi Sachchidananda
   Ashram

Kerala
17 Anandashram
18 Isalayam
19 Sree Rama Dasa Madhom
   Ashram
20 Sivananda Yoga Vedanta
   Dhanwanthari Ashram
21 Mata Amritanandamayi Math

Maharashtra
22 Meherabad
23 Divine Knowledge Society
24 Ramesh Balsekar
25 Yoga Institute of Santa Cruz
26 Gurudev Siddha Peeth Ashram
27 Vipassana International Academy
28 Kaivalyadhama Yoga Institute
29 International Meditation Center
30 Christa Prema Seva Ashram
31 Osho Commune International
32 Ramamani Iyengar Memorial
   Yoga Institute

Orissa
33 Karar Ashram

Punjab
34 Radha Soami Satsang Beas

Rajasthan
35 Brahma Kumaris World Spiritual
   University

Tamil Nadu
36 Saccidananda Ashram
37 The Krishnamacharya Yoga
Mandiram
38 A.G. Mohan
39 Krishnamurti Foundation-
   Vasanta Vihar Study Centre
40 Theosophical Society Headquarters
41 VasaviYogasram
42 Reaching the Unreached
43 Aravind Eye Hospital
44 Sri Aurobindo Ashram
45 Auroville
46 International Centre for Yoga
   Education and Research
47 Sri Ramanashram
48 Yogi Ramsuratkumar Ashram
49 Vellaiyanantha Swami Ashram

Uttar Pradesh
50 Sadhana Kendra Ashram
51 Kainchi Ashram
52 Satsang Bhavan
53 Dargah Hazrat Inayat Khan
54 Gobind Sadan Institute for
   Advanced Studies in
   Comparative Religion
55 Sawan Kirpal Ruhani Mission
56 Sri Ram Ashram and Orphanage
57 Swami Dayananda Ashram
58 Jeevan Dhara Sadhana Kutir
59 Saccha Dham Ashram
60 Sivananda Ashram
61 Tut Walla Baba Ashram
62 International Vishwaguru Yoga-
   Vedanta Academy
63 Yoga Niketan
64 The Yoga Study Center
65 Yoga Sadhana Kendra
66 International Society for Krishna
   Consciousness

West Bengal
67 Lokenath Divine Life Mission
68 Missionaries of Charity
69 Ramakrishna Math and Mission
70 Yogoda Satsanga Society of India

China

Northeastern
States

Bhutan

Brahmaputra

Bangladesh

Myanmar
(Burma)

Bengal

Andaman and
Nicobar Islands

Indian Ocean

welcome to India

India is nothing like this guidebook.

A true guidebook to India should mimic the experience of being there. The book should have a brilliant orange and green cover, with several letters transposed in the title, and the pages inserted upside down. The numbering in the Table of Contents should be slightly off, according to no discernible pattern. Certain chapter listings should prove to have no corresponding text; conversely, certain crucial chapters should not be listed in the Table of Contents at all. As you flip through the pages, your room should fill with the scent of sandalwood, camphor, and cow dung, and echo with Sanskrit chanting mixed with the brash, two-note warble of truck horns.

Information should be vague and sometimes purely invented; contradictory facts should be asserted, with supreme authority, as both being true. Peacock feathers and sacred ashes should mysteriously materialize between the pages. The authors should be credited with multiple honorific titles and degrees from specious universities. The price of the book should be fixed at several times its value, but vendors should be encouraged to bargain.

The guidebook should give elaborate directions—complete with train schedules and hotel rates—to the sites of fleeting and unrepeatable incidents: a blessing from an ash-covered sadhu by a funeral pyre; a vision of Kali in a dream on the cramped top bunk of a sleeper train. It should advertise as coming attractions events that happened thousands of years ago: the enlightenment of the Buddha under the Bodhi Tree; Krishna seducing the milkmaids on the riverbanks near Vrindaban. And in the midst of an indecipherable bus schedule, a verse from the Upanishads should be printed, so shimmeringly beautiful that it precipitates sudden enlightenment.

In short, the entire book should evoke an experience of intense irritation and frustration; but you should find yourself enchanted and unable to put it down.

This guidebook is more conventional. This book attempts to impose order on what is inevitably chaotic. It aims to give you the illusion—as you pack your bags and purchase your tickets—that you know where you are going. The illusion, we say—because a spiritual journey to India is inevitably a swan dive into the unknown.

In 326 B.C.E., when his army marched into northern India, Alexander the Great began seeking out the "naked sophists" whose repute had already spread as far as Greece. He was taken to a band of forest ascetics, sitting on rocks so hot they scorched his soldiers' feet. In one of the first recorded attempts to export an Indian guru, he persuaded one of the yogis to return to Persia with him. But when they reached Persia, the yogi asked for a funeral pyre to be built and draped in flowers. He then sat in lotus posture and burned himself alive before the silent Greek army.

Two and a half millennia later, Indian gurus have become familiar figures on the Western scene. You can find hatha yoga at the YMCA and meditation courses advertised in Forbes. You can log onto the Internet and download enough information about kundalini to keep you note-taking for your next several incarnations.

But a spiritual pilgrimage to India is not, primarily, about information. It's about initiation. And a Westerner who decides to go to the source of these spiritual traditions is entering a surreal world that's as bewildering today as it was in the time of Alexander. It's a land where wandering sadhus light ritual fires in the mountains near nuclear power plants; where corporate meetings are scheduled based on Vedic astrology; where satellite dishes beam MTV into remote mountain villages, and temple loudspeakers blare 4,000-year-old chants over gridlocked city streets. Untreated sewage and industrial waste pour into a river still worshiped daily as a goddess. A major political party offers, as a part of its platform, to adopt all of Britain's "mad cows" to keep them from being slaughtered. India is profoundly spiritual and fantastically corrupt, famous for its swindlers as well as its sages. It's a modern industrialized democracy with social norms governed by texts already ancient at the time of the Trojan War.

India will bend your mind, assault your body, flood your senses, and shred your nerves, from the moment you step off the plane into its smoky, unforgettable perfume of burning cow dung, diesel fumes, and a few thousand years of accumulated human sweat. And ultimately, if you're lucky, your old identity will break down like one of the decrepit, smog-belching autorickshaws that clog the Indian streets—and you'll have to walk on without it, through the twisting alleys of an unknown city, with cows eating empty juice cartons from streetside garbage dumps and ash-daubed mystics chanting mantras in the gutters. It's this breakdown and the attendant possibilities for transformation—more than a specific teacher or spiritual site—that's the real blessing India has to offer.

There's something ludicrous, of course, about taking a guidebook along on such an adventure—like carrying your Daily Planner with you on an acid trip (with notes reminding you to put your pants on before you walk downtown). One of the charms of India is that it incinerates your agenda—leaving in its place, like some sort of vestigial organ of efficiency, a handful of illegible hieroglyphics scrawled on the backs of tattered airmail envelopes. In India, as in life, there's no way of predicting where your teachers will show up. You may think you're going to a yoga institute to perfect your practice of Downward-Facing Dog Pose—only to find yourself trekking up a Himalayan trail, ice-tipped peaks slicing the sky around you, tracing the sacred Ganges to her source in a glacier the shape of a cow's head. You may plan for months to be in Varanasi for Shivaratri, the holiest "Night of Shiva"—only to find yourself, on that mystical evening, stalled in a broken-down train in the sweltering plains, where (shivering with fever, with amoebas throwing their high school prom in your gastrointestinal tract) you find yourself staring into the face of Shiva in person. This kind of derailment is part of the magic of India, where plans often need to be discarded like excess luggage. ("What was I thinking?" you wonder, looking, bemusedly, at your laptop computer, your three extra sets of yoga leotards, your breadloaf-sized tub of spirulina.) As many travelers learn the hard way, the things that you don't let go of freely may well be snatched from you.

But still, as you launch yourself into the dreamlike territory of your personal spiritual pilgrimage, it can be helpful to have some road signs to mark the way. That's what this book is for. It's all too easy, in India, to spend weeks just trying to find an ashram that turns out to have been right around the corner all the time; to spend three days on a hot and reeking train, heading for a yoga center in the northern mountains, only to discover that the one you really wanted was the one by the same name on the southernmost tip of the peninsula. If you yearn for an intimate, one-on-one setting, you may be unhappy being one of five thousand devotees at an ashram whose meditation hall is guarded by a metal detector. If you want information on curing asthma with hatha yoga, you may not get it from a master whose teaching is about dropping concern for the body to focus on the formless, eternal Self.

Of course, what you think you want is not always what's best for you. It could be argued that the misfires, fumbles, and wrong turns are the most important part of a spiritual journey. Still, you'll always be grateful for that old India hand you meet in a chai shop (while drinking cup after cup of achingly sweet tea laced with ginger and cardamom) who gives you the rundown on every ashram she's been to; for the pilgrim in the next seat on the bus (a baby goat trussed in his lap) who tells you, in enthusiastic though barely intelligible English, that the village where your bus's axle has just fallen off is the home of a great saint. This book, we hope, is the printed version of such an encounter.

Like travel itself, this book is inherently random. Trying to describe all the ashrams, saints, and holy sites of India would be like trying to list all the malls in the United States (with a description of the best bargains to be found at each). Instead, like a fellow traveler you meet on a train, we're simply offering you what we know about the places we've been to—with a little bit of hearsay about places we've heard of but haven't visited ourselves. We're giving you the information we wish that *we'd* had as we set out on our spiritual wanderings; and we're trying to answer the questions that people asked us, along the way, about the places we'd been.

This guidebook is not comprehensive. Spirituality is all-pervasive in India. For thousands of years, the continent has been the playground of the gods; it would require several full-length atlases just to begin to chart its mythic landscape. Every mountain and river has a sacred story associated with it. "You are seeing that hill? Across the river only?" a hotel manager will say, pointing out of a crumbling hotel doorway with a few exhausted chickens (looking like birds assembled from parts left over after an all-day sale at the deli) scratching halfheartedly in the dirt outside the lobby. "That hill is the chest of Sati, Lord Shiva's wife. Lord Shiva dropped it here when he was dragging her dead body all over India." He speaks casually, with a convivial wag of his head, as if filling you in on an incident that happened just the other day that might affect which restaurant you eat at. Or, "You know the Bhagavad Gita?" asks the computer programmer on the bus to Delhi. "This place we are passing through now is the very place where Lord Krishna and Arjuna defeated the Kaurava brothers."

For the most part, we've made no attempt to chart this voluminous sacred geography. Instead, the main section of our introductory guidebook focuses primarily on established institutions—ashrams, yoga schools, meditation centers, and places of service where you can go to formally study and practice India's ancient spiritual paths. We've chosen places where foreigners are welcome and where, for the most part, someone can be found who speaks English. Many of the centers we've featured are the Indian headquarters for groups that are already established in the West, like B.K.S. Iyengar's yoga institute in Pune and Mata Amritanandamayi's ashram in Kerala.

Naturally, these criteria have some disadvantages. Some might argue that the purest forms of Indian spirituality can only be found in the most traditional ashrams, where English isn't spoken and you must be an orthodox Hindu to enter. Others would say that you won't find true yoga in the ashrams at all—you'll have to head for the hills to track down a baba in a remote Himalayan cave.

> A wiser kind of tourist shall one day arise who will seek out, not the crumbling ruins of useless temples, nor the marbled palaces of dissipated kings long dead, but the living sages who can reveal a wisdom untaught by our universities.
>
>
>
> —PAUL BRUNTON
> (from *A Search in Secret India*)

For most travelers, though, those places aren't an option, at least when you first arrive. The centers we've selected offer an introduction to the rich and often confusing world of Indian spirituality. We hope they will help you get oriented so that—when you are ready to strike out on your own—you'll at least have some idea of what you're looking for. To enrich your travels, we've given you occasional sidebars on pilgrimage sites you can visit all over India—the holy places of several different religions, which may or may not have ashrams and practice centers associated with them.

But eventually, perhaps, the best we could hope for you is that you will lose this guidebook, drop it out the window of some lurching, overloaded bus, to be eaten by cows along with your banana peels. And that you will find yourself adrift, swept onto a train that you never meant to be on, heading for a mountain you'd never heard of before—but whose name alone, inexplicably, is enough to make the skin start to shiver on the back of your sweat-soaked neck.

how to use this book

This book is not intended to duplicate information that can be found in one of the many excellent travel guides to India. Rather, it offers specialized information about an India that's largely left out of such general guidebooks: the world of yoga, meditation, ashrams, and gurus.

The book is divided into five main sections. Why Go to India? (p. 9) gives a taste of our own personal experiences traveling through spiritual India, so you know who your guides are on this journey. Going to the Source (p. 23) supplies background information about gurus, ashrams, and pilgrimages in general. Getting There and Getting Around (p. 35) gives you practical information about packing, health, itineraries, and other logistics. The Overview of Indian Spirituality is a sort of spiritual Cliff's Notes to the major philosophies and religions that you may encounter on your travels.

The bulk of the book is a directory of ashrams, yoga schools, meditation centers, and places of service. The directory has been divided alphabetically by state. Within each state, organizations have been grouped by city. The index on page 401 will help you track down specific teachers, places, and practices. The map of India on pages xiv and xv shows the location of each center. Contact information is listed both within India and—

when available—for a U.S. branch of the organization. Many groups also have European branches—this information is generally easily obtained from the U.S. contact.

Throughout the book, Pilgrimage Sites sections—primarily compiled by our Delhi-based correspondent Lea Terhune—contain information about sacred sites all over India, with a sampling from the Hindu, Buddhist, Jain, Sikh, and Muslim religions.

Common spiritual terms used throughout the book are briefly defined in the Glossary on p. 397. We have tried to be as consistent as possible in our rendering of Indian names and honorific titles. We hope no offense will be taken at any honorifics we may have omitted in the interest of journalistic consistency and conciseness.

With only a few exceptions, each of the ashrams, yoga schools, and meditation centers listed has been visited personally by at least one of the authors within the last several years. We've done our best to ensure that the information we've provided is as up-to-date as possible; factual information was sent to each of the centers for verification prior to publication. However, the laws of impermanence are in full force: teachers move away or drop their bodies; programs are added or canceled; organizations fold; phone numbers change with almost diabolical frequency. We regret any inconvenience that may be caused by such circumstances.

Of course, the centers listed in this book represent only a tiny fraction of the thousands of ashrams and spiritual centers in India. If we've left out your favorite guru, ashram, or sacred site, please let us know. Your feedback will be valuable in preparing future editions of this book. Send all information to:

FROM HERE TO NIRVANA
c/o YOGA JOURNAL
2054 UNIVERSITY AVENUE
BERKELEY, CA 94704
FAX: (510)-841-9200
E-MAIL: INDIAGUIDE@YOGAJOURNAL.COM
WEBSITE: HTTP://WWW.PENGUINPUTNAM.COM

why go to India?

We once asked T. K. V. Desikachar, the founder of the Krishnamacharya Yoga Mandiram in Madras and a teacher well known and respected in the West, why Westerners should come to India to study yoga. "No reason at all," he responded. "Then why do they keep coming?" we persisted. "Because they are mad," he said.

Perhaps it does take a touch of insanity to set out on a spiritual quest to India. If it's meditation you're looking for, you can find ashrams and zendos in most major Western cities. If you're primarily interested in the physical postures of hatha yoga, you can find plenty of good teachers in California, where you can also drink the water. Wisdom is evenly distributed around the globe. And ultimately—as any true teacher will tell you—the real spiritual journey is into your own heart. "If you have the money, you can go to India," said the philosopher J. Krishnamurti. "But I do not know why you go, you will find no enlightenment there. Enlightenment is where you are."

And yet . . . A journey to India is its own kind of practice, offering its own unique insights and risks. And no one who goes there seeking wisdom will return empty-handed, although the gifts may not be the ones you thought you wanted—just as, in an Indian restaurant, the dishes that actually arrive may bear only a tangential relationship to the ones you thought you ordered. The menu is not the meal—in India, if you forget that fact, it will be rubbed messily in your face.

On paper, there are plenty of reasonable reasons for a spiritual seeker to go to India. You can go because it is the birthplace of four of the world's great spiritual traditions—Hindu, Buddhist, Jain, and Sikh—and the home to a profusion of others. You can go because you want to experience the teachings of yoga and meditation in their original cultural context. You can go because it's the land of the Upanishads, the Bhagavad Gita, the Mahabarata; the place where the Buddha proclaimed the Four Noble Truths to a band of ascetics in a deer park, where Krishna taught dharma to Arjuna as he prepared to drive his chariot into battle, where Shiva gave the first hatha yoga teachings to the king of the fishes. You can go because for thousands of years, its rishis and sages have devoted themselves to the pursuit of the question: Who Am I?—and because, in snowbound mountain caves and smoggy city ashrams, that question is still being asked.

But ultimately, the reasonable reasons are not why you will go. You will go for unreasonable reasons—a picture of Kali in a library book that tumbles off the shelf as you're reaching for something else, a pair of luminous eyes in a dream, a longing that quivers at the edge of your consciousness like an unscratchable itch. The real reasons will probably not be the ones you tell your mother. They may not even be the ones you tell yourself. And you may not know what they are until long after your trip is over.

In the end, every story is different. The following are the stories of why we went, and what we found there. You will write your own.

Anne's Story

I first went to India because of a leaf.

It was a heart-shaped leaf, the size of my palm, pressed and dried to a lacy, delicate translucence. When I held it up to the light, I could see the intricate whorls and branches of its veins, fragile and exquisite as the skin on a lover's fingertip.

The leaf was given to me by an Indian friend, Shantum, when I took the five Buddhist precepts in a ceremony at Plum Village, the community in France founded by Vietnamese Zen master Thich Nhat Hanh. Shantum explained that it was a leaf from the Bodhi Tree in Bodh Gaya—a descen-

dent of the actual pipal under which the Buddha had attained enlightenment. Twenty-five hundred years ago, the Buddha sat down beneath its
sheltering branches, on a cushion of kusa grass, and vowed that he would
not get up until he cut through all delusions and freed himself from the
treadmill of death and rebirth. Under the light of the full moon, he suc-
ceeded.

Back at my home in California, I set the pipal leaf in the lap of the Buddha on my altar to remind me of the Buddha's successful quest. Every day,
as the sun broke through the milky morning fog, I sat in front of it and
meditated on my breathing, according to the method the Buddha prescribed. Then I'd get up and do Sun Salutations on my bare hardwood
floor, folding into forward bends, arching into backbends, spiraling into
twists—waking the life force of *prana* and sending it pulsing through my
body, according to the ancient practices of hatha yoga.

As I practiced, sometimes I'd feel the leaf, tugging on my heart like a
magnet. And it began to occur to me that I should go to the place the leaf
came from. I'd majored in Eastern religions in college; I'd been a Buddhist
for over ten years, and a hatha yogi for eight. It seemed only fitting to make
a pilgrimage to the source of the practices that had transformed my life.
When I got a brochure in the mail, advertising a two-week tour of Buddhist
sacred sites led by the friend who had given me the leaf in the first place,
I couldn't resist.

With a band of nine other pilgrim-tourists, I visited Lumbini, where
the Buddha had been born as a prince named Siddhartha Gautama. I meditated in the tiny, smoke-blackened cave outside Bodh Gaya where Siddhartha had spent six years in ascetic practice, until his spine showed
through the skin of his belly and his buttocks looked like horses' hooves.
I sat under the Bodhi Tree—its trunk swathed in gold silk, its branches
canopied with streamers and flowers—and listened to the sonorous chanting, deep and unfathomable as the mind itself, of hundreds of Tibetan
monks. Under the light of a three-quarters moon, I circumambulated a
half-ruined stupa at the Deer Park, where the Buddha first proclaimed the
Four Noble Truths of suffering, the cause of suffering, and the path to re-
lieve it.

And then I was back in California, jet-lagged and bewildered and un-
accountably happy, with a head full of hallucinatory images dissolving like
fragments of a dream: Adolescent Tibetan monks wrestling and playing
with toy cars in the courtyard near the Bodhi Tree. Smoke rising from a

blackened corpse on the banks of a silver river. A cow standing in the middle of a Delhi intersection, watching the fume-spewing gridlock and assiduously eating the business section of the *Hindustan Times*.

I didn't know what to say when my friends asked me if I'd had any spiritual breakthroughs. Meditating in India, I had to admit, had been no different from meditating in the United States—whether sitting under the Bodhi Tree or sitting in my bedroom, my mind was still my familiar mind, lumpy and chaotic, like an unmade bed. On one level, India was everything that I disliked most: noisy and polluted and crowded and inefficient and misogynist. Breathing the air in Delhi for a day, I'd read, was the equivalent of smoking a pack and a half of cigarettes. Drinking the water was as foolhardy as rollerblading on the freeway. Travelers had told me tales of unidentifiable fevers, ravenous bedbugs, creeping fungoid rashes, tapeworms the length of their arms. "I love it," I heard myself saying. "I have to go back."

Writing has always been the off-road vehicle that takes me where I want to go, no matter how inaccessible. So, with a writer's optimism, I concocted a project to take me back to spiritual India—a guidebook that would also help other seekers go there. It seemed like the perfect solution—I'd travel around to ashrams and yoga centers all over the country, exploring the roots of the traditions I loved. Then I'd write up my findings so that other people would know where to go as well.

To bolster my illusion of knowing what I was doing, I hung up a map of India in my office and dotted it with officious-looking blue and green pins marking ashrams and yoga centers, in a sort of spiritual battle plan. ("What's that?" asked one friend. "Your strategy for taking over India?") When I teamed up with Jerry Jones—who had spent over five years researching a similar project and agreed to pool his voluminous findings with mine—I thought the book would practically write itself.

It wasn't until I got back to India—optimistically lugging my laptop computer, which I hoped to use to modem dispatches to *Yoga Journal*'s page on the World Wide Web—that I realized the magnitude of what I'd taken on. Doing research in India was like stumbling around in a dark room, trying to write about the interior design based on the shapes of the bruises the furniture left on my shins. It wasn't just that the country was so vast and its spiritual heritage so immense. It was that information, in India, didn't come in the shrink-wrapped packages I was accustomed to. The harder I pushed to get things done—the standard by which I measured my self-worth back in the West—the more India contracted, became dense and impenetrable, like a muscle stretched too hard, too fast.

The first thing I had to let go of was my laptop computer—the symbol, for me, of my identity as a writer. Back in Marin County, I had been sure it was indispensable. I had consulted with an expert travel writer on the intricacies of electronic file transfer from foreign countries. I had spent many bewildered hours in electronics shops, pondering the challenges of plug adapters, voltage conversion and regulation, surge suppression, and ungrounded outlets. ("The best thing to do," the salesman at Electronics Plus advised me, helpfully, when I told him that many Indian outlets are two-pronged and ungrounded, "is to carry with you a seven-foot copper pole.")

But my high-tech plans short-circuited at the very first ashram I went to, when I tested the grounding apparatus for my surge suppressor, a custom-made arrangement involving alligator clips and the cold-water pipe in the bathroom. Fortunately, the ensuing electrical fire was confined to the immediate vicinity of my plug; the ashram's main fuse blew, but the Bombay electrician who came to fix it was really quite kind about the whole thing. "Some person," he said, studying the blackened remnants of my surge suppressor, "was not giving you very good advice."

Ultimately, my Powerbook just seemed out of place in India—as overqualified and irrelevant as a Ph.D. at an orgy. Lying in my hotel room near the Osho Commune in Pune—in a bamboo hut on stilts, with no electrical outlets at all, that pitched whenever the man in the next room rolled over, dislodging a gentle rain of dead bugs and decayed palm leaves from the thatched ceiling—I knew it was time to let it go. The next day, I gave it to an Indian friend for safekeeping and bought a ruled notebook with the pages already coming unglued and a picture of beefy, snarling wrestlers on the cover. India, it seemed, didn't want to be captured electronically. She wanted to be scratched and scribbled into increasingly tattered pages, where she would remain illegible, mysterious, and largely unretrievable.

The next thing I had to let go of was my research agenda. The smallest task took days to get out of the way—and the India I was researching bore no resemblance to the glowing descriptions I'd read in *A Search in Secret India*. At the Krishnamacharya Yoga Mandiram in rain-swamped Madras—where the government tourist office assured me cheerfully that the monsoon was officially over—dirty sheets of rain poured down for hours, turning the road from my room to the yoga center into a shin-deep soup of mud, cow dung, human feces, dead chickens, and moldering garbage. Wet clothes draped over my rickety bedposts stayed damp for days; pasty white mold grew on my sandals. When I came home, every day the first thing I did was put my feet into a bucket of disinfectant.

I felt mired in mud in more ways than one. It was like being locked in the musty basement of a house in which I'd been told there was a fabulous party going on—a party to which I was invited—but by the time I broke down the door and emerged into the ballroom, nothing would be left but crumpled napkins and dirty glasses. I kept trying to take a rickshaw to the mystical India of my books—but, of course, the rickshaw drivers spoke no English and usually expected me to guide them to their destination. Unfortunately the roads had no signs on them, and the locals knew them only by names that were no longer on the maps—the titles of Victorian monarchs, the names of long-dried-up rivers and chopped-down forests. In such an environment, cartography proved largely irrelevant, and I found myself blundering around trying to use the landscape to decipher my map, rather than vice versa. And once I'd finally get there—and paid ten times the fare that I should—the place I was going would turn out to have closed two years ago, or to be open only in the afternoons, which is when I'd have an interview scheduled on the other side of town.

Of course, I could try to call first, but that would mean slogging through the mud to the local phone booth—just a phone on a counter in a cycle-rental shop—and it would invariably be out of order, so I'd have to go to the one at the post office, which would be closed for lunch. And once I'd get to the phone and hand over my one rupee and manage, with the help of the attendant, to produce a dial tone, I'd be connected with an official whose English was accented so heavily that at first I'd think he was speaking Tamil. After we said, "Hello?" "Hello?" back and forth about nine times, we would have a conversation that went something like this: "Could you tell me what your hours are today?" "Yes." "What are your hours?" "Yes, madame, today." "You are open today?" "Opening, yes. But tomorrow." "You are open tomorrow?" "Yes, madame." "But not today?" "Yes, opening today. Tomorrow closed." "Open today what time?" "Yes." "And where are you located?" (Moving, in desperation, from time to space.) "Today open." "WHERE?" "Ktrtntlnckrnt." "Excuse me?" "Excuse me?" "Where did you say you were?" "Ktr Llkrcskrtle." "Could you spell it?" "Madame?" "The road you are on." "Yes, we are on the road."

And then it would be too dark to go anywhere anyway, and the rain would be starting again. So I'd go back to my room and read another chapter of *Godmen of India*, with mosquitos materializing mysteriously—like the sacred ashes produced by a guru—inside my mosquito netting, and the TV haranguing me in Tamil through the floor.

I finally started to get the message when I got to the ashram founded by the saint known as Papa Ramdas on the jungly coast of Kerala. Sprawled on the cool clay floor of my bedroom, eating dripping chunks of pineapple under the lazy thump of the ceiling fan, I read the life story of Ramdas, who wandered all over India by entrusting himself to the promptings of Ram, the invisible divine force behind all things. He would get on whatever train Ram put in front of him when he arrived at the station—and disembark when Ram, in the form of an irate ticket collector, insisted it was time. "Where was the train taking him? It was none of his concern to try to know this," Ramdas wrote of his journeys. "Ram never errs and a complete trust in Him means full security and the best guidance."

Chanting drifted through my window—the lilting mantra "Om Sri Ram Jai Ram Jai Jai Ram," which is sung all day at the ashram, as a reminder to surrender to God. I walked through the steamy noon heat to the cowshed, clean-swept as a temple, and fed my pineapple rinds to a cow with luminous eyes. As she licked the juice from between my fingers with a prehensile tongue, I read the plaque on the cowshed wall: "Man, through the cow, is helped to realize his oneness with all that lives. Cow is the best companion one can have. The cow is a poem, she is the second mother to millions . . ." Ramdas had the right idea about traveling in India, I thought. While I wasn't quite ready to travel ticketless, I could tell it was time to let go of the goals I'd plotted in my Daytimer before I left.

This lesson really sank in when I got to Mt. Arunachala, the sacred red hill in Tamil Nadu believed by Hindus to be the physical manifestation of Shiva himself. One hot December morning, I hiked up through the scrub of cactus and lemongrass on a path of sun-warm red stones worn smooth by the bare feet of countless pilgrims—stopping, from time to time, to make way for a foraging pig, or a woman carrying on her head a bundle of lemongrass straw the length of a small automobile. I was headed for the tiny cave where the great teacher Ramana Maharshi had spent seventeen years absorbed in deep contemplation of the Self—the blissful, indestructible, all-encompassing consciousness that is our true nature. I paused for a moment at the entrance—where Ramana used to sit for hours, staring with open, unflinching eyes into the blazing sun—to look out at the town of Tiruvannamalai spread out in the valley below, with its turreted, ancient temple to Shiva. Then I went into the cave itself—a hot, dark, and airless chamber, about fourteen feet in diameter—and sat down in a corner on the smooth black marble floor. As my eyes grew gradually accustomed to the light, I could see five or six other people meditating, and an altar bearing a sculpted red replica of Arunachala, garlanded with jasmine.

I closed my eyes to meditate and sweat, wondering how long I would have to struggle with my own mind that day before I achieved some measure of silence. I thought of the words of Ramana: "O Arunachala! Thou doest root out the ego of those who meditate on thee in the heart, O Arunachala!" And then I heard a voice in my head—not the usual insistent commentary on my experience, but someone gentler: *There's nowhere to get to. You're already here.*

I sat there for what seemed like a long, long time, sinking into the unaccustomed quiet in my mind. Finally, as thoughts of chapattis and dal began to intrude, I opened my eyes and took a peek at my watch—to discover, to my surprise, that only a few minutes had passed since I first sat down. I went back to my meditation. After a long time more, I looked at my watch again—to find that the hands had not moved at all. A few minutes after I entered the cave, the watch had stopped, as if Ramana himself had reached out, put his hand on my wrist, and taken me out of time.

I didn't get my watch fixed (in fact, I had already put a new battery in it, just before coming to India). Instead, I set it under a hibiscus flower on the center of the portable altar I carried with me from town to town. Instead of rushing off on schedule to my next destination, I stayed for several weeks at the ashram at the foot of Mt. Arunachala, meditating on the mountain and performing the slow, ritualistic walk around its fourteen-kilometer circumference that Hindus do as a form of worship. "The act of going round Arunachala is said to be as effective as circuit around the world," Ramana Maharshi had said. "That means that the whole world is condensed into this hill."

And with that, my real journey began.

It's not that I met my guru—at least not in the form of a single person. For me, the main teachings of India were not in the ashrams and yoga schools. Instead, my teachers emerged, like wrathful and benevolent deities, from India herself: The runover dog I saw bleeding to death in a Bombay bus station, in a sludge of sewage and betel juice spit, and his mate who sat next to him, her nose tipped upward, and howled. The radiant eyes of the legless man who scooted himself with his hands down the aisle of the train, offering shoeshines.

After all, at the heart of what all the masters kept telling me—on sweat-slick yoga mats, in meditation halls sweet with jasmine and sandal-wood—was one central spiritual message: The ultimate teacher is always the present moment, whatever that happens to be. In India, this realization was unavoidable. The present moment was always intense, immediate—as insistent as a beggar knocking on a taxi window at a gridlocked intersection, as clear as the Ganges gushing over mountain granite. And I had no choice but to be where I was, when I was—if for no other reason than that it was simply so difficult to get anywhere else.

India confirmed for me that I am fundamentally a nature worshipper. I felt closer to the spirit hiking in the Himalayas—icy slopes disappearing in clouds, the bottle-green Ganges snaking through a water-sculpted gorge—than I did in the ancient temples, no matter how magnificent. Some of my deepest meditations were sitting in an ashram cowshed, contem-plating the golden eyes of the cows. (Sure, you have to watch out for the manure—but isn't that the case with any teacher?)

India is a land of bhakti—the Sanskrit word for devotion to God. In India, devotion is not just confined to the worship of the gods depicted in the temples—330 million of them, by some counts. Bhakti is showered on sacred mountains, sacred rivers, sacred rocks, sacred trees, and, of course, the ubiquitous sacred cows. In an ashram garden in Pune, I watched a sadhu decorate a tulsi bush with bright cloth streamers and bow down before it and pray. In the backyard of a one-room hut in Tiruvannamalai—the home of an Indian family, where the mother prepared non-spicy meals for visit-ing Westerners—I attended a harvest puja for the family cow in front of an altar constructed of dung and milk. The cow—named Saraswati, for the goddess of wisdom—was a young and fretful deity, who licked off the turmeric paste painted on her legs and ate her garland of hibiscus flowers; afterward, we served her a porridge made of rice, coconut, jaggery, and ghee, which we then ate ourselves off banana leaves. It was better than any Mass I'd ever been to.

A deepening of bhakti is the greatest gift I got from India—a bhakti, for me, directed not at the formal representations of the Divine, but at the spirit that illuminates all of nature. One night in the Himalayas, caught out on a hike by a sudden spring blizzard, I spent the night in the cave of a sadhu, a mountain ascetic who lived there year-round, subsisting only on potatoes and nuts. Huddled on a rock floor as cold as an ice-skating rink, shivering under a rat-gnawed blanket, I listened to the crash of avalanches cascading from the 19,000-foot peaks around us. Every time another avalanche fell, the sadhu—tucked in a nest of blankets in an inner chamber of the cave—would toss in his sleep and call out, "Jai, Sita Ram!" "Glory to God," I suppose, is the closest literal translation. I found myself echoing his sentiment. The snow would crash down; he'd sing out his mantra; and I'd hear myself whispering, "This world is astounding."

At the ashram of Mata Amritanandamayi—a radiant woman believed by devotees to be the incarnation of the Divine Mother—I felt the Mother's presence most strongly not in the darshan hall, but on the nearby beach, where I went for a walk at sunset. I walked through miles of fine black sand punctured, occasionally, by little land mines of human feces; coconut palms stooping over tiny huts woven of bamboo and palm fronds; the hot coin of the sun sinking toward the water. I tried to sit and meditate on an altar of black boulders, but the stench of excrement was too strong; so instead I spread my cotton shawl on the damp sand and watched a boy in a white loincloth, knee-deep in the silver waves, tossing his net and hauling out, only seconds later, three wriggling fish.

A soft breeze stroked my face; tiny sand crabs, legs as fine as my mother's hair, scuttled in and out out of their holes. And I thought—What temple could be more beautiful than this planet? What guru more wise? I could bow down to the human body, fragile and glorious; to the placid, generous cows. These are the teachers I want to study with.

A wave crashed in and came roaring up to the very fringe of the shawl I was sitting on. It felt like a blessing.

I suppose it's no accident that the messenger who called me to India in the first place was a leaf. Now that I'm back in California, in my house in a redwood forest, that leaf still sits in my Buddha's lap—reminding me, now, not just of Siddhartha Gautama's awakening under the Bodhi Tree, but of the awakening that is available to anyone, under any tree, anywhere.

When that leaf crumbles, I may go back to India to get another one. But to be honest, I may just pluck a spray of redwood needles from the tree outside my door. I'm pretty sure that will do the job just as well.

Jerry's Story

His hair was twelve feet long, braided, wrapped around his head, and draped across his wiry frame and protruding ribs. His equally long beard joined these matted locks in a pile of hair on the floor around him. The fingernails on one hand extended five inches from his fingertips, and his dark, penetrating eyes held me in a commanding gaze. He looked fierce yet childlike with a hint of amusement in his eyes as he contemplated his foreign guests. Vellaiyanantha Swami had taken no food or drink for ten years, his devotees told me, and had not moved from the chair he was sitting in for twenty-five.

I was on my sixth trip to India, continuing a spiritual quest that had started many years earlier. At that time, my life had been at a turning point. After years of personal and professional success, my marriage had ended and my business had suffered some major setbacks. The things that had seemed important before—like accumulating property and working sixteen-hour days—no longer brought me satisfaction. And what had once seemed like hobbies—yoga, TM, bodywork—I was beginning to see as steps on a path I was longing to explore further. When I went to India in 1986—to attend a conference in Delhi—it felt like the first leg of a spiritual pilgrimage.

I decided to take a year sabbatical, beginning in India with a visit to an ashram, followed by a meditation retreat. The peace of the ashrams and the chance to sit in the presence of gurus appealed to me. I began at an ashram in Pune and worked my way south, traveling from remote villages to smoggy cities. As I met different gurus and practiced different forms of meditation and prayer, I thought how helpful it would be to have more specific information as I made my way through the labyrinth of India's spiritual offerings. On more than one occasion, I spent days traveling to tiny towns that barely made it on to my map—only to find that the guru I was looking for was only in residence from January to April, or even (in one instance) that he had died several years before. Some ashrams I could never even locate from my sketchy directions. I began to yearn for decidedly Western information—addresses, phone numbers, schedules.

Someone should write an ashram guide, I thought. But I couldn't possibly be the one to tackle a topic so huge, about which I knew so little. And besides, if people were meant to find their spiritual teacher, wasn't it all somehow predestined? Wouldn't it happen without my Western efficiency being part of the process?

Then I met Gunther Leising at the Anandashram in north Kerala. Gunther was doing a photo book of the "god men and god women of India," and he had compiled a list of gurus and ashrams from his own travels and from the tips from swamis and sadhus he'd met along the way. With his notes as my guide, I traveled for several months, going from ashram to ashram, teacher to teacher. I recorded information about the ashrams, collected books and pamphlets of the gurus' teachings, and discussed the idea of writing a guidebook with the masters I met along the way.

"It depends on your intention," said Poonjaji of Lucknow. "If you are coming from a place of ego, it is not a good idea. If other than that, it may be useful."

"The worst thing you can do!" said Swami Krishnananda of the Sivananda Ashram. He then suggested a book that might be helpful for such a project.

And Chandra Swami, who had been in silence for fifteen years in the Himalayas, responded to my idea by wagging his head from side to side and making a clicking sound. I interpreted this as, "It's okay. You can do it."

When I had first set off with Gunther's list, I was really looking for my own guru. I was attempting to judge and compare gurus and ashrams to determine the one that would be perfect for me. But as my experience deepened, Sathya Sai Baba's advice echoed in my head. Some people have only one guru and some people have many, he'd written. Perhaps I was the "many" type, rather than the "one" type. I relished spiritual adventures like my encounter with Vellaiyanantha Swami in his tiny south Indian village. But I let go of my search for a personal master and continued my trek around this mysterious and magical country with a different focus— I had a book to research.

By the spring of 1993, I was on my fifth trip to India, with ashrams in Maharashtra, Gujarat, and Rajasthan on my agenda. At my first stop, a fellow pilgrim asked if I planned to visit Lucknow to see a guru named Poonjaji. I had heard of Poonjaji, but my plans were to head in the opposite direction, so I did. But at the very next ashram, I was asked again: Had I heard of Poonjaji? Did I plan to visit Lucknow?

That evening as I meditated, the words kept swirling around in my head: Luck Now, Now Lucky, Lucky Now, Lucknow Now. A great name for a guru's town, I thought. I contemplated my carefully crafted travel agenda, leading me in the opposite direction. After debating the logistics of an alternate route, I decided I would leave it up to the travel gods—I would go wherever I could get the best train and plane connections.

And so I found myself on a flight to Delhi and an overnight train to Lucknow. I arrived in the Lucknow satsang hall about halfway through satsang and quietly took a seat in the back. As soon as I sat down, I knew right away that something was different. I felt a heightened sense of energy and alertness, oddly similar to the feeling I felt in the real-estate business when I smelled a really good deal. After satsang, I bought a book on Poonjaji in the ashram bookstore, found a room nearby, and spent most of the day reading.

I awoke the next morning at 4 a.m., feeling wide awake and energetic. Every cell in my body seemed to be on high alert. I sat down to write a letter, which I passed to Poonjaji at satsang the next day. In the middle of satsang, Poonjaji pulled out my letter and called me up to sit with him at the front of the group. He read my letter aloud: "In your book, you say that the real master looks into your mind and heart, sees what state you are in, and gives advice which is always appropriate and relevant. Will you look into my heart and mind and give me such advice?"

Poonjaji studied my short letter for a long time. Then he began to ask me a series of questions. "You have come from where? You just came yesterday? Who was it that arrived? Who are you? Who is possessing the body that just arrived?"

Confused, I weakly answered, "I know that I am consciousness." His energy was focused on me like a laser, and I fell silent. "And why are you quiet now?" he asked.

"I don't have an answer."

"You will have an answer when there is something in front of you. What have you lost in this quietness?"

"I've lost my questions," I replied.

"With the losing of the questions, the questioner has also been lost. No I, no questions. Tell me, without I, how do you feel?"

"Warm," was all I could answer.

Poonjaji giggled. "That warmth is called love," he said. "Keep quiet now."

In that moment, I felt all my questions fall away. All I needed was to be where I was.

In the weeks that followed, I remained in a quiet, blissful state. No effort was needed—all of my actions seemed to unfold on their own. And some of that bliss and peace stays with me to this day.

"How do I know when I've met my guru?" I asked Poonjaji just before I left to return to the States. "Your true guru is inside you," he replied. "Your outside guru is the one that shows you that your true guru is inside you." I knew, as I was leaving for home, that Poonjaji was my outside guru. He had introduced me to the joy and love of the guru inside me. In the end it was not an intellectual decision for me, but rather a deep, inner knowing. I left Lucknow with a great sense of peace.

I don't know that "keep searching" is the advice I would give to others who are looking for a guru. Maybe your true guru is the parking attendant in your office garage, or your strange Aunt Mildred, as Ram Dass pointed out. What I do know is that the ten trips and twenty months I spent traveling in India have been an incredible blessing, and I still go back almost every winter to get my windshield clean. India clears my vision, focuses my priorities, shines a light on my path. So whenever people ask me about traveling to India, all I can say is simply, "Go."

going to the source

When we first set out to write this book, we called it a guide for people who wanted "to go to the source of yoga." By "yoga," we didn't just mean the system of physical postures and breathing exercises that has become America's latest fitness cult (presided over by such unlikely gurus as Jane Fonda, Sting, and Ali MacGraw). We meant the full range of mystical technologies developed in India over thousands of years to bring about the exquisitely blissful "union"—the literal meaning of the word "yoga"— of the finite Self with the Infinite.

Of course, the source of yoga is not really in India. It's in the heart and soul of each individual practitioner. You don't need to travel thousands of miles to find it; you certainly don't need to buy our book. The Infinite is as close as your own breath, your own heartbeat.

But India has spawned a wide range of practices for tapping into that inner wellspring of bliss, which are still being taught all over the country in venues ranging from mud-and-tarp shacks and Himalayan caves to government-accredited yoga universities. Many of these practices have already been exported to the West. As often happens when shipping packages from India, however, many of them have arrived in fragments. We've re-

Except in the rarest of cases, spiritual work of any real depth and duration is not possible without a teacher. . . . How does a person awaken and sustain the deepest creative flow within him- or herself without the support of someone who has experienced the process already? We would not presume to study any other extraordinarily subtle and sophisticated discipline without the guidance of a mentor. Spiritual work is no different.

Moreover, the process of inner work confronts us with so much intensity at various moments that without a guide most of us would falter, drop away, or even fall apart in the face of it. We require someone who can not only arouse within us the experience of our deeper awareness but who can also support us as we undergo the internal changes necessary to explore that awareness and establish ourselves within it.

—SWAMI CHETANANANDA
(from Dynamic Stillness,
Part Two: The Fulfillment of Trika Yoga)

ceived bits and pieces of teachings, snapped off from their cultural and philosophical roots.

In the West, our introduction to yoga may come via a *Buns of Steel* workout tape; our introduction to meditation via a corporate stress-reduction seminar at Apple Computer. A journey to India offers the chance to experience these teachings in their original context—and to sit with masters who have devoted their lives to studying and practicing them. As one Indian yoga student said, only half joking, "You are coming to India to study yoga for the same reason that we are going to Europe for open-heart surgery. Yes, we have doctors who can do it here—but if we fly to London, we know it will be done right."

Of course, an Indian letterhead alone is no guarantee of quality. In India, as in the West, spirituality is potentially big business; and swamis, like rickshaw drivers, can be quick to take advantage of a gullible foreigner. When the advaita vedanta master Poonjaji went looking for an enlightened teacher, all he found, he said, were "businessmen in robes." Holy sites are swarming with pseudo-sadhus, ranging from orange-clad, mala-wielding beggars (who will dispense a blessing in exchange for a cup of chai) to jewel-decked gurus with palatial ashrams and their own private planes

> Every sensible aspirant to higher consciousness must . . . learn to make a clear distinction between the claims of the pseudo-yogis and the sensational results they promise and the true yogic disciplines, which demand a balanced life, regulated behavior and appetites, self-subdual, devout application, and a keen power of discrimination between right and wrong or good and bad. Side by side with the counterfeit, there are noble sadhus and ascetics in India whose lives are an example of purity, saintliness, and renunciation. But since they are unpretentious and humble, choosing solitude and simplicity to ostentation and display, they are seldom known or accessible to the seeking crowds.

—GOPI KRISHNA
(from Living with Kundalini)

(whose blessings may be considerably more costly). Since the Indian government has started to require that hatha yoga be taught in the schools, "yoga teacher" has suddenly become a respectable field, and government-accredited institutions are cranking out career yogis who may be inspired less by divine summons than by job security.

But it is still possible to find genuine teachers and genuine teachings—with the help of synchronicity, discrimination, and a bit of divine guidance. Remember the advice the tantric teacher Vimalananda once gave a student: "If you want to find out whether or not a sadhu is genuine, first go to see him, but don't ask any questions. Sit quietly and don't say much; listen, and try to keep your mind blank. If when you sit near him, you find yourself forgetting the things of the world and becoming more peaceful, then he is a good saint; his halo is quieting your mind. If not, run away!"

Gurus and Teachers

In this guidebook, we'll introduce you to more than seventy ashrams, yoga schools, meditation centers, and service organizations where teachers of various persuasions can be found. Some of these teachers call themselves gurus (or are called that by their devotees); others vigorously shun the term. (In non-Hindu traditions, in fact, the word "guru" does not even properly apply, although they may have enlightened masters who serve somewhat the same function.) For our part, we've made no attempt to judge or rate teachers—we've simply laid out their teachings, in the hopes that they will speak for themselves.

Ancient texts distinguish multiple levels of teachers, ranging from God-realized masters—whose mere presence is enough to ignite the fires of enlightenment—to pious bureaucrats who can't do much but stamp your spiritual papers. It's important not to confuse one with the other. But it's also important to stay open to the possibility that the person sitting before you—whether a silk-robed teacher on a flower-draped dais or a leprous beggar in a Calcutta gutter—can be your gateway to awakening.

In traditional Hindu philosophy, the guru is the "dispeller of darkness," an enlightened being who has realized the true nature of reality and can help you do the same. An awakened consciousness can be contagious; just by sitting in the force field of a master, your own mind can be brought to rest. "Guru is God embodied in human form to liberate souls from ignorance. Guru is the divine doctor, who cures us by giving us knowledge of Self," wrote the Indian saint known as Papa Ramdas. "A God-realized soul alone can awaken and kindle another soul. Reading books alone will not do. The contact of great souls who have realized God is essential."

A fully awakened teacher is considered to be an embodiment of the Divine. In this worldview, the mere sight—or darshan—of a realized being is a powerful blessing, the equivalent of lifetimes of spiritual practices; and the profound initiatory relationship between guru and chela, or disciple, is a bond that carries over from lifetime to lifetime. In some traditions, the guru is credited with the power to transmit a jolt of shakti, or spiritual en-

> Remember that with every step, you are nearing God, and God too, when you take one step towards Him, takes ten towards you. . . . When the road ends and the Goal is gained the pilgrim finds that he has traveled only from himself to himself, that the way was long and lonesome, but that the God whom he reached was all the while in him, around him, with him, and beside him.
>
>
>
> —SATHYA SAI BABA

ergy, that can jump-start the disciple's own spiritual generator. At the very least, a good teacher is a potent role model, a guide who has walked the path ahead of you and can keep you from stumbling into potholes or blundering off the road entirely.

On a practical level, a guru often acts as a village priest or godfather, assisting his followers in all aspects of their lives. Indian devotees often seek the guru's advice on practical matters such as career decisions or the marriage of a child. Other gurus remain in silence *(mauna)*, transmitting awakening through the sheer force of their presence. While some Westerners find such silence frustrating at first, many people report that the most powerful teachings occur in the absence of words, as their own inner wisdom awakens to answer their questions.

Traditionally, gurus are divided into two types. *Mukta* gurus behave predictably and rationally and offer specific, consistent spiritual teachings. *Siddha* gurus are unpredictable, often to the point of apparent lunacy, as if drunk on God. They convey their teachings not through step-by-step instructions, but through shattering their disciples' rational, limited minds.

In reality, unfortunately, some so-called gurus may be less than fully awakened. "Many are the gurus who rob the disciple of his wealth, but rare is the guru who removes the afflictions of the disciples," lamented an eleventh-century tantric text. "There are many gurus, like lamps in house after house, but hard to find, O Devi, is the guru who lights up all like the sun." Western newspapers have reported on an epidemic of scandals involving teachers from almost every spiritual tradition. And fallen gurus are not confined to the West—*India Today* recently reported on one well-known Indian teacher who was jailed after gold bullion and two dead bodies were found at his ashram.

With the stakes this high, it's essential to use discrimination when looking for a teacher. Don't assume that someone's a master based on an orange costume and a Sanskrit name as long and curly as his beard. The Dalai Lama recommends observing a teacher for twelve years before surrendering. If your patience won't last that long (not to mention your visa), at least follow the commonsense precautions described on page 28.

It's also important to remember that you can learn a lot from someone who may not be your ultimate teacher—and that, in fact, there may not be any one "perfect master" for you. As one swami from the Sivananda Yoga Center commented, many Westerners come to India looking for enlightenment, when maybe all they're ready for is a few basic breathing exer-

Early Warning Signs of Spiritual Blight

Spiritual groups—like families, corporations, therapy groups, and marriages—are susceptible to the full range of human foibles. Wandering the spiritual path by no means protects us from the normal dose of folly that accompanies any other human endeavor. Spiritual work is perhaps all the more ripe for foibles because of the excellent cover-up that self-deception lends for the use of the spirit in the service of the ego, libido, and pocketbook.

Be wary when you notice the first signs of:

Taboo topics. Questions that can't be asked, doubts that can't be shared, misgivings that can't be voiced.

Secrets. The suppression of information, usually tightly guarded by an inner circle.

Spiritual clones. In its minor form, stereotypic behavior, such as people who walk, talk, smoke, eat, and dress just like their leader; in its more sinister form, psychological stereotyping, such as in an entire group of people who manifest only a narrow range of feeling in any and all situations.

Groupthink. A party line that overrides how people actually feel.

The elect. A shared delusion of grandeur that there is no Way but this one. The corollary: you're lost if you leave the group.

No graduates. Members are never weaned from the group.

Assembly lines. Everyone is treated identically, no matter what their differences.

Loyalty tests. Members are asked to prove loyalty to the group by doing something that violates their personal ethics.

Duplicity. The group's public face misrepresents its true nature.

Unifocal understanding. A single worldview is used to explain anything and everything; alternate explanations are verboten. For example, if you have diarrhea it's "Guru's Grace." If it stops, it's also Guru's Grace. And if you get constipated, it's still Guru's Grace.

Humorlessness. No irreverence allowed. Laughing at sacred cows is good for your health.

—DANIEL GOLEMAN, PH.D.

cises. "You don't need a Ph.D. to teach a kindergartener," he said. "And if the student isn't ready, he will not even see the real masters."

And ultimately, the real teacher will never be found outside yourself. "Going within means just listening to your own Guru. And this Guru is your own Self," said Poonjaji. "The real Guru will introduce you to the Guru within and ask 'you' to keep quiet. This is your own grace. It comes from within you. No one else can give you this grace."

About Ashrams

For the most part, gurus don't start ashrams; disciples do. An ashram—which some books define simply as "the abode of the guru"—is a community of seekers that grows up around a teacher; all of the physical facilities exist only to facilitate the transmission of the teachings.

The spiritual centers described in this book range from a tiny cave in a hillside with a few cots for devotees to a palatial personal-growth resort with a bar and an Olympic-size swimming pool; from a sylvan Himalayan retreat where you can do walking meditation in a pine forest to a city complex where you may want to wear a pollution mask as you walk to satsang. Some have a full and highly organized program; others have no structure. Some require that you stay at the ashram without leaving the premises; others have no residential facilities at all. Some insist that you work at community chores; others prefer that you use all your time for formal spiritual practices. Some follow traditional Hindu, Buddhist, or Christian rituals; others denounce all religious forms as restrictive social conventions.

They all have one thing in common, though; they're dedicated, at least in theory, to the path of self-realization. The word "ashram" comes from a Sanskrit word meaning effort, and as one ashram's rulebook explains, an ashram is not a place "for recreation or passing one's time." (This, despite the recent article on "the cosmic circuit" in *Condé Nast Traveller*, which advised, "You are there to have a good time, maybe do a little work on yourself, but primarily to relax.") Rather, it's a place for turning inward for meditation, prayer, ritual, and spiritual renewal. If there's a resident guru or teacher, the ashram gives you a chance to interact with him or her—either through darshan (the sight of the guru, which is considered to be a blessing), satsang ("sharing of truth," generally in the form of talks or question-and-answer periods), or sometimes even private interviews.

This guidebook includes not only traditional ashrams, but yoga and meditation centers offering systematic courses in the techniques of awakening. Some of these centers are associated with traditional ashrams; others are more like Western schools or retreat centers. Because many spiritual seekers are drawn to the path of selfless service—what's traditionally called "karma yoga," the yoga of action—we've also included spiritually oriented service organizations dedicated to helping India's poor. These organizations may or may not have a spiritual teacher or residential facilities associated with them.

❧ **Facilities.** Ashram accommodations vary considerably—some are much more comfortable than the average Indian hotel, while others are simply bare cells. They're nearly always clean, quiet, and well-maintained, however. Most ashrams have dormitories or shared rooms; some offer private rooms as well. Most provide beds or mattresses, bedding, and mosquito nets if necessary. However, at some you'll have to purchase these items in a nearby town. If you'll be traveling from one to another, you may want to carry along a pillowcase, a sleeping sack made from two sheets sewn together (you can get this made quite cheaply in India), and a piece of fabric (about four feet by six feet) that can serve as a bedcover, meditation shawl, and even towel.

Generally bathrooms are communal and toilets are Indian-style (floor-level, with a nearby tap or bucket of water for cleaning yourself). Toilet paper may or may not be available. Showers may or may not have hot water (although cold water is rarely a problem in the Indian climate). Showers are usually Indian-style, with a faucet, bucket, and pitcher for pouring water on yourself.

Ashram facilities often include libraries, meditation rooms, flower and vegetable gardens, temples, and walking paths. See individual entries for more details.

❧ **Meals.** Food is always vegetarian and can range from excellent to mediocre. At the very least, however, it's usually clean and plentiful. In general, ashrams are among the safest places in India to eat. Water is generally filtered; the food is prepared by devotees with care and attention to detail. Many ashrams have their own vegetable gardens and a few cows for milk and curd. Food is usually served Indian style—you'll sit on a mat on the floor and eat with your hand or a spoon from a plate or banana leaf. (Eat with the right hand only, as the left is considered unclean. If sitting on the floor is painful for you, don't give up the spiritual quest and go home—chairs are usually available upon request.)

🌀 **Dress.** Modest, practical attire is essential. Shorts are not appropriate for men or women; women should be sure that their clothes are loose-fitting and cover the shoulders and upper arms as well as the legs. For women, a scarf draped over the chest is recommended (and even required at some ashrams). Clothes should be comfortable and durable for working in the garden or kitchen, or marathon sittings at meditation, darshan, or satsang. Shoes should slip on and off easily (since it's considered extremely offensive to wear them into a home, temple, or satsang hall).

As a gesture of respect, make sure that your clothes are clean and properly mended (however challenging a practice this may seem in a land where just inhaling seems to get you dirty). One traditional story tells of a ragged man who bolted at the sight of a saint, returning only when he had fresh clothes on—it's important, the story concludes, to come to a holy person "clean on the outside as well as the inside."

🌀 **Cost.** Most ashrams do not charge for lodging or meals, although there may be a "suggested donation" to cover operating costs. Remember that ashrams are generally funded exclusively by donations—it's definitely not good karma to treat them as cheap hotels. As a relatively wealthy foreigner, you may wish to donate more than the local Indians do, thereby subsidizing the spiritual quest of someone with less money.

In addition to their services to pilgrims and devotees, many ashrams run charitable projects such as leper colonies, medical clinics, schools, and model industries. Consider giving as generously as you can. As Mother Teresa once said to a wealthy businessman, "Give until it hurts."

🌀 **Work.** A part of ashram life is community work—often described in the schedule as "seva" (service) or "karma yoga." Keeping an ashram running takes considerable effort, from preparing and cleaning up after meals to gardening to scrubbing floors. In addition, some communities run cooperative farms, cottage industries, presses, and other businesses.

At some ashrams, even short-term guests are expected—and even required—to participate in this work for several hours a day as part of their spiritual training. In fact, you may find that you spend more time chopping vegetables than singing bhajans. At others, however, work is discouraged in favor of more formal practices. As a visitor to Mother Krishnabai's ashram was sweetly informed when he asked about seva, "Mother prefers that you work on yourself." See individual entries for more information about work requirements.

❧ **Silence.** Silence as a spiritual discipline has been practiced by religious orders for centuries. Many of the most revered gurus of India—such as Ramana Maharshi, Meher Baba, and others—spent years in total silence. The practice of silence is often prescribed as a tool for quieting the mind, helping us realize our true nature.

Many ashrams advocate periods of silence in their posted guidelines, but adherence to this policy varies greatly. Be sure to respect ashram rules about when and where to talk.

❧ **Etiquette.** Your stay may go more smoothly if you remember the following points:

- It's traditional—though not obligatory—to take a small present or offering to the guru or teacher, such as fruit, flowers, or sweets. Often the guru will redistribute these gifts as prasad (food blessed by the guru that is considered to convey spiritual nutrients).
- Devotees often show their respect and devotion by prostrating before the guru or touching his or her feet. This custom often makes Westerners uneasy, although it comes as second nature to Indians, who traditionally extend this courtesy to their parents, grandparents, schoolteachers, and other respected figures. If prostrations make you queasy, you can simply acknowledge the teacher by placing your hands together as if in prayer. (In fact, some gurus actively discourage more dramatic shows of devotion.) In any interaction with a teacher, sincerity and honesty are much more important than form.
- Shoes should be removed before entering the temple, satsang or meditation hall, or dining area. In some cases the entire ashram grounds is a shoes-off zone. When in doubt—take them off.
- Most ashrams cultivate a contemplative atmosphere. It's exciting to swap enlightenment stories with visitors from around the world—but remember that too much socializing may distract others and destroy the tranquil environment that many people have come for.

- Photography may or may not be permitted—you may want to ask permission before taking pictures, especially of the guru or teacher.
- Traditional Hindu ashrams prohibit women from entering the temple during menstruation.

Finally, remember that most true ashrams are not competitive. Sincere seekers are usually welcome to stay at an ashram without professing their allegience to the resident guru. Feel free to explore any ashram with an open but discriminating mind.

Spiritual Pilgrimage

Some spiritual seekers prefer not to visit ashrams or teachers at all, but to make a pilgrimage instead to some of India's thousands of sacred sites. "The milk of the cow in reality pervades the whole body of the animal through its blood, but you cannot milk it by squeezing the ears or the horns; you can get the milk only from the teats," said the mystic Ramakrishna. "Similarly, God pervades the universe everywhere, but you cannot see him everywhere. He manifests Himself more readily in sacred temples which are full of the spirit of devotion diffused by the lives and spiritual practices of the devotees of former times."

India is bristling with such sacred sites—known in the Hindu tradition as tirthas, a word that literally means ford or crossing. A tirtha is a place where a pilgrim can cross from the mundane to the sacred, from ordinary reality to the timeless, transcendent world of the spirit. They are places where gods battled demons, saints performed miracles, great souls entered or discarded their bodies. Sometimes the land itself is considered to be an incarnation of the Divine: Perhaps the ultimate tirtha is the holy river Ganga, worshipped as a goddess, where a pilgrim can cross the waters of samsara—the endless cycle of birth and death—and arrive at the shore of liberation. A dip in the Ganges washes away sin, it's said, and a mere sip of her water drives away the Lord of Death.

A pilgrimage, or yatra, to a sacred site is not a vacation. On a yatra, you forfeit tourism and enter into a voyage of discovery of the Self. What's most important is not where you go, but your attitude: your willingness to shed the crumpled skins of your ego and open to the cosmic mysteries. Superficially, a pilgrimage site may look like any other place in India—noisy, garbage-strewn, crowded with picnickers carrying radios blaring Hindi film songs and peddlers harassing you to buy virulently dyed soft drinks and plastic statues of unrecognizable deities. What makes it mystical is your ability to look beyond the surface.

Pilgrims prepare for a yatra with fasting, worship, prayer, and—most important—study of the sacred site they are planning to visit. Traditionally, pilgrims were advised to travel on foot: "If one employs a conveyance, he will lose half of his merit," advised one text. "If he takes advantage of shoes or an umbrella, he will still further reduce his merit. If he carries on business on the way, three-fourths of the merit is gone, and by accepting a gift, he loses all merit." Modern pilgrims often travel by bus and train, but the principle remains the same: to leave the familiar comforts and activities of home and surrender to the unknown. Everything that happens on a pilgrimage is grist for the spiritual mill, and all experiences have a single purpose: to awaken the soul.

Throughout this book, we've offered descriptions of some of India's most important pilgrimage sites of several different spiritual traditions. This information is in no way comprehensive, but it offers the would-be pilgrim a place to begin. And ultimately, as with life itself, it doesn't matter so much where you go, as long as you stay awake for the journey.

getting there and getting around

At the Ramana Ashram in Tiruvannamalai, we met a yogi from Santa Barbara, California, who was prepared for every conceivable disaster. So as not to expose himself to the parasites lurking in Indian cuisine, he had brought along all his own food in a suitcase the height of a small cow, including a quart of blue-green algae, several pounds of protein powder, and a hundred individually wrapped packets of Mu's Munchies. Before he went out the door, he covered himself from head to toe in a herbal mosquito repellent that made him smell like an explosion in a Lemon Pledge factory.

Two days after we met him, we found him sitting in the meditation hall covered with angry red welts. "Bedbugs," he informed us.

India will find a way to get under your skin, no matter how many precautions you take. Nonetheless, a little forethought can make your trip infinitely more fulfilling, if only by making you better prepared to cope with the disintegration of your plans. In this book, we won't try to duplicate information that you can get in most good guidebooks to India. A particularly thorough and user-friendly guide is Lonely Planet's award-winning *India: A Travel Survival Kit*. Other useful publications include *Trains at a Glance*, available at newsstands in larger Indian stations, which gives schedules for all major train lines throughout India; and *Travel Links*, available at Indian bookstores and newsstands, which gives airline schedules and limited railway timings.

You can buy decent maps of India in most bookstores or travel stores in the United States and Europe, in bookshops in larger Indian cities, and from Indian street peddlers (who may give you a shoe-shine, tell your fortune, or clean the wax from your ears as a bonus). You can pick up detailed state maps—helpful in finding your way to ashrams in smaller towns—at the tourist offices of most Indian states. (Note that many cities in India are in the process of changing their names from the names used by the British to historically used local names: for instance, Bombay is now officially Mumbai, Madras is Chennai, etc. Most maps contain both names.)

What to Bring

If you have any doubt about the load you're about to carry with you to India, try this simple experiment before you leave. Carrying all your luggage, head downtown at rush hour in the nearest big city. Ideally, a heat wave or torrential thunderstorm should be in full swing. Have a long list of urgent errands to accomplish in disreputable neighborhoods. Use only public transportation—driving or taking a taxi is cheating, as is hiring someone to carry your bags. After five or six hours, return to your home and reevaluate: Do you still think you need your Filofax? Your blowdryer? Your sack of runestones and healing crystals?

Again and again in India, you'll need to scramble on or off a crowded bus in a hurry, walk a mile in a monsoon, or dash for a train that is unexpectedly departing on time. You'll be thankful if you can easily carry or wheel your baggage and aren't dependent on porters—who may well demand extortionate prices if they see you are at their mercy, or collude with a rickshaw driver to whisk you to a hotel-and-carpet-shop run by a entrepreneurial "cousin."

Think of packing as a spiritual practice, and prune your luggage as rigorously as your ego. Visualize your bag as a metaphor for how you live your life—only have what you really need, and use everything you have. Or tune into your past-life memory of being a sadhu. We've found it's well worth the effort to get everything you need into one carry-on size suitcase or backpack. It's quite possible to travel continuously for six months from subfreezing to tropical climates, and get by fine with one carry-on bag and a small shoulder satchel or daypack.

You can purchase clothing and most other items very reasonably in India. Indian clothes, shawls, and sandals are comfortable, practical, and colorful—as well as a bargain. Bring an Indian tailor your favorite shirt, and he will duplicate it (and perhaps add a few unique flourishes of his own) in a matter of hours. This is far easier and more entertaining than last-minute shopping at home.

Select clothes that can all be worn with each other. Don't bring a lot of duplicate clothing—remember that you'll be able to have laundry done (or do it yourself) quickly and inexpensively. A shirt or pair of pants can be washed and ironed for a few rupees when dealing direct with the "dhobi" or laundry person (hotels can be much higher), and one-day service is standard. (The India laundering method—which involves slamming wet garments against rocks with jackhammer vigor—is, admittedly, hard on clothes. It helps to soak your clothes in soapy water overnight and then entreat the dhobi to be less enthusiastic.) If you handwash your own laundry, the sun will normally dry it the same day.

People dress modestly in India, particularly in the ashrams. Normally, short pants or cut-offs are frowned on even for men. Light-weight pants and sleeved shirts are fine. Slip-on sandals are cool and convenient for both men and women. Women should not wear shorts, short skirts, low-cut blouses, or other figure-revealing clothes; the chest, shoulders, and upper arms should be covered as well as the legs. To aid in the cover-up, many women travelers buy beautiful Indian scarves and wear them around the neck, shoulders, and even head. Long cotton dresses or Indian Punjabi outfits (baggy pants with a knee-length overshirt) are comfortable and suitably modest. Wearing Indian clothes will cut down on the harassment you get. If you're really feeling ambitious, you can try to master the art of wearing a sari (to the amusement—but delight—of local women, who will hasten to tell you how much better you look now that you're properly dressed).

For moderately cold weather, layer up with a tee shirt, shirt, sweater, and windbreaker. If you're going to extremely cold areas (such as Ladakh in winter), you can purchase a heavy sweater, blanket, warm hat, and gloves and mail them home or give them away on departure. (There are a lot of needy people in India who can benefit from such gifts.)

If you're planning to study hatha yoga, remember that Western exercise wear—such as form-fitting leotard and tights—is not acceptable in most Indian yoga centers. Instead, women should wear loose-fitting cotton pants and tee shirts with sleeves (shorts are okay for men). Even if you're going to a more Westernized center—like the Iyengar Institute in Pune—you may still find that tights are too hot—instead, wear shorts with fitted legs (so you can turn upside down without offending anyone).

Periodically you can mail books home (like good karma, they seem to accumulate as you visit ashrams), taking advantage of the special low sea mail rate for a "books only" package. You can also mail parcels home to yourself if you find yourself getting overloaded. Save most of your gift shopping for the end of the trip, when you can handle a few extra bags or parcels. The major cities of departure from India feature large government emporiums where you can buy fine craftwork from all over India. This may cost a little bit more than buying locally, but it's worth it for the convenience.

India is such a visual feast that you'll probably want to take lots of photos. You can usually get the most common film types and speeds in the cities and tourist sites. If you have specific film needs or concerns about freshness, you may want to bring your own.

Film processing is available in the cities, although you can't count on speed or consistent quality. If you don't want to cart around developed photos, wait and have your film developed when you go home.

The following packing list works for a trip of two weeks or six months.

❧ Clothing (Men)

walking/hiking shoes
walking sandals
2 pair loose pants (1 lightweight)
1 longsleeve shirt
1 turtleneck
3 light cotton or knit shirts
2 tee shirts
4 pair socks (one pair should be wool)
4–5 pair undershorts

1 belt
1 windbreaker
4 handkerchiefs
1 hat
1 light wool sweater
1 white ashram outfit (buy in India)
1 meditation shawl (buy in India)
1 bathing suit

❧ Clothing (Women)

walking/hiking shoes
walking sandals
3 tee shirts
1 loose longsleeved shirt

4 pair socks (1 pair should be wool)
1 top and bottom silk long underwear

1 light wool sweater
1 windbreaker
1 hat
2 pair comfortable, loose cotton
  pants
1 loose, long dress (optional)
4–5 pair underwear, bras

1 lightweight but body-covering
  robe
1 lightweight scarf (buy in India)
1 shawl (buy in India)
1 white ashram outfit (buy in
  India)
1 bathing suit

❧ Other

inflatable travel pillow
medicine kit, including:
  electrolyte powder
  antibiotics and antidiarrheal
    medicine
  thermometer
  fungal cream
  disinfectant
  bandaids
  aspirin
  herbal remedies
    (echinacea/goldenseal and
    other favorites)
  vitamins
toiletries kit
sink stopper
earplugs
water bottle
water disinfectant drops or
  filter
flashlight
sunblock and lipscreen
sunglasses
insect repellent
small towel
handiwipes
assorted ziplock bags
notebook or journal and pens

pollution mask
travel alarm
guidebooks
maps
address book
pocket knife
money belt
credit cards
traveler's checks/U.S. cash (for
  banks that won't change
  traveler's checks)
cup and spoon
camera and film
extra batteries (for camera,
  flashlight, etc.)
scotch tape
small foldup daypack
sleeping envelope (have made in
  India) and pillowcase
mosquito netting
laundry soap and travel laundry
  line
tampons (can be hard to find in
  India)
sturdy padlock and steel cable or
  chain (essential for securing
  room and attaching luggage to
  train seat or overhead racks)

Most illnesses suffered by travelers to India have to do with contaminated food or water, so regularly chant the travelers' mantra: "If you can't boil it or peel it, forget it!" Oranges, bananas, papaya, and peeled apples are staples in India. Strictly avoid salads or other raw vegetables unless you know how they have been disinfected.

In general, it's best to eat vegetarian in India, although eggs are usually safe. Avoiding meat, poultry, and seafood lessens the risk of food poisoning associated with a lack of refrigeration. Stick with bottled, boiled, filtered, or treated water. Ashram water is almost always safe to drink, but stay away from unbottled water in hotels or restaurants, no matter how elegant.

Try to watch how people handle the food they are cooking or selling. Wash your hands regularly—especially before eating—or use handiwipes if you can't get to soap and water. Disinfect any cuts or open sores immediately.

If you feel sick for more than a few days, consult a doctor. Parasites are common in India but can be detected and eliminated easily and effectively. Medical care is widely available at reasonable prices—for the equivalent of a few U.S. dollars, you can get a consultation and some medicine. Prompt lab tests are normally available (although make sure you are going to a reputable lab—it's not unheard of for labs to make up results without doing any tests at all).

In the larger cities, air pollution can cause headaches, fatigue, and respiratory problems. A small cotton surgical-type pollution mask (available at drugstores in the West and in some Indian cities) can help, especially when walking or riding in an autorickshaw in heavy traffic. Special carbon-filter masks are available from many bicycle shops in the United States and Europe.

In general, you can minimize the health risk in India by good common sense. The Lonely Planet India guidebook includes a comprehensive overview of how to stay healthy in India, including a rundown of potential diseases and disasters (from prickly heat to meningitis) and information on recommended vaccinations. When it comes to vaccinations against contagious diseases, every traveler must make up her own mind—none are required, but many are recommended by most Western doctors. Most hospitals and clinics with a foreign traveler's immunization clinic have written information available. In the United States, you can get up-to-date recorded or faxed information from the Center for Disease Control in Atlanta, Georgia, by calling (404) 332-4565. Your doctor, travel agent, or travel bookstore may also have some useful tips. The Osho Commune International (p. 215) publishes a good booklet entitled *Staying Healthy in India,* which can be ordered from the commune office.

Making Phone Calls

The telephone numbers given in the contact information in this guidebook include the India country code (91), the city code, and the local number. If you are dialing from inside India to a city other than the one you are in, omit the 91 and dial a 0 before the city code. If you are dialing within a city, you will not use a 0 or the city code—just dial the local number (which is normally six or seven digits).

Phoning can be frustrating—telephone numbers change frequently, and often information operators are unable to give the current correct number. The best way to make calls is to go to one of the PCO (public call office) phone booths—also marked STD (for calls within India) and ISD (for international calls)—and ask the attendant to assist you. Public fax booths are widely available in larger cities.

When to Go

In general, plan your travel within India to coincide with the weather—moving from north to south as the weather cools, or vice versa. If you have the flexibility, obviously try to travel when the weather is best in the area you plan to visit. India is a large country, and the weather at any given time varies widely from the southern beaches to the northern mountains, from blistering hot to bone-stunning cold. Most guidebooks give you the maximum and minimum average daily temperatures for all months of the year.

Generally the weather is pleasant from mid-October to the beginning of April in most areas of India. In the far south, December, January, and February are the most comfortable. In the mountainous areas of the far north, the later spring, summer, and early fall are the best times to visit.

Around Christmas and New Year, a deluge of Indians and foreigners travel in India, so you may need to book travel or lodging arrangements far in advance. "High season" for foreigners visiting ashrams is normally No-vember through February. Some ashrams may be crowded at this time—writing ahead helps assure a room.

Some of the gurus who tour outside or around India are more likely to be at their ashrams during the high season, but there will also be more visitors, limiting guru-access. Many seekers report that gurus are much more available during the summer months because of the diminished crowds.

How to Travel

We have found the train system to be the most comfortable, safe, and interesting form of travel in India. A relic of the British Raj, the rail-way system crisscrosses the entire country. On the trains and in the sta-tions, vendors hawk food, bottled water, chai (Indian tea brewed with milk, sugar, and spices), coffee, and other goods and services, from cigarettes to scalp massages to three-piece suits. Train rides are also a great way to meet Indian travelers, who will enliven long journeys with everything from po-litical debates to picnics to spontaneous concerts in the aisles.

Train cars are divided into several classes—which class you choose will depend on your budget and tastes. On day trains, many people prefer coaches where the windows open to more expensive first-class air-conditioned coaches. For overnight trips, second-class AC is the most com-fortable, especially for women traveling alone (with its open berths, it's actually safer than first class, where you may be shut into a closed com-partment with an unknown male passenger). You'll need to make advance reservations for overnight sleeper trains, but not for shorter day trains, as seats are usually available and the reservation process can be time-consuming and frustrating.

Buses are the most economical and often the most reliable form of public transportation. All larger cities and towns and most villages are served by regular bus service. Riding on a full bus in India—with passen-gers including an assortment of farm animals—is an experience you ought to have at least once.

Taxis and cars (with driver) for hire are relatively inexpensive by West-ern standards and are very convenient, especially if you're going some-where that isn't served by frequent rail or bus service or you are unsure of an ashram's location or openness to visitors. Hired drivers are usually flex-

ible about schedule, route, overnight stays, and other logistics. (Be prepared for a harrowing trip, however, as the driver—his gas pedal apparently
linked to his horn—barrels down the narrow, potholed roads, weaving
through trucks, bicycles, pedestrians, bullock carts, goats, and cows with
more faith in Krishna's protection than you might be feeling.) Taxis for
longer trips normally cost about four rupees per kilometer, including the
return distance, plus waiting time and overnight charges for the driver
(waiting time and overnight costs are normally reasonable by Western
standards).

If you have more extra money than you have extra time, airlines are
an alternative to train or bus travel. Prices are comparable to Western rates.
The state-run Indian Airlines is the principal carrier, but an ever-expanding
number of new private airlines serve various cities. Inquire with a local
travel agent or pick up the *Travel Links* or other airline guide. Published
schedules are not always reliable and times change with the season, so
check with the airline and be flexible.

However you choose to get around, you will meet many other travelers along the way, and you'll normally find both Westerners and Indians
very willing to assist you. If you look even a little bit lost or confused,
you'll probably be asked if you need help. (But do be careful of your lug-

My breakthrough into Hinduism came when I stayed with a Punjabi
printer in Allahabad who took me for the customary morning bath in the
Ganga. It was winter, chilly; we stripped off. I could see flotsam and
jetsam and cigarette cartons and all sorts of muck bobbing about. He
plunged in, calling, "Come! This is Ganga Mai." "You don't expect me
to jump into this," I yelled. "It's filthy!" He replied, "It's not the water
that's filthy; it's the dirt."

Suddenly, like Zen satori, I knew he was right. I jumped in too.
And from that moment, I've never had typhoid or those things. I've had
immunity—psychic immunity. You can't stay in India on boiled water;
you have to come round to the Indian way—if you get a bug, it's for a
purpose. It's easier to live that way.

—BILL AITKEN
(quoted in Turning East: New Lives in India)

gage—especially in the Delhi railway station—as some thieves pose as good samaritans. An offer of help can be followed with a demand for payment, and you may find yourself steered in directions that you didn't want to go—like to your rescuer's marble shop.)

After a few days, you'll give up the expectation of efficient Western-style travel and slow down to the rhythm of India. Don't let the fear of the unknown keep you from hitting the road.

indian philosophies and religions

On an early visit to India, we lived for a week in a Christian ashram in Pune, while dividing our days between the Iyengar Yoga Institute and the Osho Commune. In the morning, we watched sweat-beaded yogis in damp leotards hanging in Dog Pose from wall ropes, their faces taut with anxious concentration, while a teacher roared at them to rotate the skin on their inner armpits toward their navel. In the afternoon, we bought a maroon swimsuit (all clothing worn at the commune must be maroon, by Osho's decree) and dove into the lagoon-shaped swimming pool of the commune's Club Meditation, in pursuit of Osho's ideal of Zorba the Buddha. In the evening, we attended a cross-cultural celebration of the Eucharist that included a Hindu arathi (offering of fire) and readings from both the Upanishads and the Gospel According to John.

That kind of spiritual diversity is characteristic of India, where mutually contradictory facts often coexist quite comfortably without apparent cognitive dissonance. ("But you told me the bus ran every day!" you protest, brandishing the schedule like holy scripture, after waiting for two hours past the printed time. "Yes, madame, bus is coming every day," the man behind the ticket counter assures you again. "And today bus is not

> Just as a man, having cast off old garments, puts on other, new ones, even so does the embodied one, having cast off old bodies, take on other, new ones . . . To one who is born death is certain and certain is birth to one who has died. Therefore, in connection with a thing that is inevitable, you should not grieve.

—THE BHAGAVAD GITA

coming.") But it can be befuddling to Westerners who have come to India looking for a singular Ultimate Truth.

Keep in mind that truth comes in a multiplicity of forms, as variegated and colorful as the 330 million Hindu gods. One guru will advocate a lifetime of celibacy; another will prescribe sex as a path to samadhi. One will exhort you to crank your body to ever-sweatier heights of hatha-yoga gymnastics to ignite the dormant kundalini in your spine; another will advise, gently, that you give up physical practices altogether, as they distract you from contemplating the spirit that lies beyond form. One teacher will tell you to sit cross-legged and watch your breath for eleven hours a day; another will say that meditation is unnecessary, since you already *are* the enlightenment you seek. Even within a particular path, contradictions multiply—it's rumored that one famous hatha yogi refuses to teach in any room that another well-known one from the same lineage has taught in, due to differences of opinions on such weighty matters as whether poses should be taught independently or as part of a prescribed sequence.

Whatever the teaching, the master is sure to find plenty to substantiate it in the voluminous ancient texts—and if not, gurus have been known to invent a few slokas when necessary. And everywhere you go, zealots will assure you that theirs is the only true way to happiness, and become anxious—or even belligerent—when you mention divergent viewpoints.

The following brief overview of India's spiritual paths is designed to help you sort through the bewildering multiplicity of options. (As a roadmap, it's necessarily sketchy—for more comprehensive treatments, consult the recommended reading list on page 52.) It also offers you another chance to remember that the map is not the territory. However your experience unfolds, chances are it won't fit neatly into any of the categories described below. Which is probably a good thing—otherwise, why should you bother going?

Philosophies

🌀 Vedanta

"Tat Tvam Asi—That Thou Art," proclaim the Upanishads, the esoteric concluding books of the ancient Indo-Aryan scriptures known as the Vedas. This proclamation lies at the heart of Indian spirituality: That the essence of all beings and all things is indivisible, infinite, unchanging Spirit—and that the individual soul (the atman, or the true Self) is one with this cosmic Consciousness (or brahman).

This is the fundamental teaching of Vedanta, the vast body of metaphysical speculations that originated with the Upanishads (the first of which were composed about 800 B.C.E.). By far the most dominant of the six classical systems of Hindu philosophy, Vedanta is itself divided into several different schools. The most influential of these is the advaita (nondual) Vedanta taught by the ninth-century sage Shankaracharya: It holds that there is only one underlying Reality, which appears in many forms, thus confusing the unenlightened mind.

In the words of a brochure from the Vedanta Society founded by the nineteenth-century teacher Swami Vivekananda, "The Supreme Reality, Brahman, cannot be described; the most one can say of it is that it is Sat-Chit-Ananda—Absolute Existence, Consciousness, Bliss. Vedanta recognizes, however, that the absolute Brahman becomes manifest in various aspects and forms and is known by various names. In other words, Brahman, or God, is both formless and with form, impersonal and personal, transcendent and immanent. Vedanta declares that one can realize God in whatever aspect one wishes, and, further, that one can realize him directly and vividly in this life, in this world." All of the gods and goddesses worshipped in Hinduism are simply manifestations of this one, unchanging Brahman. So, too, is the Self that is contacted through meditation and yoga.

Vedanta philosophy shapes the teachings offered at most of the ashrams and yoga centers in this book. Two ashrams explicitly dedicated to the study of Vedantic texts are the Chinmayananda Mission (p. 106), which has branches all over India, and the Dayananda Ashram in Rishikesh (p. 331).

❧ Yoga

When the Bhagavad Gita was composed over two thousand years ago, the art of yoga was already ancient. In fact, some scholars detect evidence of yogic beliefs and practices in such venerable texts as the Rig Veda, which dates back to the third millennium B.C.E.—hence the claims on the boxes of bestselling yoga workout videos that their product depicts a "five thousand-year-old exercise system." However, it's unlikely that the ancient seers were particularly concerned with tightening their tummies or sculpting their inner thighs. In fact, it's unlikely that they were practicing any of the physical postures that have come to be viewed as synonymous with yoga in the West, but which were probably not developed until around a thousand years ago (just the other day, by yogic time standards). Rather, they were engaged in yoga in the truest sense—the quest to realize the unity of the individual Self with cosmic Consciousness.

Most of the paths described in this book can fit under this broad category. The word "yoga" comes from a Sanskrit root meaning both "union" and "discipline"—thus, yoga can be defined as both the state of union with our true Self, and the bewildering variety of disciplines (featuring disparate and often conflicting methods and philosophies) for bringing about that joyful Self-realization.

In the words of one ancient text, "Yoga is ecstasy." Yoga offers a variety of paths for putting us in touch with our true blissful nature. In some philosophical frameworks, this process is depicted as a sort of spiritual garage cleaning, a laborious process of clearing away the accumulated debris that obscures our soul—in yogic terms, separating prakriti (matter) from purusha (spirit). In other models, there is no duality between matter and spirit—it's simply a matter of waking up to the true nature of who we already are. In either case, the end result, on a practical level, is the same. As the god Krishna explains to the warrior Arjuna in the sixth chapter of the Bhagavad Gita, "When the restlessness of the mind, intellect, and self is stilled through the practice of yoga, the yogi by the grace of the Spirit within himself finds fulfillment. Then he knows the joy eternal which is beyond the pale of the senses, which his reason cannot grasp. . . . He has found the treasure above all others. There is nothing higher than this. . . . This is the real meaning of yoga—a deliverance from pain and sorrow."

We are what we think.

All that we are arises with our thoughts.

With our thoughts we make the world.

Speak or act with an impure mind

And trouble will follow you

As the wheel follows the ox that draws the cart . . .

Speak or act with a pure mind

And happiness will follow you

As your shadow, unshakeable.

—DHAMMAPADA,
the sayings of the Buddha

Different systems of yoga use very different techniques to bring about that fundamental transformation of consciousness. Like an old banyan tree, yoga has sprouted countless branches over the centuries, with each limb supporting a full load of gurus, texts, and techniques. Each approach appeals to a different personality type, ensuring a road for everybody—for example, emotional people often gravitate to the devotional practices of bhakti yoga, whereas highly physical people are drawn to the hatha-yoga path. In practical terms, the systems overlap and merge—yogis are pragmatic creatures, and tend to pick up whatever tool is useful for the job at hand. However, for purposes of discussion, we can divide the river of yoga into five main currents: jnana, bhakti, karma, raja, and hatha.

Jnana Yoga, the Path of Wisdom: Jnana yoga is not, as is sometimes thought, primarily devoted to the study of ancient texts. Rather, jnana yogis use the mind to dismantle the mind—working with keen discrimination (viveka), they sort out the real from the unreal, the true Self from the illusions thrown up by the ego. All that is illusory is discarded—in the words of the Upanishads, "Neti, neti"—"not this, not this." According to Ramana Maharshi (p. 286), a great twentieth-century jnana yogi, "The thought 'Who am I?' will destroy all other thoughts, and, like the stick used for stirring the burning pyre, it will itself in the end get destroyed. Then, there will arise Self-realization."

If you're drawn to the jnana yoga path, places you might want to visit include the Ramanashram in Tiruvannamalai (p. 286), Satsang Bhavan in Lucknow (p. 313), and the home of Ramesh Balsekar in Bombay (p. 183).

Bhakti Yoga, the Path of Love and Devotion: "Children, knowledge without devotion is like eating stones," says the contemporary south Indian yogini Mata Amritanandamayi (p. 168). As Krishna points out in the Bhagavad Gita, it is hard for a human being still in physical form to commune with the Divine—who is none other than the true Self—as pure, formless spirit. Instead, in the heart-centered path of bhakti yoga, the devotee surrenders to the Divine in whatever form It assumes—Krishna, Rama, Radha, Sita, or any one of a host of other gods and goddesses. The devotee invokes and celebrates the Spirit through ritual, chanting, singing, and dancing.

In the words of the ecstatic mystic Ramakrishna (p. 382), "You have taken birth in this beautiful human form to worship, experience, and eventually merge with Divine Reality. Taste God's Love. Kiss the fragrant Lotus Feet of the Lord. Do not become distracted by attempting to analyze Divine Mystery. . . . A few sips of the precious wine of Love will thoroughly intoxicate you. Why leave the full glass untouched on the table while inquiring how the wine was produced or estimating how many gallons may exist in the infinite wine cellar?"

In most traditions, devotion is also extended to the person of the guru, who is considered a gateway to God; therefore, most guru-led ashrams will have some bhakti component. For a full-fledged bhakti experience, visit the Mata Amritanandamayi ashram (p. 168), the Anandashram (p. 153) in northern Kerala, or the Sai Baba ashram in Puttaparthi (p. 69).

Karma Yoga, the Path of Selfless Service: When you see the words "karma yoga" on an ashram schedule, get ready to start chopping vegetables or scrubbing floors: in this context, it generally means "work." Ideally,

---

Yoga is the calming of the disturbances of the heart.

—THE YOGA SUTRAS OF PATANJALI

---

it has a loftier meaning as well—it's a chance, in the words of the Bhagavad Gita, to "act without attachment to the fruits of your actions." Rather than renouncing the world, the karma yogi works for the service of the world, without attachment to the outcome. In this way, he or she relinquishes attachment to the ego and begins to identify with the larger Self. "Whoever lets go attachment to the fruits of his actions, and instead dedicates his actions to God, is not touched by sin, like the lotus leaf is not touched by water," Krishna tells Arjuna. "By steadily letting go the fruits of his actions, the yogi attains peace. . . . By mentally renouncing the fruits of his action, the yogi's mind becomes disciplined. Thus, he knows himself to be the Atman [soul], happily abiding in the city of nine gates (the body). He knows that he is not the doer who acts or causes to act."

Karma yoga can be explored in any ashram setting or at places of service such as the Aravind Eye Hospital in Madurai (p. 268) or Mother Teresa's Missionaries of Charity in Calcutta (p. 379).

Raja Yoga, the Path of Meditative Awakening: Also known as ashtanga (eight-limbed) yoga, this is the path codified by the sage Patanjali around the second or third century A.D., which pundits categorize as one of the six orthodox systems of Indian philosophy. As outlined in Patanjali's Yoga Sutras, raja yoga—the "royal" path—is an eight-pronged system for stilling the turbulent waves of the mind, so it can reflect the true Self without distortion.

Raja yoga begins with moral restraints and disciplines (yama and niyama), such as truthfulness, nonviolence, sexual restraint, and devotion to God. (These guidelines are based not on abstract notions of purity, but on the practical observation that it's hard to have a quiet mind after a day spent lying, killing, and stealing.) The next two steps are asana (posture) and pranayama (breath control)—the yogi assumes a stable and comfortable position and focuses attention on the breath. (These two steps are greatly elaborated in the system of hatha yoga, which is generally practiced in conjunction with raja yoga.) Then follow the meditative techniques of pratyahara (withdrawal of the mind and senses from the distractions of the outside world); dharana (concentration on a single point); and dhyana (complete absorption in the object of meditation). The result of these practices is samadhi—the ecstasy of Self-realization.

The practices of raja yoga—as well as the associated practices of hatha

Recommended Reading

India by Richard Waterstone (Little, Brown). A handbook to all aspects of Indian spiritual life that's small enough to fit in your daypack.

Travels Through Sacred India by Roger Housden (HarperCollins). An informative personal journey through India's sacred landscape.

The Shambhala Guide to Yoga by Georg Feuerstein (Shambhala). A succinct overview of yoga history and philosophy.

Light on Yoga by B. K. S. Iyengar (Schocken). The classic illustrated manual of hatha-yoga postures.

What the Buddha Taught by Walpola Rahula (Grove). Cogent summary of essential Buddhist teachings.

Old Path White Clouds: Walking in the Footsteps of the Buddha by Thich Nhat Hanh (Parallax). A retelling of the Buddha's life and teachings by a Vietnamese Zen master.

The Hindu Religious Tradition by Thomas J. Hopkins (Wadsworth). A concise scholarly overview of Hinduism.

The Living Gita by Sri Swami Satchidananda (Holt). Translation and commentary of the Bhagavad Gita specifically for Western seekers, by one of the West's most popular Indian gurus.

Sadhus: India's Mystic Holy Men by Dolf Hartsuiker (Inner Traditions). A beautifully photographed exploration of the mystical life of sadhus.

Dancing with Siva: Hinduism's Contemporary Catechism by Satguru Sivayay Subramuniyaswami (Himalayan Academy). A hefty tome for would-be practitioners.

The Mahabarata (South Asia Press) and *The Ramayana* (Viking Penguin) by R. K. Narayan. Masterful and readable retellings of the great Indian epics.

yoga—are taught in such schools as the Yoga Institute of Santa Cruz (p. 187) near Bombay, the Bihar School of Yoga (p. 89), Ananda Ashram in Pondicherry, the Vivekananda Kendra Yoga in Bangalore (p. 134), the Krishnamacharya Yoga Mandiram in Madras (p. 247), and Kaivalyadhama in Lonavala (p. 202).

Hatha Yoga, the Path of Energy: "As a mountaineer needs ladders, ropes and crampons as well as physical fitness and discipline to climb the icy peaks of the Himalayas, so does the Yoga aspirant need the knowledge and discipline of hatha yoga . . . to reach the heights of raja yoga," wrote the contemporary hatha-yoga master B. K. S. Iyengar. Hatha yoga is almost always practiced in conjunction with raja yoga—in fact, it's usually not considered a separate path at all. The ancient hatha yogis knew what Western science is just beginning to recognize: The state of the body affects the mind, and the state of the mind affects the body.

Hatha yoga's elaborate physical postures (asana), breathing techniques (pranayama), and cleansing practices (kriya) were developed to relax, detoxify, and strengthen the body and nervous system in preparation for the rigors of meditation. Asana practice is also a form of meditation-in-motion in its own right, calming the mind and cultivating a state of relaxed but alert concentration.

The earliest hatha-yoga texts—such as the classic Hatha-Yoga Pradipika and Gheranda Samhita—were written between the ninth and the fourteenth century A.D., although the techniques they describe may be considerably older. At their highest levels, hatha-yoga practices are designed to awaken the kundalini-shakti—the potent (and sometimes dangerous) energy that lies coiled at the base of the spine—and conduct it upward to the crown chakra, where it brings about Self-realization. (If the body and nerves have not been properly prepared, this kundalini awakening can cause severe physical and mental problems, so it's important to have a qualified teacher.) On a more mundane level, hatha yoga is frequently employed as a system of physical therapeutics, due to its positive effects on blood pressure, cardiovascular efficiency, the endocrine system, and the nervous system.

In addition to the places listed under Raja Yoga—which include hatha yoga to varying degrees—hatha yoga is the primary practice taught at the Ramamani Iyengar Memorial Yoga Institute in Pune (p. 221) and the Ashtanga Yoga Research Institute in Mysore (p. 142).

✿ Tantra

In the West, the term "tantra" usually conjures up images of "sacred sex" in redwood hot tubs. However, tantra actually refers to a sophisticated stream of teachings that arose within both Buddhism and Hinduism in India around two thousand years ago and were widespread by about 1,000 C.E. Prominent features of most schools of tantrism include initiation and spiritual discipleship with a master; the use of ritual and mantra; a focus on the feminine spiritual power (shakti), which manifests in the body as kundalini energy; a negation of the split between matter and spirit; and the belief that enlightenment can be attained within—and through— the physical body. In what are called the "left-hand" (i.e., somewhat unorthodox) schools of tantra, sexual energy is used as a tool for spiritual progress.

For a taste of the teachings of a controversial modern tantra teacher, visit the Osho Commune (p. 215). For a more conservative approach, try the Bihar School of Yoga (p. 89).

Religions

✿ Hinduism

Vedanta, yoga, and tantra—while they can be practiced as nonsectarian philosophies—all arose within the embrace of Hinduism, which Hindus themselves refer to as Sanatana Dharma, or the Eternal Truth. Practiced by 80 percent of all Indians—or about 700 million people—Hinduism is perhaps the world's oldest living religion. Its roots stretch back to the ancient Indus Valley civilization, which flourished in the third millennium B.C.E. in what is now Pakistan and western India, and to the Aryan nomadic tribes that moved into the region in the second millennium B.C.E. Its kaleidoscopic beliefs and practices—governing every detail of life, from what hand to eat with to how to cremate the dead—are based on four books of ancient scriptures called the Vedas, said to have been revealed to seers known as rishis in states of deep meditation. (The concluding portions of each of those books are known as the Upanishads and contain the profound metaphysical musings of Vedanta, which literally means "the end of the Vedas.")

Central to Hinduism is the belief in karma, the cosmic law of cause and effect, in which each person creates his or her destiny based on his or her own actions. Karma is carried over from lifetime to lifetime, as the individual soul reincarnates again and again. When all karma has been resolved, the soul achieves moksha—liberation from the cycle of rebirth.

Entwined with beliefs in karma is the painful doctrine of caste, the social station determined by birth. Traditionally, castes were divided into four groups according to their function in society: Brahmins, the literate priests, who perform intellectual and ritual functions; Kshatriyas, the warrior caste; Vaishyas, the merchants and farmers; and Shudras, the menial servants and artisans. (In reality, of course, caste laws are far more complex than this, and vary from region to region, with thousands of intricate subcastes and rules.) Outside the caste system are the untouchables (whom Gandhi renamed Harijans, or "children of God," and who now are called Dalits, or "the downtrodden")—they perform such "unclean" tasks as washing latrines and doing laundry. To an orthodox Hindu, untouchables pollute whatever they touch. In recent years, caste has become a highly politicized issue, with affirmative action programs for Dalits, and lower castes wielding increasing political clout.

Hindus believe in a single, all-pervasive Supreme Being—or Brahman—who manifests in a multiplicity of gods and goddesses, with whom human beings can communicate through the rituals of puja, or worship. The three main manifestations of god are Brahma, the Creator; Vishnu, the Preserver; and Shiva, the Destroyer. Brahma is rarely worshipped—in fact, there's only one Brahma temple in all of India. Instead, most Hindus are either Vaishnavites (worshippers of one of the forms of Vishnu); Shaivites (worshippers of Shiva); Shaktas (worshippers of Shiva's female consort); or Smartas (liberal Hindus who leave the choice of deity to the devotee).

In addition to the Vedas, the most important texts of Hinduism are the epic poems known as the Mahabharata and the Ramayana. The Mahabarata is an epic 100,000-verse poem—about four times as long as the Bible—that was composed over the period from 600 B.C.E. to 500 C.E. It interweaves sophisticated philosophical musings with juicy dramas of romance, dynastic feuds, and supernatural cataclysms as it recounts the fortunes of the five Pandava brothers and their rival cousins, the Kauravas. The most famous portion of the Mahabharata is the Bhagavad Gita, the "Song of the Lord," in which the god Krishna proclaims the ideals of duty, service, and love of God to the warrior Arjuna as he prepares to do battle.

The Ramayana recounts the adventures of the warrior deity Rama (an

The Hindu Pantheon

In Hinduism, the Supreme Being manifests in a bewildering multiplicity of forms—330 million, by some counts. However, the five principal deities you'll see depicted in temples and ashrams are Shiva, Vishnu (in his many incarnations), Devi (also in countless forms), Ganesh, and Hanuman.

Shiva is the Lord of Yoga—the ascetic destroyer god who haunts the cremation grounds and smears his body with the ashes of the dead. Shiva lives high in the Himalayas or in the sacred city of Varanasi; the river Ganges is said to have sprung from his matted hair. He can be recognized by the bull that he rides on or by the trident he carries. This god of renunciates is mainly worshipped in the form of the Shiva lingam, the phallic image of creative power embedded in the vulvic yoni.

Vishnu has ten different avatars, or incarnations—forms in which he has (or will) appeared to rescue a floundering universe. The first six are a fish; a tortoise; a boar; a man-lion who saves the world from a demon; a dwarf; and an axe-wielding warrior named Parashurama. The seventh is the superhero Rama, the star of the epic poem the Ramayana, who can be identified by his bow and quiver of arrows. The eighth incarnation is the beloved cowherd and flute-player Krishna.

The consummate lover, Krishna is renowned for his seduction of the gopis, the milkmaid wives and daughters of the other cowherds—his flute music drove them mad with desire, and in the course of a thirty-three-day dance he ravished all 900,000 of them. However, he's

incarnation of Vishnu) and his consort Sita, whose adventures serve as a morality tale and guide to the laws of dharma. Sita, the emblem of purity, is kidnapped by the demon-king Ravana; Rama rescues her with the aid of the loyal monkey-god Hanuman, only to banish her, despite his overwhelming love, because of the time she spent in the company of another man.

With every rickshaw dashboard sporting an assortment of deities, you don't have to strain to get a taste of Hinduism in India. The Hindu cosmology shapes the teachings at most traditional ashrams, although some also the dispenser of cosmic wisdom in the Bhagavad Gita, in which he reveals himself to the warrior Arjuna as the supreme Lord of the universe.

For Hindus, the Buddha is the ninth avatar. The tenth is Kalki, who has not yet appeared—he will reveal himself at the end of the world, when he will appear on a white horse to dispense judgment to the wicked and reward the righteous.

The goddess, or **Devi,** is worshipped in various forms, many of whom are consorts of the gods. Brahma's consort is Saraswati, the goddess of learning. Vishnu's is Laxmi, the goddess of wealth and beauty, whose four-armed image often appears near the cash register in shops. Shiva's feminine power, or Shakti, is expressed as a variety of incarnations: in her peaceful form as Sati or Parvati, or in the ferocious forms of Durga and Kali (who is generally depicted with a blood-red tongue and a garland of skulls hanging around her neck). Rama's consort is Sita, exalted as the ideal woman. Krishna's main consort is Radha, the queen of the milkmaids.

Shiva and Parvati's son is the popular elephant-headed god, **Ganesh,** whose original head was chopped off by Shiva in a jealous rage when he mistook his son for a rival lover. Ganesh is invoked to remove obstacles and presides at the entrance of every Hindu temple.

Hanuman, the monkey servant of Rama, is widely worshipped in north India. He is traditionally depicted as a bright orange monkey with a long tail, carrying a mountain in one hand and wielding a mace in the other.

modern yoga centers opt for a more secular, scientific approach. Overview courses in Hinduism—designed for Westerners—are offered at the Ved Niketan ashram in Rishikesh (p. 350). For a guide to a few of the thousands of Hindu sacred sites, see the Pilgrimage Sites sections throughout the guidebook.

Buddhism

Asked whether he was a god or a saint, the Buddha responded simply, "I am awake." The word "Buddha" literally means "the Awakened One"—and

Festivals of India

No matter what date it is, chances are good that somewhere in India, it's a festival day. Through fasting, prayers, and rituals as well as music, poetry, processions, and feasts, devotees make the leap from the mundane world to the timeless realm of the sacred. The following are just a few of India's major religious festivals:

Kumbh Mela. With more than 15 million pilgrims in attendance—including hundreds of thousands of sadhus—the Khumbh Mela has been called "the world's most massive act of faith." This mammoth celebration—held every three years, with the largest and most important one occurring every twelve years—commemorates an ancient altercation of the gods and demons, who fought over a vessel, or khumbha, which contained the nectar of immortality. The demons won, but in the fracas four drops of the nectar spilled to Earth at Allahabad, Hardwar, Nasik, and Ujjain. The festival is held every three years at each of the four places in rotation. The next Kumbh Mela will be in Allahabad in 2001.

Shivaratri. Literally "the night of Shiva," this festival usually falls in February or March. Fasting devotees spend all night in meditation, kirtan, puja, and recitation of sacred texts. The Shiva lingam is worshipped with milk, curds, honey, and ghee.

Holi. Particularly in the north, you can't avoid this springtime "festival of color," in which riotous crowds fill the streets squirting colored water on passersby. Wear clothes that you'd like to see decorated. The festival celebrates the burning of the demon Holika, who was persecuting her devout nephew to keep him from worshipping Vishnu.

Ganesha Chaturthi. This festival, which falls in August or September, honors the birthday of Ganesha, the popular elephant-headed god of new beginnings. Clay figures of Ganesha are worshipped with music and dancing—in some regions, the worship goes on for days—and then immersed into a river, lake, or sea.

Dussehra. This ten-day fall festival celebrates the god Rama's victory over the demon king Ravana, who kidnapped Rama's wife, Sita. Scenes from the epic Ramayana are performed (complete with dancers, musicians, and fireworks), effigies of demons are burned, and spectacular processions weave through the streets and markets. In some parts of India, this festival is also known as **Navratri,** or "nine nights"—each night is dedicated to a different manifestation of the goddess Durga, who helped Rama in his combat. Devotees fast and worship the goddess; in some regions, girls below the age of ten are also worshipped and given gifts.

Diwali. Diwali or Deepawali, the joyful "festival of lights," honors Lakshmi, the goddess of prosperity and good fortune, who is said to roam from house to house on this day in October or November. Every home is cleaned, whitewashed, and decorated with flowers, banners, and twinkling clay oil lamps so as not to be overlooked by the goddess; friends and family exchange sweets, and businesses begin a new financial year.

Janmashtami. During this festival, which falls in August or September, Krishna's birthday is celebrated with fasting and reenactments of Krishna's childhood pranks. Beginning at dawn, the festival reaches its climax at midnight, when Krishna was born—conches blare, bells ring, and an image of Krishna is dunked in the river. This festival is particularly colorful in Krishna's hometowns of Mathura and Brindavan.

the goal of Buddhist practice is to achieve the same luminous awakening ourselves.

The Buddha was born 2600 years ago as Siddhartha Gautama, the prince of a small kingdom in what is now northeastern India. Unable to ignore the painful realities of suffering, old age, and death, he abandoned his palace to take up the life of a wandering ascetic in pursuit of spiritual liberation. After years of meditation, study, and ascetic practices, he sat down under a pipal tree in what is now Bodh Gaya, vowing not to get up until he had achieved enlightenment. That night—perceiving how ignorance of their impermanent and interconnected nature binds all people in an endless loop of craving and misery—he cast off the chains of that ignorance forever. "Oh jailer, I see you now," he proclaimed. "How many lifetimes have you confined me in the prisons of birth and death? But now I see your face clearly, and from now on you can build no more prisons around me."

After his awakening, the Buddha proceeded to Sarnath, just outside the already ancient city of Varanasi, where he first proclaimed the Four Noble Truths that are the bedrock of Buddhist practice: that life contains suffering; that suffering arises from our craving or attachment to things that are by their nature impermanent; that it is possible to release this craving and thereby liberate ourselves from suffering; and that the way to do that is to follow the Noble Eightfold Path, a spiritual course known as the "Middle Way" because it avoids the two extremes of asceticism and hedonism. The components of this Eightfold Path are Right Understanding, Right Thought, Right Speech, Right Action, Right Livelihood, Right Effort, Right Mindfulness, and Right Concentration.

Buddhism flourished in India for centuries, largely due to the patronage of the third-century B.C.E. Emperor Ashoka, who converted to Buddhism in a spasm of remorse after slaughtering 100,000 people in a battle. He propagated the faith all over his vast empire—in fact, historical reconstructions based on ancient records indicate that at one time there were more Buddhists and Jains than Hindus in India. However, by the thirteenth century, Buddhism had gradually been reabsorbed into Hinduism, and India's network of temples and monasteries had been wiped out by invading armies, overgrown by forests, buried in humus, and forgotten. Two thousand years after the Buddha's enlightenment, there was hardly a Buddhist left in India.

However, in modern times Buddhism is trickling back, due largely to the influx of tens of thousands of Tibetan refugees fleeing the Chinese occupation of their country. Many of those refugees were important Buddhist teachers who survived persecution and death by escaping over the same mountain passes over which the great Buddhist teachers of the past had borne Buddhist philosophy to Tibet. The government of India has allotted land for Tibetans in both south and north India, and around those refugee camps permanent Tibetan Buddhist communities have grown up. The town of Dharamsala in Himachal Pradesh is the home of the exiled ruler of Tibet, the Dalai Lama, and the center of the Tibetan Government-in-Exile, and the route between Dharamsala and Manali is scattered with Tibetan monasteries built since the Tibetans fled their homeland in 1959 (see p. 108). Buddhism also got a boost in 1956, when almost a half million of India's outcastes converted en masse to Buddhism under the leadership of an outcaste politician named Dr. B. R. Ambedkar.

For a guide to Buddhist pilgrimage sites, see p. 93. Buddhist teachings are offered at meditation centers in Bodh Gaya (p. 78) and Dharamsala (p. 100) and in Tibetan monasteries in north and south India (p. 108). Also popular are the vipassana meditation centers—dozens of them all over India—established by meditation teacher S. N. Goenka (p. 197).

꩜ Jainism

The Jain religion was founded in the sixth century B.C.E. by a teacher named Mahavira, a contemporary of the Buddha. Jains believe that Mahavira was the last of twenty-four great teachers known as "thirthankaras," or "ford-makers"—realized beings who show the way across the sea of ignorance.

There is no external Supreme Being in Jainism. Rather, Jains believe in liberating the jiva—the radiant energy of the soul—through individual effort, including ethical vows, ascetic practices, and meditation. Absolute nonviolence and reverence for life are the key pillars of the Jain religion. The universe itself is seen as a living organism—even elements like air and water are not to be unnecessarily disturbed. Jains are strict vegetarians. Jain monks, called munis, wear masks to avoid inhaling insects, carry brooms to sweep away small creatures before sitting down, and limit their bathing to minimize the death of microorganisms in the water. Some sects dress in white robes; others go naked ("sky-clad") to eschew all attachments. Whether renunciate or layperson, the aim of life is to transcend karmic entanglements, follow the example of the tirthankaras, and strive for liberation.

All About Sadhus

In Hindu tradition, "sadhu" is the term that refers to a renunciate doing spiritual practice to attain Self-realization. Sadhus live a highly ritualized life outside the social norms of caste Hindus, renouncing material possessions and all worldly interests. Their ascetic lifestyle is essential to the fabric of Hindu society.

The numerous sects of sadhus differ in their clothing and their tilaks, the sectarian markings on their foreheads and upper bodies. Sadhus wear lungis, a traditional cloth tied and wrapped in countless variations. They never shave and their hair is often in long matted locks. Sunnyasi sadhus, who worship Shiva, wear ochre cloth and three horizontal lines across their foreheads. Vaishnava sadhus, who are devoted to Vishnu and his incarnations, generally wear white or brown cloth and three vertical lines on their foreheads. Nath and Aghora sadhus often wear black clothes, but these sadhus are fewer and less visible. Though some women become sadhus, their numbers are few—it's a Hindu belief that austerity is not a woman's path to God.

A sadhu's life begins when he is initiated by a guru and receives a name and mantra, thus becoming a member of a particular sect and its established hierarchy. A sadhu's name indicates his sectarian affiliations and, with prestige, other titles are added to indicate his status or residence. It is appropriate to address a sadhu with the title Baba or the more formal Baba-ji ("respected old man"), regardless of his age.

Across sectarian lines, sadhus embrace common values and practices. Many sects worship fire, which represents the burning away of ego, leaving only ashes. In certain rites, sadhus cover their bodies with ashes, which has the practical effect of keeping them warm in the cold season. In the hot season, wearing ashes increases the heat, or tapas, in the body, a practice that is performed to develop self-mastery and psychic powers. Sadhus often ritually smoke chilam—a mixture of tobacco and hashish or marijuana—to achieve euphoria.

Sadhus value the itinerant lifestyle, and their travels are shaped by the Hindu liturgical calendar. Though a sacred place, or tirtha, is always worthy of pilgrimage, specific dates on the lunar calendar render certain holy places particularly auspicious. During such times sadhus gather for immense festivals, or melas. Though train authorities are becoming less tolerant of sadhus traveling without tickets, most maintain the older tradition of no-ticket transportation. Sadhus can be seen on trains and station platforms all across the pilgrimage routes of India.

Sitting among sadhus can be rewarding. On a nonverbal level, you can observe an ancient culture that has refined simplicity to a spiritual art. The disciplines of a sadhu's daily routine and rules of purity cultivate a state of calm inspiration. Few real sadhus speak English, and it would require years of study to acquire enough of their language to receive verbal teachings. However, though it is useful to know a little Hindi, sadhus are quite accessible—the lack of a common language need not keep you from encountering their world.

It is essential to approach sadhus with humility and respect. While sitting around a sadhu's dhuni, remember that their fire is sacred: it is not a receptacle for burning paper wrappers, cigarette butts, or other discarded items. Be careful not to touch them or their possessions, because of their rules of ritual purity.

Sit among them with a quiet mind, but be aware that some sadhus are charlatans. You can recognize great souls, or mahatmas, by their humility. The prior life of genuine sadhus is of no relevance, and they are not inclined to discuss their past, their personal history, or their achievements.

In the company of foreigners, a sadhu may compromise his rules of conduct. An inferior sadhu may have ambitions of being recognized as a guru by foreigners. Filled with visions of future ashrams in the West, he may forgo adherence to the more strict rules. When the exotic lifestyle of an ascetic meets the naive fascination of a foreign woman, trouble may ensue. Though celibacy is a highly regarded state for a sadhu—and in the strictest traditions even looking at a picture of a woman is considered unworthy—many sadhus have no reservations about enjoying sex with a foreign woman. This form of cultural exchange is best avoided, as it will likely leave the sadhu with years of reparation in his sadhana. To avert a sexual encounter with a sadhu, it may help to visualize him walking around in your hometown wearing short hair and jeans. Quite ordinary!

Sadhus are often pleased to share their spiritual knowledge or simply to serve chai to Western visitors. They may even welcome you to live with them and share their food and intoxicants. Their generosity is usually genuine, and, with proper sensitivity to decorum, living with them can prove valuable. If you do remain for some time, it's appropriate to contribute money toward expenses and present blankets as a gesture of gratitude. Before leaving, it's traditional to present an offering of money to the presiding sadhu. And singing a small chant in their language is a gracious gesture that will leave you all with the best kind of memories.

—SITA SHARAN

Since agriculture and trades where animals are sold for food are considered to generate negative karma, Jains have become strong in the business and professional community. There are only about 4.5 million Jains in India, but their high ethical standards have made them respected and influential.

A contemporary Jain teacher well known around the world is Gurudev Shree Chitrabanhu in Bombay (p. 179). The ancient Jain temples in Mt. Abu, Rajasthan, are a major pilgrimage site (p. 243).

✺ Sikhism

Sikhism was born in the early 1500s from the vision of the first Sikh guru, Guru Nanak. After first rejecting his family's Hindu religion, then trying and rejecting Islam, he had an ecstatic vision while bathing in a river. Claiming to have been taken to God's kingdom, he returned pronouncing, "God is neither Hindu nor Muslim, and the path I follow is God's."

Born at a time when corrupt rulers held sway in India and oppression of the people was severe, Guru Nanak founded a practical religion based on social responsibility and responsibility to God. Like Hinduism, Sikhism posits the laws of karma and reincarnation; however, it rejects image worship, Vedic rituals, and discrimination based on caste and sex. The Sikh scripture begins with the basic declaration Ek Onkar Satnam—"There is One God whose Name is Truth."

The name Sikh comes from the Punjabi word "sikhna," which means study or learning. As a spiritual discipline, Sikhism has two basic components: a daily discipline of meditation and prayer combined with social service and action. Guru Nanak taught the importance of earning a livelihood and supporting your family while living an honest, moral life. He emphasized the importance of charity to the poor, the sick, and the old. Sikh beggars are very rarely seen in India because beggary is considered a sin.

The Sikh holy book is the Guru Granth Sahib, a compilation of the teachings of the ten Sikh gurus who lived and taught from the late fifteenth to the early eighteenth century. The last guru, Guru Gobind Singh, formed a Sikh brotherhood to fight against the Moghul invaders, which was known as the Pure Order, or Khalsa. Male members took the last name Singh, or Lion; women took Kaur, or Princess. Members adopted what were to become the five marks of Sikhism, known as the five K's: Kesh, or unshorn hair and beard; Kanga, or comb; Kara, the steel bangle; Kach, or underdrawers; and Kirpan, or steel sword. The five K's each have spiritual as

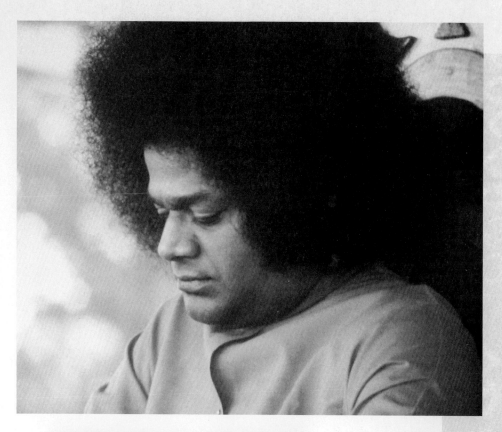

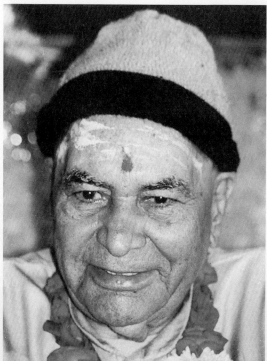

Sri Sathya Sai Baba

Sri H. W. L. Poonjaji

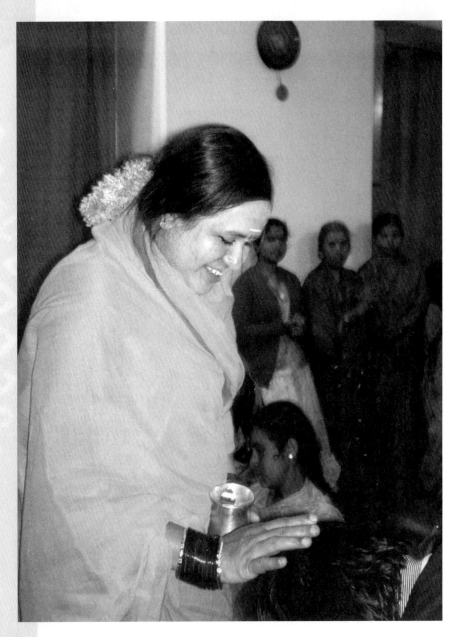

Sri Karunamayi

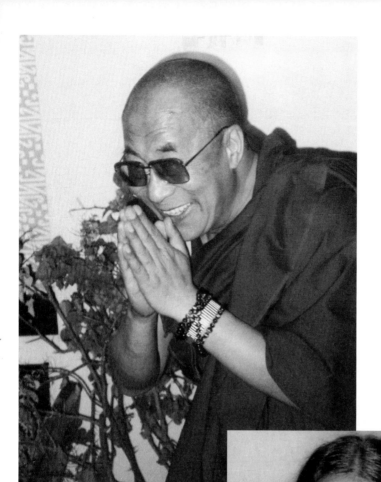

His Holiness
the Dalai Lama

Mata
Amritanandamayi

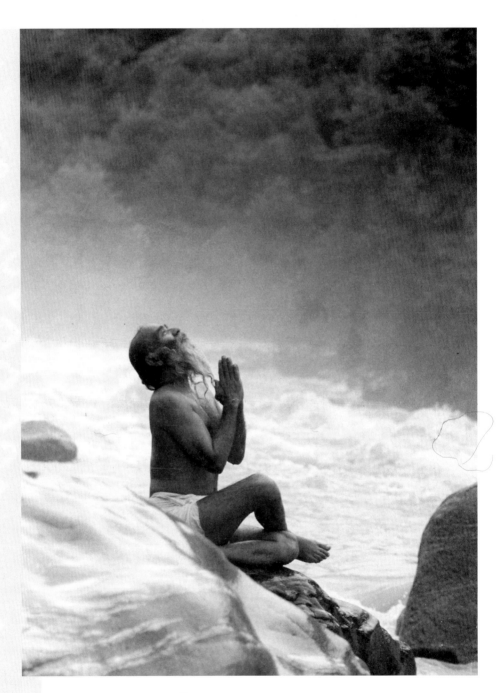

Swami Shyam

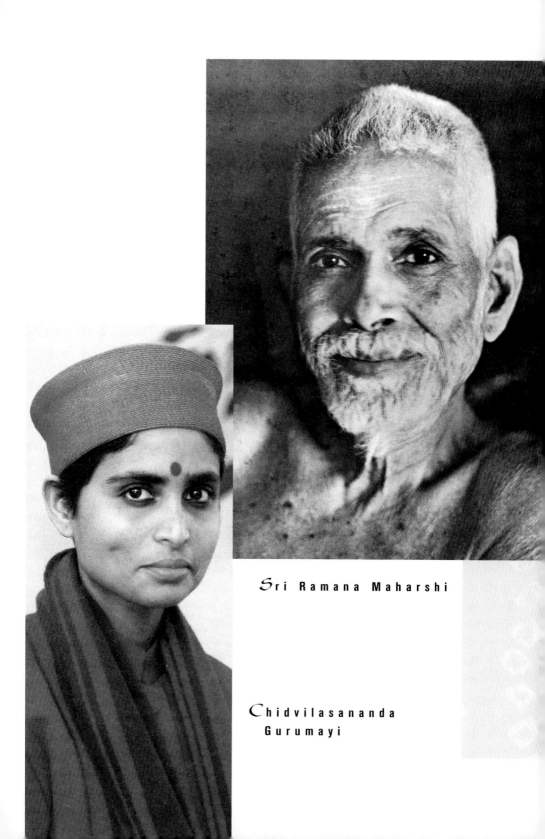

Sri Ramana Maharshi

Chidvilasananda
Gurumayi

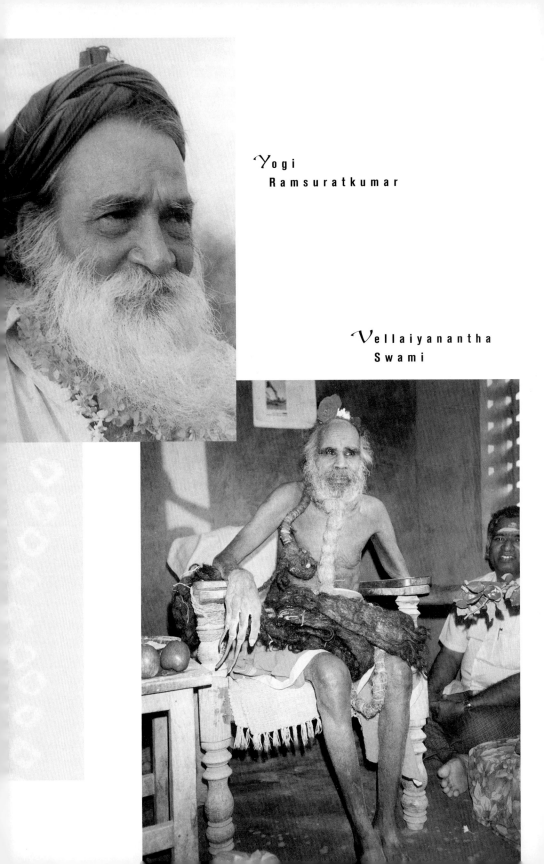

Yogi
Ramsuratkumar

Vellaiyanantha
Swami

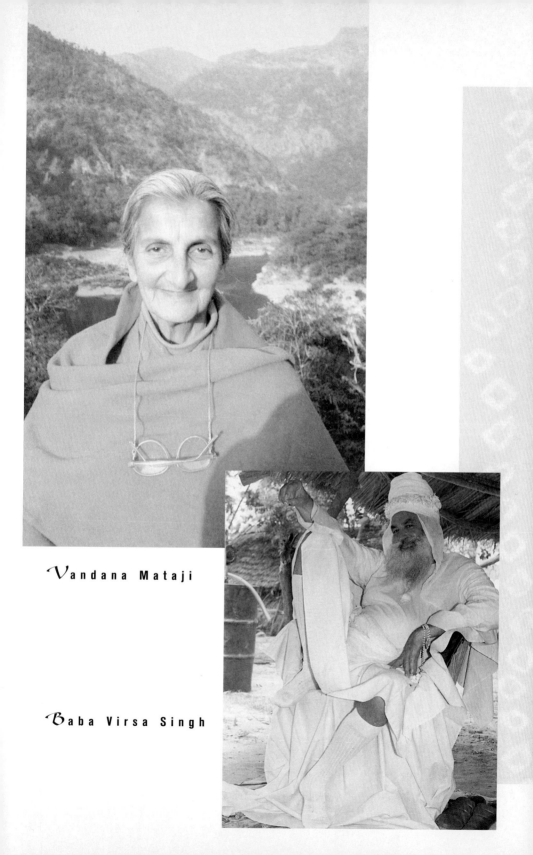

Vandana Mataji

Baba Virsa Singh

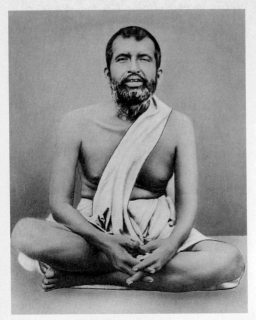

Sri
Ramakrishna

Sri B.K.S.
Iyengar

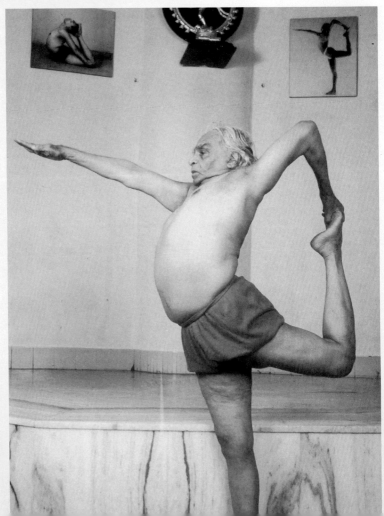

well as practical significance, and contribute to self-respect and strong community identity.

For information about Sikh pilgrimage sites, see p. 237. A contemporary Sikh spiritual master is Baba Virsa Singh at the Gobind Sadan center near Delhi (p. 320).

✺ Islam and Sufism

Islam—an Arabic word that means "submission to the will of God"—began in 610 C.E. when an Arab trader born in Mecca became a prophet after having visions of the Angel Gabriel. The prophet Mohammed is believed by Moslems to be the last of a line of prophets featured in the Old and New Testaments, beginning with Abraham and including Jesus Christ.

"There is only one God, Allah, and Mohammed is his Prophet," proclaims the basic tenet of Islam. Islam's holy book is the Quran, which contains the prophecies received by Mohammed; it is supplemented by the Hadith, a collection of his instructions and sayings. Formal worship is conducted in mosques, where namaaz, or prayer, is chanted five times a day.

With a population of about 105 million Moslems, India is one of the largest Islamic nations in the world. Islam entered India within a hundred years of the death of Mohammed, brought by Arab seamen and raiders. Islam made a more aggressive advance during the eleventh century with a wave of Moslem invasions, and Moslem rulers held sway over much of India for almost eight hundred years. However, Hinduism remained the dominant religion of the populace.

Of greatest interest to most Western spiritual seekers in India is Sufism, the mystical branch of Islam, a tolerant and nondogmatic path that emphasizes direct personal communion with God. Sufis emphasize the path of love, using music (qawalli) and dance to induce ecstatic trance. A flow of enlightened teachers of Sufism began from the Near East in the thirteenth century, and Sufism has a strong influence to this day, particularly in Kashmir.

For information about Moslem sacred sites in Kashmir, see p. 119. Sufi teachings are given at the Dargah of Hazrat Inayat Khan in New Delhi (p. 317).

✺ Christianity

According to legend, St. Thomas the Apostle arrived in India in 54 A.D. and is buried on a hilltop in what is now a suburb of Madras. In fact, some people will tell you that Jesus himself spent time in India mastering yogic powers, although there's little scholarly evidence to back up that claim. Today, there are 22 million Christians in India, mainly concentrated in Nagaland, Kerala, and Goa.

From the point of view of the Western spiritual seeker, the most interesting aspect of Christianity in India are the "Christian ashrams"— Christian communities organized like traditional Hindu ashrams and committed to interfaith dialogue. Good places to start are the Christa Prema Seva Ashram in Pune (p. 211) and the Saccidananda Ashram in Tamil Nadu (p. 244). If you're interested in undiluted Christianity, try the late Mother Teresa's Missionaries of Charity in Calcutta (p. 379).

nirvana

Prasanthi Nilayam Ashram
Puttaparthi, Andhra Pradesh

Bhagavan Sri Sathya Sai Baba (1926–   )

With over ten million devotees worldwide—and 1,638 centers in 137 countries—Sathya Sai Baba is undoubtedly the most famous of India's living gurus. He's believed by his disciples to be an avatar, a human incarnation of God, and his plump, frizzy-haired visage can be spotted on rickshaw dashboards, cash registers, phone booths, and altars all over India, alongside more traditional deities like Krishna and Ganesh. His main ashram in his birth town of Puttaparthi has grown to the size of a small, well-regimented city, where thousands of people come every day in quest of miracles and blessings.

Teacher and Teachings

Sai Baba is best known for his alleged miracles, which include mind-reading, healing people of cancer, blindness, paralysis, and other diseases, and materializing Swiss watches, Shiva lingams, and a variety of other coveted gifts with a wave of his hand. As a divine being, he is said to be in command of the laws of nature; he himself has explained that "Swami creates some objects in just the same way that he created the universe." While such powers, or *siddhis*, are frequently attributed to Indian saints, Sai Baba is remarkable for the frequency and consistency of these phenomena, which have continued unabated for over forty years and been witnessed by millions of people (although some have challenged them as clever magician's tricks).

The miracle stories fill volumes and run the gamut from cosmic to comical. A distant devotee prays to Baba's picture and a layer of *vibhuti* (sacred ash) appears on the glass like a fungus. Baba materializes surgical instruments and operates on a boy's tumor—the boy is healed and bears no scars. The empty gas tank of a devotee's car spontaneously refills itself to overflowing. A devotee cables Baba about her lost traveler's checks and they mysteriously reappear in her handbag. People come to darshan in wheelchairs and walk away on their own feet; people come blind and leave sighted. And, of course, there's the endless rain of materialized objects showering into the hands of deserving devotees: candy, rings, statues, malas, showers of marigolds. If you don't like the gift you've been given, Baba can simply blow on it, and before your eyes it transforms into something different.

However, more serious devotees insist that the miracles are not the point—they're simply Baba's way of getting people's attention so that he can transmit his real message of love and devotion to God. Many devotees are initially drawn to Baba because he has appeared to them in a dream or a vision—often before they have even heard of him. In most of the Sai Baba stories, external miracles simply precipitate the recipient's inner spiritual awakening.

"It is Bhagavan Baba's mission to help humanity wake up to the innate divinity (atma) within all creation and to see that the principles of satya (truth), dharma (righteousness), shanti (peace and equanimity) and prema (selfless love) govern all human relations and activities," explains an ashram publication. "The principal method prescribed by Bhagavan Baba for this purpose is constant loving remembrance of the Supreme Divine and consecration of all activity as offering to the Lord." In recent years, Sai Baba's emphasis has been on education (he has founded schools and universities all over India), health care (charitable hospitals and dispensaries), and rural development.

Sai Baba is very much a figurehead guru for the masses—so many people came to his seventieth birthday celebration (over five million, by the ashram's count) that the state had to run extra trains from Bangalore for the occasion. (All of the devotees were fed at the ashram, which devotees say is just another one of Baba's miracles.) With thousands of pilgrims always present, don't expect much personal attention at Prasanthi Nilayam, at least on the external plane. (The tone is set by the airport-style metal detectors that guard the entrance to the darshan courtyard.) On the subtle levels, though, devotees claim that Baba watches over everyone there—everything that happens to you, externally or internally, is said to be unfolding according to Baba's master plan.

The main attraction is the twice-daily darshan, in which Sai Baba walks through the crowd—to the tune of his tinkling flute theme song—radiating blessings and distributing sweets and vibhuti. (Vibhuti, or sacred ash, is said to be symbolic of the immortal spirit, that which is left when everything worldly has been burnt away.) "Never underestimate what is being accomplished by the act of darshan," Sai Baba has said. "My walking amongst you is a gift yearned for by the gods of the highest heaven and here you are receiving this grace." Sometimes he accepts handwritten letters containing devotees' questions and prayers, which he reportedly responds to via dreams and other telepathic communications. Many people report miraculous healings and spiritual breakthroughs, although you are officially cautioned not to feel punished or rejected if that doesn't happen: "Baba has said that he does not interfere with people's karmic decisions, made before birth, about what will bring them most quickly to enlightenment. The ego may be asking for something that the soul, for its own higher reasons, does not want."

During darshan, Sai Baba generally selects individuals or groups to come see him for private interviews at a later time. These choices are made by Baba alone—based, it is said, on your past-life karma—and you're warned not to try to improve that karma by bribing or cajoling ashram officials. However, old-timers hint that you can improve your chances if you're part of a group from the same country, all identified by country flags—if you've come on your own, you might want to look around for a group you can join.

With so much riding on darshan, it's not surprising that it can sometimes be a somewhat tense affair. People start lining up hours beforehand and, once seated, guard their places ferociously. (Stand up to look around, and you may find that your spot has been nabbed from beneath your rump.) Most of the day is spent in waiting for darshan, darshan, postdarshan singing, and meals. The rest of the spiritual teachings take place on the inner planes, with everything that happens—since it's all decreed by Baba—viewed as grist for the spiritual mill.

Facilities and Food

The ashram is a massive complex of domed and turreted buildings in pastel shades of peach, baby blue, and pale yellow. Thousands of people can be housed in unfurnished four-person rooms (with attached toilet and shower) or dormitories with communal toilets and showers. Men, women, and families are housed separately; there are separate dorms for Indians and Westerners. Expect to share your room with several others; if the ashram is especially crowded, you may be assigned to a dormitory.

Mattresses, bedding, and mosquito netting are not provided. You can buy a mattress and pillow in town for about Rs 150 (try to be sure you're getting a new one, although with so many pilgrims passing through, there's bound to be a brisk recycling business). Mosquito nets are available in the ashram's general store.

Meals and snacks are available at two inexpensive canteens (one Western, one Indian)—you must stand in line to purchase meal tickets in advance (it's best to get at least Rs 20 worth of 1- and 1.5-rupee tickets as soon as you arrive). Other facilities include a bookstore, a museum featuring exhibits on world religions, a 20,000-person auditorium, a large hospital complex, and a university.

On arrival at the ashram, you must register and show your passport at the Public Relations office. Modest dress is required—long pants for men, floor-length skirts or pants for women. Women must drape a scarf across their chest.

Schedule

Foreigners are only welcome at Prasanthi Nilayam when Baba is there. He has no definite schedule, so call in advance to find out where he is. During the hot season (March to June), he is generally at the hill station of Kodaikanal; there are no accommodations at the ashram there, but plenty of hotels. He also often stays at a smaller ashram called Brindavan in Whitefield village just outside Bangalore. There are few accommodations at the Whitefield ashram; however, it's easy to make daily visits from Bangalore.

When Baba is in residence, the usual schedule begins with chanting of Omkar (twenty-one Oms) and a song to the dawn at 5:20 A.M. (to get into this event, you'll have to start lining up around 3 A.M.), followed by Nagarsankirtan (chanting of devotional songs while walking around the ashram). Darshan and interviews begin at 6:45 A.M., but you'll need to start lining up around 5 A.M. Devotional singing (bhajans) begins at 9 A.M. In the afternoon, darshan begins at 3:45 P.M. (start lining up around 2), followed by bhajans at 5:30. Lights out is at 9 P.M.

Special festivals—when unusually large crowds converge—include

Sivarathri (February or March), the sacred night of Shiva; Ramanawami (March or April), Rama's birthday; Guru Purnima (July or August), dedicated to the sage Vyasa; Janmastami (August–September), Krishna's birthday; Deepavali (October–November), the festival of lights; Sai Baba's birthday (November 23); Christmas Day (December 25).

Fees

The dormitory is free. If there are three or more in your party, you can get a room with attached bath for Rs 55. Meals cost about Rs 6 to 10, depending on what you order.

Contact Information

PRASANTHI NILAYAM ASHRAM
P.O. DIST. ANANTAPUR
ANDHRA PRADESH 515 134
TEL: 91-8555-2036
FAX: 91-8555-2190

BRINDAVAN (WHITEFIELD VILLAGE ASHRAM)
KADUGODI P.O.
BANGALORE 560 067
TEL: WHITEFIELD 33

U.S. Contact:
SATHYA SAI BOOK CENTER OF AMERICA
305 WEST FIRST STREET
TUSTIN, CA 92780
TEL: (714) 669-0522
FAX: (714) 669-9138

How to Get There

Puttaparthi is located in Anantapur District of Andhra Pradesh, about 180 kilometers north of Bangalore (which is in Karnataka). Buses or taxis go directly to Puttaparthi from Bangalore (the trip takes three to five hours). By train, go to Dharmavaram or Penukonda (stations on the

Bangalore-Secunderabad line) or to Mudigubba (via Bukkapatnam); then take a bus or minibus to Puttaparthi.

Other Services

Puttaparthi is a major tourist center offering all services, including lodging, STD/ISD and fax booths, shops, and restaurants.

Books and Tapes

Books by and about Sai Baba are available in the spirituality section of most major bookstores or through the Sathya Sai Book Center (see Contact Information). A recommended introductory book is *The Holy Man and the Psychiatrist* by Samuel H. Sandweiss, M.D.

Dr. Y. J. Rao, Head of the Geology Department, Osmania University, Hyderabad, was an appropriate person to witness the transmutation of solid rock to another substance—with a valuable spiritual lesson thrown in for good measure.

One day at Puttaparti, Baba picked up a rough piece of broken granite and, handing it to Dr. Rao, asked him what it contained. The geologist mentioned a few of the minerals in the rock.

Baba: "I don't mean those—something deeper."

Dr. Rao: "Well, molecules, atoms, electrons, protons . . ."

Baba: "No, no—deeper still!"

Dr. Rao: "I don't know, Swami."

Baba took the lump of granite from the geologist, and holding it up with his fingers, blew on it. It was never out of Dr. Rao's sight, yet when Baba gave it back to him its shape had completely changed. Instead of being an irregular chunk it was a statue of Lord Krishna playing his flute. The geologist noted also a difference in color and a slight change in the structure of the substance.

Baba: "You see? Beyond your molecules and atoms, God is in the rock. And God is sweetness and joy. Break off the foot and taste it."

Dr. Rao found no difficulty in breaking off the "granite" foot of the little statue. Putting it in his mouth as directed, he found that it was sugar candy. The whole of the idol, created instantly out of the piece of granite, was now made of candy.

—HOWARD MURPHET

(from *Sai Baba: Man of Miracles*)

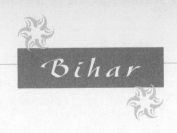
International Meditation Centre
Bodh Gaya, Bihar

Venerable Dr. Rastrapal Mahathera (1930–)

The oldest Buddhist meditation school in Bodh Gaya, the International Meditation Centre actually consists of two separate sites: an older, rural retreat about five kilometers outside of Bodh Gaya, where experienced meditators can stay for longer retreats, and a newer place in the considerably noisier center of town, which offers ongoing instruction for newcomers to Buddhist practice. Both centers provide training in vipassana (insight meditation), which their founder, the Venerable Dr. Rastrapal Mahathera, describes as "the only way to the Highest Bliss, and as proclaimed by the Great Teacher, Lord Buddha, the one and the only way to destroy the mental defilement and also the Cycle of Birth, Decay, Death, and Rebirth."

Teachers and Teachings

Dr. Rastrapal is a Buddhist monk and scholar from Bangladesh who studied meditation with a number of Thai and Burmese masters and wrote a Ph.D. thesis on "the psychological approach to the Buddhist Meditation." His courses are strictly based on the classic teachings of the Satipatthana Sutta, the foundation text of the vipassana technique, which teaches that insight into the transitory nature of existence—and thus liberation from the painful bonds of craving and attachment—can be achieved through meditation on the four foundations of mindfulness: the body, the feelings, the mind, and the objects of the mind.

At the newer center, training is continuous year-round—you can start the program at any time and continue for as long or short a period as you wish. Normally you'll begin with three or four hours a day of instruction and meditation, supplemented by recommended reading. Once you've received basic instruction, you can start a full-time program of meditation at the new or old center. The full schedule includes seven or eight periods of sitting meditation every day, alternating with walking meditation, light meals, and an evening discourse. The atmosphere is strict, and you must maintain silence except for discourses, discussions with the teacher, and necessary inquiries.

Most courses are taught by Dr. Rastrapal himself, although a Western teacher also leads some ten-day retreats at the old center during the winter. The meditation training begins by focusing on the rising and falling movements of the abdomen during breathing, as a means of focusing the mind. If thoughts or sensations arise, you're instructed to simply note them—as "seeing," "hearing," "tasting," "thinking," etc.—and return your attention to the rising and falling abdomen. This process of concentrated awareness and mental noting is extended throughout the walking and eating meditations as well, so that walking is accompanied by a stream of notes like "lifting the foot, lowering the foot" and eating by "opening the mouth, placing the food," etc. "Meditators are supposed to abide by the strict observance of each and every material and mental phenomena with arduous zeal and strong determination to experience and enter into the stream of sanctification," Dr. Rastrapal writes. "Having faithfully, earnestly, and diligently followed the instructions with full awareness and mindfully, the meditator will enter into the stages of Insight one after another."

Facilities and Food

The old center is a restful, rural place on expansive grounds with lots of trees and a few wandering cows. About fifty people can be accommodated in dormitories and two- to three-person rooms with attached baths. The center includes a library, a post office, a free primary school for children, and a health clinic. The new center near the Mahabodhi temple is more modern and compact, accommodating up to 300 meditators at a time in dormitories and two- and four-person rooms. Simple meals are provided at both centers. You will need to supply your own sleeping bag, blankets, pillows, bed sheets, mosquito netting, and meditation cushion. (These supplies can be purchased in Bodh Gaya if you don't have them already.)

Schedule

The daily schedule for the full-time course begins at 6 A.M. The rest of the day consists of alternating, forty-five-minute periods of sitting

In and Around Bodh Gaya

Bodh Gaya is the crown jewel of Buddhist pilgrimage sites—the place where the Buddha attained enlightenment while sitting under the shade of a pipal tree 2,500 years ago. Today, Bodh Gaya casts its own spell, set in the midst of ancient farm fields hardly touched by modernity. Dotted around the towering Mahabodhi Temple, which marks the site of the Buddha's enlightenment, are temples representing nearly every Buddhist country. During the active winter season, the temple grounds are a sea of saffron, black, and maroon robes, as monks and nuns from all traditions circumambulate the stupa and meditate and chant under the spreading branches of the Bodhi Tree, a descendant of the actual tree that sheltered the Buddha.

The tree itself is protected by a locked gate, but it's possible to get permission to enter the compound and sit before the vajrasana—the "diamond throne"—where the Buddha awakened. You can also sit on a grassy knoll beside the large pool where the Snake King is said to have protected the meditating Buddha during a storm. A pathway of carved lotus blossoms alongside the temple marks the path where the Buddha did walking meditation after his enlightenment.

The ancient temple itself—whose original structure was probably built around the seventh century C.E.—is covered with exquisite sculptures of the Buddha and bodhisattvas. Adjacent to the Mahabodhi Temple compound is a complex of Hindu temples overseen by a priest.

Winter—November through February—is the active time in Bodh Gaya. Teachers and disciples, both Western and Eastern, arrive to pray, meditate, and conduct or attend courses in Buddhist philosophy and meditation (pp. 57–61). Tibetan Buddhist lamas often teach in Bodh Gaya, and there are two Tibetan Buddhist temples, in addition to Bhutanese, Chinese, Japanese, and Vietnamese shrines. Some offer accommodations, and most have resident monks or nuns. One of the oldest and best-known temples is the Burmese Vihar, established in 1936, located at the entrance to town. Rooms are available, as is advice on meditation from the bhante, or abbot. Another option is the Mahabodhi Society guest house, tended by Sri Lankan monks.

Bodh Gaya is also a good base from which to visit some other important Buddhist sites. A half an hour leisurely walk from the Mahabodhi temple will take you to the place where legend says a young girl named Sujata offered a bowl of milk and rice to the Buddha just before he achieved enlightenment. (In accepting her food, he ended years of harsh ascetic practices and symbolically proclaimed the wisdom of "the Middle Way.") Although the actual site has not been located with certainty, the peaceful spot with its small Hindu shrine is worth visiting. Also within hiking distance is Pragbodhi, or Mora Pahar as the hill is now called. Here a small Tibetan temple marks the cave where the Buddha lived for six years doing ascetic practices before his enlightenment. Any local child will guide you to these sites for a few rupees.

A day trip by road from Bodh Gaya is Rajgir, where you can walk to the top of Vulture's Peak, where the Buddha delivered—and some say is still delivering on subtle levels—the teaching on Prajnaparamita, or Perfection of Wisdom. Many interesting ruins, caves, and stupas in the area testify to Rajgir's ancient eminence, including one stupa that is said to have been built by the Emperor Ashoka. There's also an enormous modern stupa built by Japanese Buddhists, a number of hot springs, and several hotels. It's best to go to Rajgir in daylight because this area is plagued by banditry.

On the road from Bodh Gaya, about thirteen kilometers from Rajgir, are the ruins of the great Buddhist university of Nalanda. Early references to it are found from the fifth century B.C.E., and its last gasps were some time in the mid-thirteenth century C.E. Nagarjuna, Aryadeva, Asanga, Vasubandhu, and Dharmakirti are among the famous philosophers who studied and taught there. The extensive ruins of monasteries and temples, so meticulously laid out with their long-gone sophisticated amenities, offer a good place to think about the impermanence of all phenomena.

—LEA TERHUNE

and walking meditation, with brief breaks for meals. Every evening there is a discourse by the teacher.

Fees

Suggested donation is Rs 50 per day for food and lodging.

Contact Information

INTERNATIONAL MEDITATION CENTRE
Attn: THE GENERAL SECRETARY
BUDDHAGAYA P.O.
BODH GAYA 824 231
DIST. GAYA
BIHAR
TEL: 91-631-400707
FAX: 91-631-400707

How to Get There

The "old center" is near Magadh University, about 5 kilometers from Bodh Gaya, and can be reached by autorickshaw. The "new center" is in Bodh Gaya proper about .5 kilometers from the Mahabodhi Temple, across the road from the Thai temple.

Bodh Gaya is about 10 kilometers from Gaya, which is on the main railway line between New Delhi (16 hours by express train) and Calcutta (10 hours). From Gaya station, take a taxi, autorickshaw, or bus to Bodh Gaya. Traveling this road after dark is not recommended, as banditry is common.

You can also fly into Patna, which is 100 kilometers from Bodh Gaya, and then take a train or bus to Gaya or a bus or taxi directly to Bodh Gaya.

Other Services

Although Bodh Gaya is a relatively small town, it is a major pilgrimage center. Most services are available, including restaurants, shops, and fax.

The Burmese Vihar, the Mahabodhi Society, and the Bhutanese Temple offer basic accommodations. The Ashok Travellers Lodge and Tourists Bungalows offer more expensive facilities.

Books and tapes are available at the new center.

When Ignorance is shattered, Light overfloods, Wisdom arises, the meditator becomes Fully Delivered and Freed from the bondages of cycles of Birth, Rebirth, Decay, and Death.... Herein, lies the sole object and the very purpose of meditation.

—VEN. DR. RASTRAPAL MAHATHERA
(from *A Guide to the Mind Purification*)

Root Institute for Wisdom Culture
Bodh Gaya, Bihar

Lama Thubten Yeshe Rinpoche, Founder (1935–1984)
Lama Thubten Zopa Rinpoche, President (1946–   )

A combination meditation retreat, cultural center, and social service organization, the Root Institute for Wisdom Culture was founded by two Tibetan lamas as a gesture of gratitude to India for giving a home to the exiled Tibetan people. Meditation courses in the Tibetan Buddhist tradition are offered from November through March at the Institute's lush three-acre center in the farmland near Bodh Gaya. You can also volunteer year-round in the Institute's service projects, which include a leprosy clinic, a tree-planting campaign, and a home for the destitute.

Teachers and Teachings

The Root Institute was founded in 1984 by Lama Thubten Yeshe Rinpoche and his disciple Lama Thubten Zopa Rinpoche, who also founded the Kopan Monastery in Nepal and the Tushita Centre in Dharamsala (p. 103). The Institute is a member of the Foundation for the Preservation of the Mahayana Tradition, a worldwide network of Buddhist centers, monasteries, and affiliated groups that Lama Zopa has headed since Lama Yeshe's death in 1984.

Lama Zopa himself is rarely at the Institute, whose current director is European and which is staffed by a combination of Indians, Westerners, and Tibetans. Courses are taught by Tibetan lamas—including some highly respected elders who normally live in strict seclusion—and experienced Western teachers. Courses range from ten days to one month; there are introductory courses in meditation and Buddhist philosophy (with titles like "How to Put Happiness and Satisfaction into Your Life"), courses for experienced students that focus on specific Tibetan texts, and occasional meditation intensives (such as a one-month *samatha* [concentration] retreat led by a strict ascetic). Most courses include discourses, guided meditation, and group discussions.

Because of the considerable emphasis on service work, a stay at the Institute—even if you're just there for a meditation course—provides the opportunity to get in touch with both the enormous suffering that can be found in India and the relief that can be offered through compassionate action. Not far from the meditation hall is the newly built Destitute Home, which houses people who have been picked up off the streets, such as a boy who was found in a local train station being offered for sale for his body parts, and a child with amnesia found in a local park. Other projects include five village schools; a number of irrigation and farming projects; and the Maitri center for the prevention, treatment, and rehabilitation of leprosy. Volunteers—especially long-term—are welcome.

Facilities and Food

The Institute is currently surrounded by fields of lentils, mustard, and chickpeas, but with the building boom that's going on in Bodh Gaya, that probably won't last long. The heavily planted grounds are thick with bougainvillea, palm trees, and hibiscus—and also, unfortunately, with mosquitoes attracted by the moisture and vegetation.

The Institute can accommodate about seventy guests in six-person dormitories, double rooms, and a few individual huts. Bedding and mosquito nets are provided. There's a meditation hall, a small library, and a laundry facility. Plans are under way to construct a 170-foot Maitreya Buddha statue in the middle of a "meditation park" featuring various educational audiovisual programs, meditation pavilions, flower gardens, and a picnic area.

Schedule

Schedule varies according to the specific teacher and program.

Fees

Rs 150 per day for three meals, dormitory accommodations, and course. Costs are slightly higher for a semiprivate room or hut.

Contact Information

ROOT INSTITUTE FOR WISDOM CULTURE
Attn: RECEPTION MANAGER
BODH GAYA
DIST. GAYA 824 231
BIHAR
TEL: 91-631-400714
FAX: 91-631-400548 (C/O GPO GAYA)

U.S. Contact:
FPMT CENTRAL OFFICE
DIRECTOR HARVEY HARROCKS
P.O. BOX 1778
SOQUEL, CA 95073
TEL: (408) 476-8435
FAX: (408) 476-4823

How to Get There

Bodh Gaya is about 10 kilometers from Gaya, which is on the main railway line between New Delhi (16 hours by express train) and Calcutta (10 hours). From Gaya station, take a taxi, autorickshaw, or bus to Bodh Gaya. Traveling this road after dark is not recommended, as banditry is common.

You can also fly into Patna, which is 100 kilometers from Bodh Gaya, and then take a train or bus to Gaya or a bus or taxi directly to Bodh Gaya. Ask in Bodh Gaya for directions to the Root Institute.

Other Services

Although Bodh Gaya is a relatively small town, it is a major pilgrimage center. Most services are available, including restaurants, shops, and fax.

The Burmese Vihar, the Mahabodhi Society, and the Bhutanese Temple offer basic accommodations. The Ashok Travellers Lodge and Tourists Bungalows offer more expensive facilities.

Books and Tapes

Books and tapes are available at the Root Institute or in the United States through Wisdom Publications, 361 Newbury Street, Boston, MA 02115, Tel: (617) 536-3358; Fax: (617) 536-1897; Orders (800) 272-4050.

The Destitute Home opened in January 1994 with the arrival of Balajee. He was found at Gaya railway station where he had lived for one year. Balajee was found lying motionless in a pool of excrement. He had not moved for four or five days. . . . Apart from the usual stomach problems of India, Balajee had a chest infection and severe weakness from emaciation. But his major problem seemed to be that he had lost all interest in life and had given up the wish to live. He spent most of each day sleeping wearing an expression of disgust with life. I thought I had better speak to him

about future lives and within hours received a letter from Lama Zopa to the same effect.

It was the solution. The thought that he might be reborn in an even worse situation was enough to wake him up. . . . He began walking around and taking an interest in life. He now often bows and prays to the small Buddha on our verandah and offers fresh flowers and incense.

—from the *Root News* (May 1994)

Wat Thai Bodh Gaya
Vipassana Retreats
Bodh Gaya, Bihar

 Christopher Titmuss (1944–   )

It may seem odd to go to India for a meditation course led by a British Buddhist—but for hundreds of foreign travelers, Christopher Titmuss's annual vipassana retreats in Bodh Gaya are one of the highlights of the spiritual circuit. A monk in Thailand and India from 1970 to 1976, Titmuss is the cofounder of Gaia House, a vipassana (insight meditation) retreat center in the South Devon countryside. He is also an internationally known teacher of "engaged spirituality," which emphasizes not only cultivating inner peace, stability, and awareness but also manifesting those qualities through social action.

Teachers and Teachings

Titmuss taught his first meditation retreat in Bodh Gaya in 1975, when he was still a monk in the Thai Buddhist tradition. Every January since then, he has led retreats at Bodh Gaya's Thai monastery, a few minute's walk from the Bodhi Tree. Assisting at the retreats are other well-known Western dharma teachers.

Generally attended by about 150 people, the ten-day retreats are based on the principles of the Buddhist meditation technique known as "vipassana," or "insight meditation," as well as the associated body of spiritual and ethical teachings set out by the Buddha himself. Vipassana teaches the cultivation of "choiceless awareness" of the body, feelings, and mental states. "Experience what is felt Here and Now, and be aware of any description or label of it," Titmuss instructs in one of his handouts. "Neither detach oneself from feelings nor indulge in them. Neither fight difficult emotions nor flee from them.... Allow claims and possessiveness over existence to fade away. Permit a palpably transforming silence and stillness to pervade one's being."

Retreats are held in silence except for daily talks by the teachers, personal meetings with the teachers, and occasional group discussions and question periods. They follow a rigorous schedule of sitting, walking, standing, and reclining meditation, including comprehensive meditation instruction and regular guided meditations. Eating is also performed as a meditation, with "initial reflection on worldwide interdependency that makes a meal possible" and mindful tasting, chewing, and swallowing of food. In regular periods of "loving kindness meditation" (metta), you focus on cultivating kindness and compassion in your heart and extending this warmth outward to others.

Titmuss particularly emphasizes the cultivation of awareness in daily life, including tips on recycling and conservation and advice to "be clear about the number of hours weekly facing a screen (television, computer, cinema)." In keeping with his emphasis on engaged spirituality, he encourages social action; however, he stresses that it must be "free from the narrow political ideology of the left, right, and center." Instead, he advises practitioners "to ask 'Where is the commitment to end suffering?' and to support this priority."

Facilities and Food

Constructed in 1957 by the Thai government as a symbol of friendship between Thailand and India, the Wat Thai Bodh Gaya temple complex includes a replica of an ancient marble temple in Thailand. The temple walls are decorated with paintings of the life of the Buddha, and there's an immense Buddha made from a combination of seven different metals.

Accommodations are in dormitories, which tend to be crowded during Titmuss's popular retreats; be prepared to meditate with choiceless awareness on the sound of your neighbor snoring. You will need to provide your own sleeping bag or blankets; it's also good to bring your own meditation cushion and mosquito net (available in the local market), as supplies are limited. A shawl is useful in the cool evenings.

Vegetarian meals are eaten in silence as a form of meditation.

Schedule

Retreats are held each year from January 7 to 17, January 17 to 27, and January 28 to February 4. To register before mid-November, write to Gaia House in England; after mid-November, write to Thomas Jost in Bodh Gaya (see Contact Information). It's not necessary to send a deposit.

The day begins with early morning yoga, followed by an intensive schedule of meditation that lasts until 9:30 P.M. Breakfast and lunch are the only two substantial meals; there's a light afternoon snack of tea and fruit, and a hot drink is served before bed. Evening talks are open to the public.

Fees

$50 (U.S.) for lodging, meals, and course fees. Additional donations for the teachers are accepted.

Contact Information

WAT THAI BODH GAYA
BODH GAYA
DIST. GAYA 824 231
BIHAR
INDIA
TEL: NONE
FAX: NONE

For Registration/Information:
Until Mid-November
THE MANAGERS
GAIA HOUSE TRUST
WEST OGWELL, NEAR NEWTON ABBOT
DEVON TQ12 6EN
ENGLAND
TEL: 0044 (0)1626-333613

After Mid-November:
THOMAS JOST
BODH GAYA POST OFFICE
DIST. GAYA
BIHAR 824 231
TEL: NONE

How to Get There

Wat Thai is about .5 kilometers from the Mahabodhi Temple in Bodh Gaya. Bodh Gaya is about 10 kilometers from Gaya, which is on the main railway line between New Delhi (16 hours by express train) and Calcutta (10 hours). From Gaya station, take a taxi, autorickshaw, or bus to Bodh Gaya. Traveling this road after dark is not recommended, as banditry is common.

You can also fly into Patna, which is 100 kilometers from Bodh Gaya, and then take a train or bus to Gaya or a bus or taxi directly to Bodh Gaya.

Other Services

Although Bodh Gaya is a relatively small town, it is a major pilgrimage center. Most services are available, including restaurants, shops, and fax.

The Burmese Vihar, the Mahabodhi Society, and the Bhutanese Temple offer basic accommodations. The Ashok Travellers Lodge and Tourists Bungalows offer more expensive facilities.

Books and Tapes

Christopher Titmuss is the author of *The Green Buddha, The Profound and the Profane,* and *Freedom of the Spirit.* All are available from Gaia House (see Contact Information).

Practice includes equally the social, religious, and political features of existence. We influence the world in the course of practice with the willingness to challenge abuse of power.

Practice includes working with various challenges so that all experiences and situations belong to practice.

—CHRISTOPHER TITMUSS

Bihar School of Yoga
Monghyr, Bihar

🌀 *Swami Satyananda, Founder (1923–)*
🌀 *Swami Niranjanananda Saraswati, President (1960–)*

The Bihar School of Yoga feels disconcertingly like a college campus, complete with a glittering concrete and steel administration building (topped with a giant Om sign) and roll-call taken at the start of each yoga class (with students answering to their names with a brisk "Hari Om!"). But perhaps that's appropriate for an ashram—already known for its intensive yoga training programs—that's in the process of launching the world's first "yoga university," a two-year master's program in yogic arts and sciences. Modeled on the ancient Buddhist university of Nalanda and the tantric university of Vikramshala, both of which flourished not far from here hundreds of years ago, the program aims to blend practice with scholarship in a traditional "gurukul" setting.

Teachers and Teachings

The ashram was founded in the early 1960s by Swami Satyananda, a disciple of the great Rishikesh yoga master Swami Sivananda (p. 343). Prior to studying with Sivananda, the young Satyananda was initiated by a female adept in tantra (p. 54)—a path that holds that the awakening of Shakti, or energy, is an essential step in the transformation of Shiva, or consciousness. Unlike other schools in the Sivananda lineage, the Bihar School teachings incorporate tantric elements, which awaken and redistribute prana through guided visualizations and kriyas (integrated sequences of asanas, pranayamas, mudras, and bandhas [energy locks]).

As Swami Satyananda said, "This physical body is a storehouse of pranic energy, a dynamo, with infinite types of electrical currents passing through it." At the Bihar School, asana, pranayama, mudras, and bandhas are viewed as a means of tapping into this storehouse. "Unless you understand how energy and consciousness work together, you can't awaken the higher levels of the mind," explains Swami Satyadharma, a senior American teacher who has been living at the ashram for almost twenty years.

Definitely, this is not a California-style tantra. This ashram is about discipline, surrender, and self-control—not hot tubs, heart sharing, and "sacred sex." Days are tightly scheduled from 5 A.M. to 8 P.M. with one day off a week. Students dress in white kurta pajamas, and the staff (about half Westerners, half Indians) wear the orange robes of sannyasins, or renunciants. The grounds are surrounded by sixteen-foot brick walls, topped with barbed wire, to keep the world out and the students in. Once you've entered through the giant gates, you can't leave the premises without a "gate pass" signed by two or three swamijis; student passports are confiscated, and getting them back—to go into town to change money, say—can require extensive negotiations. These measures are intended to cultivate an atmosphere of concentration by shielding you from the chaos of the outside world so you can concentrate on your studies in a traditional ashram setting.

The actual practices that are taught here were largely developed by Swami Satyananda himself—and modified to suit modern practitioners—based on hints and references in ancient tantric texts; classical yoga and samkhya teachings; and modern scientific research into anatomy, physiology, and psychology. If you're already a serious hatha-yoga practitioner, be forewarned that the asana practice here is very basic and minimal—and it's hard to find time elsewhere in the densely scheduled day for physical exercise, unless you create it, as some students do, by skipping a meal.

The Bihar School's "signature practice" is "yoga nidra"—literally, yogic sleep—a guided, supine meditation in which the entire body is progressively relaxed and the awareness withdrawn from the external world. In this relaxed state, says Satyananda, the mind is receptive to suggestions about removing unwanted habits and tendencies; and you can receive intuitive information from the unconscious that can help you solve all your problems. "In fact, yoga nidra can be used for directing the mind to accomplish anything," Satyananda wrote. "This is the secret of the extraordinary accomplishments of great yogis and swamis."

Courses are offered through two programs: the well-established Bihar School of Yoga and the newly launched Bihar Yoga Bharati (the yoga university). BSY offers one-month residential teacher training courses; fifteen-day yoga health management courses; advanced training in tantric practices for graduates of the teacher training program; and a sannyas introduction course that lets you (temporarily) explore the monastic life without giving up the world altogether. (The Bihar School has drawn some criticism from more traditional schools for its system of initiating students into different levels of "sannyas," which do not necessarily entail traditional lifestyle restrictions like celibacy.) BYB offers a four-month certificate in yogic studies; a one-year diploma program, and six two-year master's degrees: yoga philosophy; Sanskrit and other Indian languages; yoga psychology; Indology; applied yogic science; ecology and environmental studies. Courses are intensive and include exams and written papers.

Swami Satyananda left the Bihar School in 1988, first to become a wandering saddhu, then to found a service organization in another village. The ashram is now under the spiritual guidance of Satyananda's successor, Swami Niranjanananda, the son of one of Satyananda's devotees, who has been living at the ashram since he was four years old.

Facilities and Food

The campus sits in a crook of the Ganges River, which wraps around its terraced, immaculate lawns and gardens. According to local lore, this hill was the site of the palace of Karna, a king who fought against Kushna and Arjuna in the great Indian epic the Mahabarata. Five residential buildings contain 163 clean, well-appointed single and double rooms with private or shared baths; all bedding is provided. The seven-story main building contains classrooms, offices, and a research library.

Food is basic, non-spicy Indian vegetarian. No private cooking is permitted.

Schedule

Schedules vary from program to program, but generally begin with a 5:30 a.m. asana class, followed by a light breakfast; the rest of the day consists of alternating lectures, periods of karma yoga, and yoga nidra, with meals at 10:30 A.M. and 5:30 P.M. In the evenings there is kirtan or sat-sang.

Fees

At the Bihar Yoga Bharati, the four-month program is $1,000 (U.S.) for foreign students (Rs 4,000 for Indian nationals); the one-year program is $3,000 (U.S.) (Rs 12,000 for Indian nationals). The one-month teacher training program offered by the Bihar School is $300 (U.S.). Food and lodging are included.

Contact Information

BIHAR SCHOOL OF YOGA
GANGA DARSHAN, FORT
MONGHYR, BIHAR 811 201
TEL: 91-6344-22430
FAX: 91-6344-23169

How to Get There

Monghyr is accessible by trains from Delhi, Calcutta, Varanasi, and Bombay that stop at Jamalpur Junction station. The ashram is six miles from Jamalpur and can be reached by taxi.

Other Services

There are some services in Monghyr—which is a good-sized industrial town—but it's hard to get permission to go into town, even on your days off.

Books and Tapes

Dozens of books by Swami Satyananda and Swami Niranjanananda are available through the ashram store. A good introduction to the practice of the Bihar School is *Prana Pranayama Prana Vidya*, by Swami Niranjanananda Saraswati.

Tantra is essentially a practical science rather than an intellectual one, and only practice leads to true experience and real understanding.

—Swami Satyananda

BUDDHIST PILGRIMAGE SITES IN *Bihar and Uttar Pradesh*

Twenty-five hundred years ago the man who was to become the Buddha was born in Lumbini, located on modern maps just across the Indian border in Nepal. Lumbini is the first of the four chief Buddhist pilgrimage sites. The other three are in northeastern India in the states of Bihar and Uttar Pradesh: Bodh Gaya, the place of the Buddha's enlightenment (p. 78); Sarnath, the place where he gave his first teaching; and Kushinagar, the place where he left his body and achieved mahaparinirvana, or final liberation. According to the Mahaparivirvanasutra, the Buddha himself recommended pilgrimage to these four shrines, which are fairly accessible and are visited annually by thousands of pilgrims from around the world. Other frequently visited sites mark places where important events in the life of the Buddha occurred.

Thanks to the efforts of the Mauryan Emperor Ashoka, who was converted to Buddhism about two hundred years after the Buddha's death, we are able to recognize the most important pilgrimage sites today by the stone pillars he erected at each. Inscribed on each pillar, in several languages, are texts proclaiming the significance of the site.

Lumbini. The Buddha was born Siddhartha Gautama, the son of Suddhodana, king of the warrior Sakya clan, and Queen Maya. Their capitol city was Kapilavastu, and Siddhartha was born in nearby Lumbini.

In winter Lumbini is lushly beautiful, but in summer it can be unbearably hot, and the monsoon often brings treacherous floods. Although there are plans to develop the area into a kind of religious park, with forests, shrines, and pilgrim hostels, little has been done so far. Monks may be found in residence at the small Tibetan temple or the Theravadan temple, but, ongoing archeological investigation aside, activities in Lumbini revolve around prayer, meditation, and visits to the sacred park where Queen Mayadevi is believed to have given birth to her son. The centerpiece of the Lumbini park is the restored Mayadevi temple, dedicated to Queen Maya, mother of Buddha. Nearby is an Ashokan pillar and a bathing tank said to be where the baby prince had his first bath.

From Lumbini it is a short trip to the ruins of what is thought to be Kapilavastu, the royal city where the Buddha spent his life before renouncing his princely birthright. It is primarily an archaeological site.

Accommodations range from a simple guest house to the rather splendid Japanese-built Lumbini Hokke Hotel, where you can, if you choose, wash the road dust off in a traditional Japanese bath and sleep on a futon in a Japanese-style room.

Lumbini is a few kilometers from the border checkpost at Saunali (Naugarh on the Indian side). The nearest airport on the Nepal side is Bhairawa, and there is a well-traveled road to Kathmandu (about eight hours). On the Indian side, Gorakhpur or Lucknow are the nearest airports. From India, Lumbini may be approached by road or rail to Naugarh in Uttar Pradesh. Lumbini is only a few kilometers beyond the border. Taxis, scooters, and buses are available.

🌀 **Sarnath.** After the Buddha achieved enlightenment, he walked toward the sacred Hindu city of Kashi or Benares, now called Varanasi (p. 358). Near the city, in a Deer Park at Sarnath, he shared for the first time the truths he had realized, in what Buddhists call the "first turning of the wheel of dharma."

For those with an interest in Buddhist art, archaeology, or scholarship, Sarnath is a treat. A Tibetan Buddhist college features a library that is fast becoming computerized. The archeological museum houses priceless treasures.

The chief monuments of Sarnath are the Dhamekh and Dharmarajika stupas. Sadly, the Dharmarajika stupa—built by the Emperor Ashoka around 300 B.C.E. to preserve the relics of the Buddha—was destroyed by Jagat Singh, an official of the Raja of Banaras, who poached it for building materials in the late eighteenth century. Inside the stupa he found a green marble box containing relics of the Buddha, which he threw in the river. No human relics have been found in the Dhamekh stupa, although there is evidence that an earlier stupa had been raised in the same spot, probably also by Ashoka, to commemorate the actual site of the first teaching.

Surrounding the stupas are ruins of cells and courtyards of monasteries, shrines, and an Ashokan pillar. Sarnath is a tranquil place to walk and consider the Four Noble Truths first taught here by the Buddha: the truth of suffering; the causes of suffering; the cessation of suffering; and the path to enlightenment.

Sarnath is ten kilometers from downtown Varanasi which, as a city holy to Hindus, is a hub of pilgrimage tourism. Places to stay in Varanasi range from five-star on down. In Sarnath there are a few basic hostels, and it is far quieter than bustling Varanasi.

Flights and numerous trains arrive daily in Varanasi. From Varanasi take a taxi or autorickshaw to Sarnath. Although there are a few guest houses in Sarnath, there is greater choice of accommodation in Varanasi.

Kushinagar. The Buddha died in a remote village called Kushinagar. There, it is said, he achieved his parinirvana, or ultimate liberation. Kushinagar lies between Lumbini and Sarnath, near Kasia in the Indian state of Uttar Pradesh, and is easily accessible by road from Gorakhpur. Like other Buddhist sites, it has a mystic charm that tempts the visitor to stay awhile. Unfortunately, accommodations in Kushinagar are probably the worst on the main Buddhist circuit. Even in the time of the Buddha it was so much off the beaten track that some of his disciples reportedly complained to him about his choice of such a place to die.

After his parinirvana, the Buddha's body was cremated near Kushinagar and his relics distributed and enshrined in eight places, including Kushinagar. The shrine of the parinirvana houses a huge and quite beautiful image of the reclining Buddha. Behind the Nirvana Temple is the main stupa which is believed to contain relics of the Buddha. The surrounding park is populated by long-tailed langur monkeys and dotted with ancient monastic remains. Within a two-kilometer radius of the Nirvana Temple are another temple and the cremation stupa. Unless a tour group with a megaphone is present, it is a picture of serenity.

Kushinagar is about fifty-five kilometers east of Gorakhpur, and the best way to get there is by bus or taxi. One popular means of doing this circuit is taking a taxi from Varanasi to Lumbini, stopping overnight at Kushinagar at the government-run Traveller's Lodge.

🦋 **Vaishali.** Located near the town of Basarh about fifty kilometers north of Patna in Bihar, Vaishali was the scene of many incidents recounted in the sutras. It was, for years, the place of the "rainy season retreat" of the Buddha and his disciples. The Buddha announced his approaching death at Vaishali, and a hundred years after that event the Second Buddhist Council was held here. The relics of one of Buddha's main disciples Ananda were enshrined at Vaishali.

Now visitors can see an Ashokan pillar and the ruins of a number of stupas, some of which are believed to have contained relics of the Buddha. There are three bathing tanks and several temples. There are three hostels near Vaishali—including a youth hostel and a tourist rest home—and a Jain dharamsala where you can stay.

🦋 **Sravasti.** Not far from Gorakhpur in the state of Uttar Pradesh, Sravasti, like Vaishali and Rajgir, was the setting for important teachings, debates, and incidents in the life of the Buddha. Subsequently monasteries thrived there into the thirteenth century. The Buddha spent twenty-five rainy seasons in Sravasti at the Jetavana, a monastery and temple complex built by a wealthy benefactor, and performed some of his more astonishing miracles here.

Today there are remains of two monasteries, six temples, and five stupas, which evoke the feeling of the profound teachings given on the spot. One of the Sravasti stupas marks the place where the Buddha sat during his discourses. Another is said to be the stupa of Angulimala, a murderer who wore a necklace made from the fingers of his victims—he was converted by the Buddha and became a model monk. There is even a well where the Buddha drew water for daily use.

There are rest houses at the Burmese temple, the Chinese temple and the Jain dharamsala. Sravasti is reachable by road from Lucknow via Balrampur or Bahraich.

🦋 **Sankissa.** Sankasya—now Sankissa—is where the Buddha is said to have descended from Tushita Heaven where he had spent a rainy season teaching his mother, Queen Mayadevi. A flight of golden stairs is said to have appeared, down which the Buddha came. The stairs sank into the ground except for upper steps. The emperor Ashoka is said to have dug around the stairs and been unable to find their end, so he had a temple built above them.

A Hindu temple that superseded the Buddhist one marks the spot of the descent. There is an Ashokan pillar and a modern Buddhist temple built by a Sri Lankan monk. There are a few small guest houses in the vicinity. Sankasya is about 300 kilometers from Delhi, or 175 kilometers from Agra.

—LEA TERHUNE

The Library of Tibetan Works and Archives
Dharamsala, Himachal Pradesh

From the outside it looks like a Tibetan temple, but once you pass through its imposing red-varnished gates, the Library of Tibetan Works and Archives is very much a school, complete with the smell of chalk dust and the hum of visiting scholars' portable computers. Founded as a repository for cultural artifacts, books, and manuscripts from Tibet, the Library of Tibetan Works and Archives has become an international center for Tibetan studies, which to date has attracted more than five thousand research scholars and students from over thirty countries.

Teachers and Teachings

The LTWA has eight departments: research and translation, publication, oral history and film documentation, reference, Tibetan studies, Tibetan manuscripts, a museum, and a school for thangka painting and wood carving. A resident team of Tibetan scholars is engaged in research, translation, instruction, and the publication of books.

The LTWA offers regular courses in Buddhist philosophy and practice and the Tibetan language, taught by lamas in Tibetan and translated into English. Courses generally last from one to two months—with two one-hour meetings per day—and cover such topics as "Merit Accumulation, Pure Morality, and Bodhissatva Conduct"; "The Heart Sutra"; "The Seven Points for Mind Training"; and "The Thirty-Seven Bodhi-Factors." This is not the place for a dilettante—without a serious interest in Tibetan Buddhism (and a strong foundation in personal practice) you may find yourself lost and bored long before you've reached the thirtieth bodhi-factor. However, it's a great place for an experienced practitioner with academic inclinations.

You can only live at the LTWA if you are a bonafide "research scholar"—with a letter of recommendation from your university or other institution—or are enrolled in a minimum of two courses. However, anyone can sign up for courses and use the reference library (after registering and paying a nominal membership fee).

Facilities and Food

The foreign language reference library has over 7,000 titles in English and other languages on Buddhism, Tibet, and related subjects. The manuscript department has over 70,000 Tibetan books and manuscripts dealing with Tibetan Buddhist philosophy, psychology, history, medicine, etc. The museum houses about 1,000 Buddhist artifacts from Tibet.

Residential rooms are limited—only twenty-five to thirty people—so you may not be able to stay there even if you qualify as a research scholar or enrolled student. However, there is plenty of lodging and food in the immediate vicinity. Rooms generally have an attached kitchen.

Schedule

The usual schedule consists of a lecture from 9 to 10 A.M. and 11 A.M. to 12 P.M. and a Tibetan language class from 10 to 11 A.M. On Mondays a meditation class is often offered.

There are no classes on second and fourth Saturdays and Sundays or on Tibetan holidays. Dates and times may change due to scheduled and unscheduled public teachings given by His Holiness the Dalai Lama.

Fees

Registration: Rs 20. Buddhist philosophy: Rs 100 per month each class. Tibetan language: Rs 200 per month each class.

Room rents range from Rs 500 to Rs 2,000 per month.

Contact Information

THE LIBRARY OF TIBETAN WORKS AND ARCHIVES
(CENTRE FOR TIBETAN STUDIES)
GANGCHEN KYISHONG
DHARAMSALA 176 215
HIMACHAL PRADESH
TEL: 91-1892-22467

Around and About Dharamsala

Turn in one direction, and you see snow-frosted peaks shooting up to a height of nearly 17,000 feet; turn the other way, and you're looking out over the fertile green plains of the Kangra Valley. A favorite hill-station and summer resort for the British, Dharamsala was virtually abandoned after India achieved independence in 1947. But it attracted international attention in 1960, when His Holiness the Dalai Lama, fleeing the Chinese occupation of Tibet, made it his home and the seat of the Tibetan government in exile.

Today, tourist brochures promote Dharamsala as a kind of "Little Lhasa," home to more than 5,000 Tibetan refugees. In recent years, the town has become a Mecca for pilgrims from all over the world, both Tibetan and non-Tibetan, who come here to seek the blessings of the Dalai Lama and to study and practice Buddhist teachings. It has also become, more and more, a favorite traveler's hangout—a standard stop on a circuit that includes Goa, Pushkar, and Kathmandu.

Dharamsala consists of two separate settlements, about ten kilometers apart. The Tibetan part of town is Upper Dharamsala, also known as McLeod Ganj.

Aside from its sheer physical beauty—including some great hiking trails—the real appeal of Dharamsala, of course, is the chance to experience Tibetan religion and culture. Some opportunities include:

Audiences with His Holiness the Dalai Lama. The Dalai Lama's residence is opposite the Tsuglagkhang (Central Cathedral), about a ten-minute walk from McLeod Ganj. His Holiness regularly receives visitors for public audiences—apply at the Branch Security Office in McCleod Ganj near Hotel Tibet. For an appointment for a private audience with the Dalai Lama, try writing in advance to The Office of Tibet, 241 E 32nd Street, New York, NY 10016 (Tel: (212) 213-5010; Fax: (212) 779-9245).

Teachings by the Dalai Lama. Each March the Dalai Lama gives ten days of free public teachings (in Tibetan, with simultaneous translation into English and several other languages) at the Tsuglagkhang (Central Cathedral). There's no need to register in advance but the town tends to be absolutely packed at this time, so it's best to reserve a hotel room in advance if you can.

Traditional Tibetan Medicine. Fifty students a year study traditional Tibetan medicine at the Tibetan Medical and Astro Institute (TMAI), which also has a dispensary, an in-patient unit, and a surgical ward. A popular resource for travelers—who go for consultations on everything from "Delhi belly" to chronic health complaints—the TMAI is located in Ganchen Kyishong, about a ten-minute walk below the Tibetan Library. It has a branch clinic in McLeod Ganj, where there are also two other clinics for traditional Tibetan medicine: Dr. Yeshi Dhondhen's clinic and the Dr. Lobsang Dolma Khangar Memorial Clinic.

Tibetan Institute of Performing Arts (TIPA). About a fifteen-minute walk from McLeod Ganj, TIPA gives public performances of the musical, dance, and theatrical traditions of Tibet, including *lhamo,* or Tibetan folk opera.

Norbulingka Institute. Named for the Dalai Lama's summer residence in Tibet, the Norbulinka Institute was established to preserve Tibetan art and literature in exile. The Institute trains refugee Tibetans to use authentic methods, tools, and materials. The beautifully landscaped grounds include a temple (with an immense gold-plated Buddha hammered by master craftsmen), a museum, a shop, and a guest house. It's located in the valley below Dharamsala and can be reached by bus or taxi.

Namgyal Monastery. Founded in Tibet by the Third Dalai Lama in the sixteenth century, the Namgyal Monastery is a tantric college that performs rituals for His Holiness. Located next to the Central Cathedral in McLeod Ganj, the monastery is home to more than 180 monks, who perform prayers and rituals of all the major schools of Tibetan Buddhism.

Nechung Monastery. Just below the Tibetan library in Gangchen Kyishong, this is the seat of the State Oracle of Tibet (who, working through trance mediums, has guided the Tibetan government since the eighth century). The oracle plays a key role in the search for incarnations of each Dalai Lama.

Dolma Ling Nunnery. Located just behind the Norbulinka Institute in the valley below lower Dharamsala, this is the base for the Tibetan Nuns Project, which provides housing and education for over 350 refugee nuns who have fled persecution and torture in Tibet. Volunteer opportunities are available.

Tibetan Women's Association. The TWA works for the political freedom and social upliftment of Tibetan women, especially the rehabilitation and education of nuns escaping from Tibet. Their office is in the Delek Clinic building in McLeod Ganj. Volunteer opportunities are available.

For further information about sights in and around Dharamsala, an excellent booklet entitled *A Guide to Little Lhasa in India* is available from the Department of Information and International Relations, Central Tibetan Administration, Dharamsala 176 215, Himachal Pradesh, India. If ordering from overseas, a $10 (U.S.) donation should cover the costs of the booklet and postage.

For information on the current situation in Tibet, contact the Department of Information and International Relations, Center of Tibetan Administration, Dharamsala 176 215. In the United States, write to The International Campaign for Tibet, 1735 Eyei Street NW, Suite 615, Washington, D.C. 20006 (Tel: (202) 785-1515; Fax: (202) 785-4343).

How to Get There

The LTWA is about 1.5 kilometers below upper Dharamsala (McLeod Ganj). Dharamsala is 850 kilometers from Delhi. From Delhi, take the train to Pathankot, then take a bus or taxi about 100 kilometers to Dharamsala (two and a half to three and a half hours). You can also go by train or airplane to Chandigarh, then take a bus or taxi to Dharamsala (about 250 kilometers); or take take a bus directly from Delhi to Dharamsala.

Books and Tapes

All books and journals published by the LTWA are available for sale.

Tushita Meditation Centre
Dharamsala, Himachal Pradesh

🐚 *Lama Thubten Yeshe Rinpoche, Founder (1935–1984)*
🐚 *Lama Thubten Zopa Rinpoche, Spiritual Director (1946–   )*

The name "Tushita" means "the Joyful Heaven"—it's the name given to the celestial abode where Buddhas reside just prior to manifesting in the world. Perched in a forest of evergreens and rhododendrons above McLeod Ganj—high enough for the traffic sounds to fade away—the Tushita Meditation Center offers introductory and continuing courses in Buddhist meditation and philosophy in the Tibetan Mahayana tradition. Personal retreat facilities are also available for people with prior meditation experience.

Teachers and Teachings

The Center was founded in 1972 by Lama Thubten Yeshe Rinpoche and his disciple Lama Thubten Zopa Rinpoche, who fled Tibet in the wake of the Chinese invasion. (The two monks also founded the Kopan Monastery in Nepal, the Mount Everest Centre for Buddhist studies at Lawudo, and the Root Institute in Bodh Gaya (p. 81).) Since Lama Yeshe's death in 1984, Lama Zopa has been the spiritual director of the Foundation for the Preservation of the Mahayana Tradition, a worldwide network of Buddhist centers, monasteries, and affiliated groups. A Spanish boy has been recognized as the reincarnation of Lama Yeshe; now in his teens, he has begun monastic training in Dharamsala and can frequently be seen at the Tushita Institute.

Lama Zopa himself is rarely at Tushita; courses are taught instead by a variety of Western and Tibetan teachers (many of them drawn from local monasteries). If you're a beginning meditator (or just new to Tibetan Buddhism), the eleven-day introductory courses—one offered every month, except during the monsoon season—are an excellent way to ease into the practice. (As one staff member put it, "We'll hold your hand as you learn to meditate.") The attitude is more relaxed and flexible than you might find at other meditation centers; perhaps for that reason, the courses tend to be particularly popular among younger Western travelers.

During the first eight days of the course, there are three daily one-hour meditation periods each day, with at least part of each session guided by the instructor. The morning session focuses on awareness of breath and body. The afternoon session is more analytical—you'll be given specific Buddhist ideas to contemplate in the light of your own experience, such as the observation that everything is subject to change, or the best way to live to prepare yourself for your inevitable death. In the evening session, you'll work with simple visualization techniques. In the morning there will be a talk by an experienced Western practitioner; in the afternoon, by a Tibetan lama (with translator if necessary). The last three days of the course consist of silent meditation.

All visitors are required to abide by the five Buddhist precepts: no killing (even of small insects); no stealing; no lying; no alcohol, cigarettes, or other intoxicants; no sex.

Facilities and Food

The Center is rustic and somewhat spartan, with spectacular views of the Himalayas and the Kangra valley. About sixty-five people can be accommodated in dormitories, semiprivate, and private rooms. Couples must stay in separate rooms. The Center also has two meditation halls, a library, a yoga room, a small bookshop, and a small shop for daily necessities.

The food is vegetarian (with eggs and dairy products); no special diets are provided.

Schedule

Courses run ten days, beginning with meditation at 6:30 A.M. and continuing until 9 P.M. During the first eight days of the course, there are three daily one-hour meditation periods each day, alternating with teachings and discussion. The last three days of the course are silent (except for the meditation instructions) and consist of seven 45-minute or one-hour meditation periods.

During the monsoon season, Tushita holds a three-month Vajrasattva retreat—a tantric purification method—for experienced practitioners.

Fees

Course: Rs 100 per day; double room Rs 55 per person; dormitory: Rs 35; three meals per day: Rs 90.

TUSHITA MEDITATION CENTER
P.O. MCLEOD GANJ
DHARAMSALA, DIST. KANGRA
HIMACHAL PRADESH 176 219
TEL: 91-1892-21866

U.S. Contact:
FPMT CENTRAL OFFICE
DIRECTOR HARVEY HARROCKS
P.O. BOX 1778
SOQUEL, CA 95073
TEL: (408) 476-8435
FAX: (408) 476-4823

How to Get There

The retreat center is about one kilometer (up a steep hill) from the bus/taxi stand in McLeod Ganj (upper Dharamsala). Dharamsala is about 850 kilometers from Delhi. From Delhi, take the train to Pathankot, then take a bus or taxi about 100 kilometers to Dharamsala (two and a half to three and a half hours). You can also take an overnight bus directly from Delhi to Dharamsala.

Other Services

Despite its small size (population 17,000), upper Dharamsala (McLeod Ganj) has plenty of restaurants, hotels, shops, faxes, and other facilities.

Books and Tapes

Especially recommended are *Wisdom Energy* by Lama Yeshe and Lama Zopa (Wisdom Publications) and *The Door to Satisfaction* by Lama Zopa (Wisdom Publications). You can order books and tapes by Lama Zopa and Lama Yeshe in the United States through Wisdom Publications, 361 Newbury Street, Boston, MA 02115. Tel: (617) 536-3358; Fax: (617) 536-1897; Orders: (800) 272-4050.

Rejoicing is another important practice that prevents pride, jealousy, or anger. Whenever you hear that somebody has been successful, rejoice. For example, if you hear that someone has been successful in business, you should rejoice. When you hear that someone—whether your friend or your enemy—has found a partner, again rejoice: "How wonderful it is that they have found the happiness they were seeking!" Feel as happy as you do for yourself when you find something that you have been wanting . . .

If you cherish only yourself, you cannot experience happiness, but if you cherish others as you cherish yourself, it arises naturally.

—LAMA ZOPA RINPOCHE,
from *The Door to Satisfaction*

Chinmaya Mission
Sidhbari, Himachal Pradesh

🌀 *Swami Chinmayananda (1926–1993)*
🌀 *Swami Tejomayananda (1950–   )*

Tucked in a wooded valley against a backdrop of snow-tipped Himalayan peaks, this upscale ashram is the regional center for the Chinmaya Mission, a Vedantic organization with eight major centers in India and over 150 smaller centers around the world. The Chinmaya Mission teaches classical Vedanta in the tradition of the ninth-century sage Adi Shankaracharya—tailored primarily for modern, educated Indians who are interested in getting back in touch with their country's ancient spiritual heritage.

In India Hinduism has come to mean nothing more than a bundle of sacred superstitions, or a certain way of dressing, cooking, eating, talking, and so on. Our gods have fallen to the mortal level of administration officers at whose altars the faithful Hindu might pray and get special permits for the things he desires; that is, if he pays the required fee to the priests!" wrote the Mission's founder, Swami Chinmayananda, a former journalist who became a disciple of Swami Sivananda of Rishikesh, then spent seven years studying with a guru in the Himalayas. "But Hinduism is not this external show that we have learned to parade about in our daily life. . . . True Hinduism is the Sanatana Dharma [Eternal Truth] of the Upanishads."

The central teaching of Shankaracharya's advaita (nondual) Vedanta is that the individual soul or consciousness is, in essence, identical with the Supreme Consciousness. The Sidhbari ashram is a training center for renunciates, who enroll for a three-year residential program studying Vedanta and the Upanishads, and then go and teach in Chinmaya Mission centers around the world. However, it also offers regular eight- to ten-day "camps" for laypeople—sometimes in English and sometimes in Hindi—focusing on Vedanta in general or some particular Vedantic text. These popular courses are generally attended by about 150 to 200 people (primarily Indians, although Westerners are welcome). It's best to write ahead as camps often fill up.

Between camps (which occupy about half the schedule), you're welcome to stay as a guest at the ashram and participate in the daily round of meditation, kirtan, lectures, and discussions. At this particular ashram, lectures are usually conducted in Hindi, except when there's an English-language camp going on. (The Chinmaya Mission in Bombay is the place to go for English-medium instruction.) However, Swami Tejomayananda—the resident teacher and Swami Chinmayananda's successor as head of the Mission—speaks excellent English and is generally available for private consultations.

Swami Tejomayananda was a postgraduate student in physics when he became a Vedanta student, and his assignments have included heading the Chinayananda Mission in San Jose, California. As gurus go he's on the young side—but he's a highly educated and articulate teacher with a quick sense of humor, who speaks equally fluently in Hindi, English, and

Exploring Tibetan Buddhism

Shortly before Buddhism disappeared from India, some of the greatest Indian Buddhist teachers brought Buddhist philosophy to Tibet. Tibet became an isolated stronghold that preserved these teachings for more than a thousand years, until the Chinese invasion of Tibet in the 1950s. Tibetan high lamas and their followers who escaped Chinese atrocities and persecution then brought Buddhism back to India in a big way.

Tibetan Buddhism now has a firm foothold in Indian soil after decades of struggle by Tibetan refugees. Donors from all over the world—particularly Southeast Asia—have given money to build monasteries and fund schools.

Tibetan Buddhist monasteries are to be found mainly in northwest, northeast, and south India, clustered around traditional Tibetan trading routes or the areas given by the Indian government to the refugees when they escaped from Tibet. The following are some of the monasteries open to foreigners interested in meditation practice:

HIMACHAL PRADESH

Tilokpur Nunnery—on the way from the railhead at Pathancot to Dharamsala, a very short distance outside Pathancot—is located on a site blessed by the great saint Tilopa, who meditated in a cave here. The thriving nunnery welcomes guests.

Not far from Dharamsala, about twelve kilometers from Palampur, is **Tashijong**, a Drukpa Kagyu Monastery, headed by the ninth Khamtrul Rinpoche. Tashijong has accommodations for guests. Though courses are not formally taught, it is possible to arrange instruction with one of the lamas.

A little further down the road to Manali, near Baijnath, is **Sherab Ling Monastery**, headed by the 12th Tai Situpa. Western students have been part of the Sherab Ling scene since the 1970s. There are ample accommodations, including some isolated retreat cabins. The retreat cabins are rustic, in most cases with no plumbing or electricity, but the guest rooms have essential facilities. Tai Situpa gives meditation advice to small groups or individuals at his monastery when he is there. Down the hill from Sherab Ling, in the Bir Tibetan Camp, are several other monasteries, including the **Nyingmapa Cho Ling Monastery** and the **Sakya Monastery**.

Near Mandi on the Dharamsala-Manali road is a turnoff that takes you to Rewalsar—called **Tso Pema** by Tibetans. Here is a small lake surrounded by meditation caves where the great teacher who established Buddhism in Tibet, Padmasambhava, is said to have meditated and performed miracles. A Drikung Kagyu monastery has guest rooms. Lamas are often to be found meditating in caves around the lake. Accommodations are limited, but there are hotels twenty-four kilometers away in Mandi.

From Mandi you can continue on to Manali where there is a thriving Tibetan community and a number of small monasteries, including the Drukpa Kagyu monastery of **Abo Rinpoche**. Abo Rinpoche's monastery is small, but does have a few guest rooms, and there are places to stay nearby. There are no formal courses here, but it is possible to arrange instruction.

LADAKH

Ladakh is a former Western Tibetan kingdom with some of the oldest extant monasteries, since the destruction of most of the monasteries in Tibet by the Chinese. **Hemis, Lama Yuro, Phyang,** and **Tikse** are all important monasteries, but most of them do not cater to foreign meditators. It is always possible to make your own arrangements, however. The monasteries are generally in remote locations, and supplies are minimal. For more information about Tibetan Buddhism in Ladakh, contact the Jammu and Kashmir State Tourism Office or read Lonely Planet's guide to Kashmir, Ladakh, and Zanskar.

UTTAR PRADESH

A large community of Tibetans lives near Dehradun in Uttar Pradesh. The monastery of the erstwhile head of the Nyingmapa lineage, Mindroling Trichen, is at Clement Town. Although Mindroling Trichen does not teach, his daughter Khandro Rinpoche does. She speaks excellent English and has quite a few foreign students.

Also near Dehradun, in Rajpur near Mussorie, is the **Sakya College** and seat of the head of the Sakyapa lineage, Sakya Trizen, who has had a large following in the West for many years.

KARNATAKA

To seriously study Buddhist philosophy, visit Mundgod, in Karnataka, where the Gelugpa monasteries of **Drepung** and **Sera** have been rebuilt. There are busy monastic colleges here and even some Westerners studying for the geshe degree, the Tibetan equivalent of a Master of Buddhist Philosophy. Bylekuppe, near Mysore, also has a few monasteries, including that of the current head of the Nyingmapa order, Penor Rinpoche.

WEST BENGAL

Darjeeling is situated on an ancient trade route between India and Tibet. The great Tibetan trading families had establishments there from which they did business, and monasteries naturally sprang up in the area. One is the seat of the **Gyalwang Drukchen**, head of the Drukpa Kagyu sect, who has quite a few foreign disciples.

    Kalu Rinpoche's monastery is about eight kilometers outside of Darjeeling at Sonada. It has a long tradition of meditation retreat practice and there is usually a place to stay. The previous Kalu Rinpoche was a great meditator and was the first to set up centers for Western students to do

Marathi. An unpretentious man, he's always available to answer questions. Many of the other forty to fifty resident swamis also speak English; if you're interested in Vedanta, you can generally find someone to answer your questions and guide you toward appropriate books and practices. The residents seem genuinely warm and friendly; the contemplative atmosphere is conducive to doing your own spiritual practice, even when the talks are in Hindi.

The Chinmaya Mission stresses the traditional values and practices of self-control (brahmacharya), honesty (satyam), nonviolence (ahimsa), and the purification of the mind through meditation and mantra. Although the teachings revolve around the interpretation of classical texts, the presentation is generally far from dry—Tejomayananda is dedicated to the rejuvenation of Hinduism, and talks tend to be both practical and inspirational. The emphasis, always, is on the slow transformation of the mind through the transformation of the life. As Swami Chinmayananda the traditional three-year meditation retreat. The present Kalu Rinpoche is still a child, but it is possible to get instruction from Bokar Rinpoche or one of the other lamas at the monastery.

SIKKIM

Numerous monasteries dot the mountainsides and lush valleys of Sikkim. (A permit is necessary to enter Sikkim. It may be obtained at the Sikkim Tourism office in New Delhi, Calcutta, or in Siliguri, but you must have it before you go up the road to Gangtok. The permits are valid for two weeks and may be extended.) The former Kingdom of Sikkim was a Buddhist state before it was annexed by India in 1977. The capitol, Gangtok, has the **Tsuk Lhakhang,** or palace monastery, as well as an **Institute of Tibetology.** Across the valley is **Rumtek Monastery,** seat in exile of the 17th Gyalwa Karmapa, head of the Karma Kagyu lineage. It is possible to stay at Rumtek. A number of incarnate lamas of the Karma Kagyu lineage reside there, and there is a monk's college. **Pemayangtse** is an important Nyingmapa monastery about eight hours from Gangtok.

—LEA TERHUNE

wrote, "It is not possible that for six days you live a foul life and on the seventh day, you dash into the presence of the Lord and say 'Hi' to Him."

Facilities and Food

The ashram is beautiful and impeccably maintained, with solid stone buildings (trimmed in swami-orange), flower gardens, and great views of the mountains. There are about 100 private rooms, three dormitories, and floor space for about 350 mattresses during some of the larger camps. Bedding is usually available, although it's suggested you bring your own during the more crowded camps. An adjacent forest of long-needled pines is ideal for meditative walks.

Meals are traditional Indian vegetarian, served Western-style with tables and benches. (Serving and eating are generally accompanied by singing, which adds to the pleasure.) Other facilities include a meditation hall, satsang hall, library, and small medical clinic. A store sells books and clothing made by villagers as part of the ashram's training program in garment-making. Other ashram service projects are a village school, a twelve-step alcoholism program, and a nurses' training program.

Schedule

The day begins with meditation from 5:30 to 6 A.M., followed by tea and a class before breakfast. The morning is spent in discussions and classes; afternoon is generally free time, before arati (the offering of fire) in the late afternoon. Evenings frequently feature some sort of cultural program.

Fees

Donation.

Contact Information

CHINMAYA MISSION
CHINMAYA TAPOVAN TRUST
SANDEEPANY HIMALAYAS
SIDHBARI 176 057
HIMACHAL PRADESH
TEL: 91-1892-22121; 24951
FAX: 91-1892-24956

U.S. Contact:
CHINMAYA MISSION WEST
P.O. BOX 129
PIERCY, CA 95587
TEL: 707-247-3488

How to Get There

The ashram is in the village of Sidhbari, about 10 kilometers from Dharamsala and 18 kilometers from the Kangra airport. It can be reached by taxi or bus.

Dharamsala is 850 kilometers from Delhi. From Delhi, take the train to Pathankot, then take a bus or taxi about 100 kilometers to Dharamsala. You can also go by train or airplane to Chandigarh, then take a bus or taxi to Dharamsala (about 250 kilometers); or take an overnight bus directly from Delhi to Dharamsala.

Other Services

The village of Sidhbari has no services; the closest town is Dharamsala (10 kilometers), which is a major tourist center with STD, hotels, fax, and restaurants.

Books, Tapes, and Affiliated Centers

Books and tapes are available at the ashram or from the headquarters in the United States. There are Chinmaya mission branches all over India, including one in Uttar Kashi, Uttar Pradesh, which will house pilgrims en route to the source of the Ganges at Gangotri.

> Question: Swamiji, are you able to read our minds?
>
> Swamiji: God forbid! Who would want to waste their time raking through the garbage in your minds?
>
> Q: But there are times when we have a question in our minds and you do answer it, either in the satsang or the lectures, before we even have enough nerve to ask it.
>
> S: Yes, that will happen. That's the way the universe works. When a lesson is to be learned, the appropriate situation arrives. A question is there, then the answer comes.
>
> It's not from an effort or some trick on my part; I'm an instrument. Sometimes the solution could come from a stranger on the bus. But because I'm a swami, everyone thinks I'm using some special power.
>
> —NANCY PATCHEN
> (from *The Journey of a Master: Swami Chinmayananda*)

🌀 *Swami Shyam (1924–   )*

Over the past twenty-odd years, Swami Shyam—described in his informational brochure as an "enlightened being who has attained the perfection of the Vision of Oneness"—has attracted a sizeable flock of primarily Canadian and European disciples, who form a tight-knit expatriate community in the Kullu hills around his International Meditation Institute. Before you get too excited about Swami Shyam, you should know that you probably won't get to join his community—with about 180 full-time students, the center is officially closed to drop-in visitors. However, every Sunday morning his satsang is open to the general public, and—with prior permission—you can stop by for one of his lively talks and question-and-answer sessions.

Teachers and Teachings

Swami Shyam's teachings are basically a popularized form of advaita vedanta, the nondual philosophy that holds that the individual soul, or atman, is identical with Brahman, the eternal ground of pure universal consciousness. He teaches a nonsectarian meditation technique he calls "shyam dhyan," or "meditation on space." Devotees are instructed to meditate on the mantra "Amaram Hum Madhuram Hum"—which means "I Am Immortal, I Am Blissful"—while focusing on "the Knower, the Pure Existence, Consciousness, and Bliss, infinite, immortal, eternal, unchanging, One without any second name . . . considering that this Self or I or Knower is at the Source of everything and everyone."

The Swami looks like an elfin magician, with a wavy white beard, a round, mischievous face, and magnificently fringed and swirling robes. His lectures are generally playful and warm—he speaks in free-associating spirals, flinging words exuberantly at his subject with a sort of joyful imprecision, like an artist splashing random handfuls of paint on a blank canvas. Satsang is a highly interactive affair, as Swami Shyam encourages devotees to develop public speaking skills (even very young ones—you'll hear stories of two-year-olds being called to the microphone, where they expound on "tree . . . bird . . . mama . . ." to uproarious applause). Even if you're just visiting for a day, be prepared to be called to the microphone to share your thoughts on the lecture.

Born in 1924, the young Shyamcharan—a name he was given by his family guru—began his spiritual journey at age seven, when the guru told him that if he meditated everyone would love him, he would enjoy perfect health, and he would pass all his exams. Married at age eighteen, he continued his spiritual pursuits, and eventually realized what he refers to as "Shyam Space"—a state of pure existence and pure consciousness, a disidentification with the world and identification with the pure Self.

While pursing a government career as a clerk in the Indian legislature—in addition to his spiritual aptitude, he was a champion speedwriter—he began teaching his spiritual vision to others, and was eventually discovered by a pair of Canadian tourists who met him in Rishikesh in the early 1970s. They invited him to teach meditation in Toronto; he intended to stay there only a few months, but a few days before he was to return to India, his passport, plane ticket, and all his money was stolen from his hotel room while he was down the hall in the bathroom. He ended up staying for over a year, and when he returned to India, it was with a small band of enthusiastic devotees—who gave him the unofficial title of Swami, a nomenclature that he has retained, although he remains a married householder with five grown children.

Today, Swami Shyam's disciples live in independent group houses near the meditation center, which they visit daily for satsang and meditation. To join this spiritual fraternity—or even to visit for a few months—you must have been practicing meditation for at least five years; other requirements include an in-depth study of Shyam literature; regular attendance at classes in an affiliated Shyam center in Canada, the United States, or Europe; and a recommendation from a senior Shyam. You also have to have an independent source of income, as the ashram has no money-generating businesses. Brahmacharya, or celibacy, is "encouraged" as an aid to spiritual growth, but not required—some of the devotees are married, and the community includes about a dozen children, who are home-schooled and tutored by fellow Shyams. Devotees tend to be a well-educated, friendly group—although it's difficult to join the community, serious seekers are welcomed with genuine warmth.

Facilities and Food

There are no accommodations at the Institute; you can stay at the nearby Greenwood Hotel or the more expensive and luxurious Hotel Vaishali, which is also a good place to have meals. (There's a separate vegetarian menu just for Shyams, who form a good part of the restaurant's clientele.) There are also plenty of nearby dhabas where you can get vegetables, dahl, and chapatti cooked to Western tastes.

The center is set on a hillside overlooking the Beas River, with lovely grounds and gardens. It has a meditation hall, a small library, and a bookstore. When the weather is nice, satsang is held outdoors on an outdoor terrace fringed by apple trees.

Schedule

Satsang is available to outside guests only on Sundays, unless approved in advance by Swami Shyam. There's no fixed time for satsang, because, as one devotee explained, "Swamiji believes that the quest for freedom begins with freedom." However, it's a good bet that the Sunday satsang will begin sometime between 10:30 A.M. and 12 noon.

Fees

Donation.

Contact Information

INTERNATIONAL MEDITATION INSTITUTE
KULLU 175 101
HIMALAYAS
TEL (C/O HOTEL VAISHALI): 91-1902-4225
FAX (C/O HOTEL VAISHALI): 91-1902-3073

In North America, contact:
INTERNATIONAL MEDITATION INSTITUTE
2542 MONTCLAIR AVENUE
MONTREAL, QUEBEC
CANADA H4B 2J1
TEL: (514) 489-1968

The meditation center is in the Gandhinagar area of Kullu, very near the Hotel Vaishali on the main road into Kullu. Kullu is accessible by air and bus from Delhi; trains from Delhi go to Chandigarh and Simla, from which you can take a bus or taxi to Kullu.

Other Services

Although Kullu is a small town (population 15,000), it is a major tourist center, so most services are available.

Books and Tapes

Books and tapes are available through the Institute or its affiliated groups in Canada, England, the United States, Switzerland, Norway, Germany, France, New Zealand, Israel, Japan, Holland, and Taiwan. A recommended introduction is Unfolding Oneness: The Vision of Swami Shyam.

An hour or so into satsang, Swami Shyam called for a song. "We are one . . . We have always been one," the crowd began singing, swaying happily back and forth. "No duality can put us apart . . . We are one." Meanwhile, Swami Shyam was scribbling away on a pad of yellow paper. When the non-duality chorus ended, he held up the paper and proclaimed with a delighted smile, "I have written a NEW song!"

The crowd sat forward, expectantly awaiting the words of their guru. Swami Shyam cleared his throat and began to warble:
"I woke up this morning and found that I exist!
I woke up this morning—what a hit, what a hit!
I felt not only joy but bliss—
what a hit, that I exist!
Oh yeah I woke up this morning
and found that I exist . . ."
He caroled through the song several times, then stopped, put

his palms in namaste, and bowed to his audience. "Thank you very much," he said, and walked away, to thunderous applause.

—ANNE CUSHMAN (from India journal)

PILGRIMAGE SITES IN *Himachal Pradesh and Jammu and Kashmir*

HIMACHAL PRADESH

Jwalamukhi. This shrine sacred to the fire goddess—probably the most visited temple in the region—is not far from Kangra in the Beas River valley south of Dharamsala. The shrine commemorates the spot where the tongue of Sati fell as Shiva carried her around India (p. 333). The goddess appears here in the form of flames emerging from rock crevices. The main flame is framed by silver in front of the mandir entrance.

Jwalamukhi can be reached by bus from Kangra. There are some government and Himachal Tourism guest houses in and near the town of Jwalamukhi.

Kulu-Manali Temples. The Kulu-Manali area is spectacularly beautiful and boasts many old temples. It is a land of gods and goddesses—each village has its own special divinity—and the images of these devas are brought out on festival occasions, particularly during the feast of Dusshera in October, when the goddess Hidimba is brought to Kulu from her temple in Manali. The Ragunathpura temple is a focal point of the ceremonies. Visits to small temples around Kulu often require strenuous walking.

A few hours drive from Kulu, Manali's chief temple is the Dhungri temple of the demon goddess Hadimba, or Hirma Devi. It's built on a hill in the midst of an ancient cedar forest, in the wooden, tiered style typical of Himachal Pradesh. Hidimba, sister of a powerful demon, appears in the Hindu epic the Mahabharata. She married Bhima, one of the Pandava brothers. Her temple dates from the sixteenth century, but it is thought to have been a sacred site before that. Also in Manali are the hot sulpher springs at Vashist village, where many people come for healing.

Both Kulu and Manali have plenty of hotels—particularly Manali, which is a summer resort for people from the plains. Transportation in Himachal Pradesh is mostly by road. A narrow-gauge train runs from Kalkaji to Simla and from Pathankot to Jogindernager. There are flights into Simla and Kulu (Bhuntar), but these are sometimes unreliable due to weather and other reasons. Buses and taxis run from Delhi and Chandigarh.

JAMMU AND KASHMIR

While you're in northern India, you may want to travel to the state of Jammu and Kashmir, although check with authorities first—political unrest often makes travel in this area unadvisable. The region has been unsafe for trekking since armed separatist militancy began in 1990. Check with reliable sources—like the U.S. State Department or foreign office of your country—before going there. Don't listen to travel agents or Indian Tourism. A number of people who did have been kidnapped by militants.

However, if you can get there, the area is rich with sacred sites, including:

🌀 **Amarnath.** Located in Kashmir near Pahalgam, in the mountainous area south of Srinagar, Amarnath is a sacred Shiva cave. Tens of thousands of people make a pilgrimage, or yatra, every August to view the ice lingam that forms in the cave. Symbolic of Shiva's role as restorer, the lingam is worshipped throughout India—it is considered a bad omen if the ice lingam fails to form.

Amarnath is a few days trek from Pahalgam, through some of the most beautiful scenery in Kashmir. Halfway there is Sheshnag, a lake said to be inhabited by a snakelike creature also called the Sheshnag, after the the great thousand-headed cobra deity sacred to Vishnu. Sheshnag is king of the Nagas, or serpent gods, who rule the subterranean regions, particularly water. According to tradition, the Sheshnag participates in the destruction of creation by vomiting fire at the end of each age. He also becomes the couch on which Vishnu sleeps between bouts of creation. Some people claim to have seen the Sheshnag racing around the lake, à la Loch Ness monster.

Going along with the pilgrims in August presents its own challenges, with tens of thousands of ill-equipped people queuing up the mountainside, where there is poor infrastructure and unpredictable weather. Casualties due to negligence are not uncommon. In 1996 several hundred people died from exposure when the weather suddenly turned cold.

Pahalgam is located about 100 kilometers south of Srinagar and may be easily reached by taxi or bus from Srinagar. Along the way are some interesting temple ruins, such as the ninth-century Hindu temples at Avantipur and Martand near Mattan. But again, until militancy is fully contained, it is better not to wander far afield in this area. There are hotels in Pahalgam, although many closed during the unrest. For trekking, bring your own tent and gear.

🌀 **Vaishnodevi.** This cave shrine—located not far from Jammu, the winter capitol of Jammu and Kashmir state—is one of the "shakti peeths" or "seats of the goddess" that dot north India. These shrines mark the various places where Shiva dropped body parts belonging to his wife, Sati, as he carried her dead body around India, mad with grief. (See sidebar p. 333). Vaishnodevi is where the left arm of Sati was dropped. Pilgrims clamber through a small passageway into the main cave, where they worship the three forms of the Mother goddess: Kali, Laksmi, and Saraswati.

Vaishnodevi is more accessible than Amarnath, being a thirteen-kilometer uphill hike from the road that leads from nearby Katra. Jammu may be reached by air or express train from Delhi. Accommodations in Jammu range from the upscale Hari Niwas Palace on down. Maps and other information about these and other sites in the region may be obtained from the Jammu and Kashmir Tourism offices located at the Kaniska Shopping Plaza in New Delhi or in the Tourist Reception Center in Srinagar.

🌀 **Sufi Shrines.** For centuries Kashmir has been the home of saints from various Sufi orders, and there are sacred shrines throughout the valley. The most famous of these is the Hazratbal shrine on the shore of Srinagar's Dal Lake, housing a hair of the Prophet Mohammed, which is shown to the faithful several times a year.

The most revered Kashmiri saint was Sheik Nooruddinat Charar-i-sharief. The fourteenth-century wooden shrine and surrounding neighborhood was burnt down in 1995 in politically related violence, but people still visit the tomb. The feast of a Sufi saint is a good time to visit any Sufi shrine if you want to see the festive celebrations, including Sufiana music—a distinctively Kashmiri form of devotional music featuring Sufi poetry.

—LEA TERHUNE

Karnataka

| Sri Kailash Ashram |
| Bangalore, Karnataka |

🌀 *Sri Tiruchi Swamigal (1929–   )*

This prosperous, traditional ashram is the ideal place for the serious seeker who wants an immersion into Hindu spirituality with few other Westerners around. In order to stay there, you'll have to prove your dedication with a lengthy interview—first with an ashram official, then with the guru himself. Once you've been accepted, though, you'll get lots of individual attention and will be not only invited, but encouraged, to participate in every aspect of ashram life.

Teachers and Teachings

The ashram includes a busy temple complex and a school for twenty-five to thirty children. The resident guru is Sri Tiruchi Swamigal, a cordial man who speaks virtually no English but is available to answer questions through a translator. He always has the faintest shadow of a smile on his face; when something particularly amuses him, he claps his hands and laughs with unrestrained delight. He has a phenomenal memory, effortlessly recalling the faces of each of the hundred or so devotees who visit him each day (as many as a thousand on Sundays), as well as the time and purpose of each of their previous visits.

The central theme of his teachings is the worship of the Divine Mother in the form of Sri Raja Rajeswari. The daily life of the ashram includes plenty of elaborate pujas and other rituals—complete with drums, bells, and horns—in which you'll be encouraged to participate. According to his biographer, "This is the main task that the Swamiji has undertaken . . . Firstly, to preserve the core of Hindu worship and ritual as before, and secondly, to loosen the knots of exclusiveness so as to make Hindu religion more inclusive."

Although the ashram is busy, it has only six or seven permanent swamis (who answer a steady stream of telephone calls on cellular phones). Sri Tiruchi Swamigal spends about six hours a day giving individual darshan—just join the line. Most devotees are local Indians—by all appearances, an affluent, upper middle-class crowd—who come for the day, but don't stay overnight. There are, however, a number of devotees who come from a distance—some of them swamis and teachers in their own right, who may take you under their wings and give you additional teachings. Just recently, the ashram has started to receive occasional groups of visitors from the United States, Italy, and other Western countries.

Facilities and Food

The ashram is on about eleven acres with brightly painted temples covered with carvings, gold-leafed domes, and shrines in a setting of gardens and palm trees. An aviary houses peacocks and other birds and there's even a rabbit hutch (popular with visiting families). About fifty guests can stay in double rooms (with attached bath–bedding and mosquito-netting provided). Sri Tiruchi Swamigal eats with residents in the communal dining hall, where meals are served in traditional style on banana leaves on the floor. The ashram has its own cow herds and coconut plantations, as well as several model industries in the surrounding villages.

Schedule

The temple opens at 6 A.M. and closes at 8:30 P.M.; it's also closed from 1:30 to 4:30 P.M. The daily schedule includes five pujas, some of them quite elaborate; the goddess is bathed twice daily. Sri Tiruchi Swamigal is available for darshan from 8 A.M. to 1 P.M. and from 5 to 6 P.M. Call for day-to-day information.

Fees

Donation.

Contact Information

SRI KAILASH ASHRAM
KENCHANAHALLI
SRI RAJESWARI NAGAR

MYSORE ROAD
BANGALORE
KARNATAKA 560 039
TEL: 91-80-8600888 OR 8600377
FAX: 91-80-8600633

How to Get There

The Kailash ashram is about 25 kilometers from the airport and about 10 kilometers from the center of town. From town, take Mysore Road about 3 kilometers past the Mysore checkpoint to a large, pink, ornamental archway. Turn left through the arch, go about 1 kilometer and turn right on 25th Cross. A few hundred meters further on the right is the entrance to the ashram.

Other Services

All services are available in Bangalore.

Books and Tapes

Books are available through the ashram office.

Sri Mathrudevi Vishnas Shanti Ashrams
Bangalore, Karnataka and
Penchila Kona, Andhra Pradesh

🌀 *Sri Vijayeswari Devi (Karunamayi) (1958–   )*

Sri Vijayeswari Devi, better known as Karunamayi, or "the Compassionate One," is often compared to Ammachi (p. 168), the world-famous "hugging saint" of south India. Like Ammachi, Karunamayi is an earthy, exuberantly maternal woman believed by devotees to be an incarnation of the Divine Mother. But, unlike Ammachi, she speaks fluent English, and although her fame is on the rise among Westerners, it's still possible to meet with her in small informal groups (or even arrange a private appointment with her) at her forest retreat in Andhra Pradesh or her city center in Bangalore, Karnataka.

Teacher and Teachings

There is no need for another lamp to see the Sun. It is enough to remove the curtain between the sun and ourselves," Karunamayi says. "If the curtains of mind, intellect, ego, the good and the bad thought forces in man are removed, then the natural self-effulgent glow of the soul is revealed."

This glow is palpable at Karunamayi's two main ashrams—the "forest ashram" in the hills of Andhra Pradesh and the administrative center in Bangalore. You can't go to the forest ashram directly—you have to first make arrangements through the center in Bangalore. But it's well worth the effort to visit this remote retreat, surrounded by waterfalls and wild mango and gourd trees, in a forest where rishis and sages have practiced for hundreds of years (including, according to legend, the poets and seers Vashista and Valmiki, the authors of the great Hindu epics). Otherwise, you can see Karunamayi at her Bangalore ashram, where she spends half of her time when she's not on tour in India or abroad.

Now in her early forties, Karunamayi is called "Amma" (or Mother) by her devotees, who believe her to be an incarnation of the goddess Lalitha Devi. According to her official biography, Karunamayi's mother was a devotee of the great advaita vedanta master Ramana Maharshi (p. 286), who predicted that she would give birth to "the Mother." Drawn to spiritual practice even as a child, Karunamayi left home shortly before her college graduation to spend ten years meditating and practicing austerities in the forested hills of Penusila. In the early 1990s, she founded her first ashram on the outskirts of this forest.

"The goal of life is Self-realization—to know the Self alone," says Karunamayi. But unlike many other teachers of advaita vedanta (the nondual philosophy that holds that pure consciousness is all that exists), she stresses the importance of meditation and other spiritual practices as a way of attaining this goal. "By effort, you can attain realization. Meditation is purification, nothing but purification," she says. The program at her forest ashram includes regular seven- to ten-day meditation courses, featuring about six hours a day of meditation and two hours of yoga asanas. Daily meditations are also held at her Bangalore ashram.

The mood at Karunamayi's ashrams is casual. There's lots of informal contact with her, and you won't find the devotional hysteria that sometimes erupts around gurus. Most devotees are Indian, although the number of Westerners is increasing. As part of her teachings, Karunamayi gives the Saraswati (goddess of knowledge) mantra to anyone who requests it. If you wish to receive the mantra, you prepare for the ceremony—which can take several hours, depending on how many people show up—by abstaining from food for the day and arriving freshly bathed and dressed in white clothing. Karunamayi will sit in meditation for about five minutes with each devotee, send you energy, and painlessly inscribe the mantra on your tongue.

Karunamayi's teachings emphasize compassion: "The heart of any person which gets stabilized through constant thinking of God will overflow with divine love, and such a heart will weep for the welfare of the distressed," she says. "A mother experiences immense pleasure when she loves her child. If that is so, an illumined soul enjoys greater pleasure when he considers all beings as reflections of his own self, and loves them." In keeping with this philosophy, she has an active service program, including free medical camps, a free school for tribal children, food distribution, and a rehabilitation center for the mentally handicapped.

Facilities and Food

🌀 **Forest Ashram.** This is Karunamayi's retreat center, and all arrangements to visit must be coordinated through the Bangalore center. About 100 people can stay in twenty private rooms and forty shared rooms with attached baths. A large meditation and prayer hall can accommodate about 700 people.

🌀 **Bangalore Ashram.** Karunamayi's communication and administrative center, this ashram consists of a large meditation hall, an office, and a small store for pictures, books, and tapes. There are no residential facilities for devotees, but there is a good-sized hotel nearby (the Anand Sager Lodge) where most Westerners stay. (The address of this hotel is Dinesh Complex No. 52, Subbarama Chetty Road, Nettakallappa Circle, Basavanagudi. Tel: 91-80-6616626.)

Karunamayi tours in India and the West for about two months every year. When she's not on tour, she divides her time equally between her two ashrams.

🌀 **Forest Ashram.** Meditation courses are held once or twice a month—check with the Bangalore ashram for the exact schedule. The daily course schedule includes about six hours of meditation, two hours of yoga asanas, and two discourses by Karunamayi.

🌀 **Bangalore Ashram.** The meditation hall is open each day for individual practice. When Karunamayi is there, the evening schedule is as follows: personal interviews from 5 to 6 P.M.; prayers and bhajans from 6 to 7 P.M.; meditation from 7 to 7:30 P.M., a discourse from 7:30 to 8:30 P.M., and individual blessings from 8:30 P.M. on.

Fees

Donation.

Contact Information

All contact should be through the Bangalore ashram.

Bangalore Ashram
SRI MATHRUDEVI VISHNAS SHANTI ASHRAM
14/5, 6TH CROSS, ASHOKNAGAR
BANASHAKARI, 1ST STAGE
BANGALORE 560 050
KARNATAKA
TEL: 91-80-609-588
FAX: 91-80-660-0518

Forest Ashram:
SRI MATHRUDEVI VISHNAS SHANTI ASHRAM
SRI PENUSILA KSHESTRAM, PENCHILA KONA AREA

RAPURE MANDAL
DIST. NELLORE, ANDHRA PRADESH
TEL: NONE

U.S. Contact:
c/o MR. JOHN ROBERTS
TEL: (718) 898-2841
FAX: (718) 458-8583

How to Get There

🌀 **Forest Ashram.** The forest ashram is about 70 kilometers from Nellore in Andhra Pradesh. The closest airport is Madras. Take a train from Madras to Nellore Station. From there you can take a bus (which stops at the ashram gate) or a taxi to the ashram. The ashram can also be reached by bus from Bangalore or Hyderabad—verify directions with the Bangalore ashram.

🌀 **Bangalore Ashram.** The ashram is in the southern part of the city, not far from Lal Bagh Gardens and Basavanagudi. It's about 20 kilometers from the airport and 5 kilometers from the city center. You can get fairly near the ashram by bus. If you go by taxi or rickshaw, tell the driver to go to N.R. Colony. From there he can get directions to Ashoknagar, 6th Cross Street, which is less than one kilometer away.

Other Services

All services are available in Bangalore. From the forest ashram, it's 30 kilometers to the closest village with a phone or any services.

Books and Tapes

A biography of Karunamayi is available at the Bangalore Ashram or through the U.S. contact. There's also a magazine, *Poorna Pragna*, and a videotape of one of her American tours.

When the mental plane becomes as clean as a mirror, God himself will write on the mental screen His own form. As the sun clearly appears on a cloudless sky, so also the divine light radiates through the pure heart of a person.

In this world, one might have become a scholar of scriptures. One might have performed in seclusion many hard penances. One might have visited holy places and taken baths in several sacred rivers. He might be able to perform many a miracle. But when such a person has no compassion towards the poor, the unhealthy, and the suffering, all the achievements are useless. The real abode of God lies in such a heart which radiates love with equanimity towards every one.

KARUNAMAYI
(from *Karunamayi: A Biography*)

Shri Shivabalayogi Maharaj Trust
Bangalore, Karnataka

Shri Shivabalayogi Maharaj (1935–1994)

Every evening, devotees gather at Shri Shivabalayogi's Bangalore ashram to sing bhajans and lose themselves in "bhava samadhi"—a spiritual trance in which they sway and flail to the beat of the music, convulsed in an ecstasy of devotion. Although Shri Shivabalayogi is no longer in his body, his devotees say his spirit still uses bhava samadhi to inspire, heal, and instruct them, just as he did when he was physically present. For another forty years, they say, he has promised to stay with his disciples—giving darshan, blessing vibhuti, and answering questions and prayers through the medium of various devotees who serve as "channels" for his spirit.

Shivabalayogi has always used four main methods to bless his devotees: giving darshan while in samadhi; distributing blessed vibhuti (sacred ash); bestowing bhava samadhi; and initiating anyone who's interested—regardless of their spiritual path or teacher—into a nonsectarian "dhyana meditation." To date, his followers claim, he's initiated over ten million people (in a low-maintenance ceremony that involves no commitment to him as a guru other than simply receiving his blessings as an aid to meditation).

While kirtan and bhava samadhi raise the spiritual energy, daily meditation is by far the most important part of the path he advocates. Other than teaching dhyana, he has never given any verbal teachings—everything else we need to know, he says, we will learn on our own by meditating. "Know Truth through meditation. Then you will yourself know who you are, your religion, your caste, and your nature," he teaches. "Do not believe what others say and become a slave to religious prejudices." Followers are instructed simply to sit quietly for one hour, with the eyes closed and the attention directed at the point between the eyebrows. Swamiji, it's said, will take care of the rest.

According to devotees, Shivabalayogi's own awakening began as a boy of fourteen, when he and some friends were swimming in an irrigation canal of the Godvari River near the small south Indian village where he was born. The boys found some fallen palmyra fruit, and Sathyaraju, as he was then called, sat down on the banks of the canal and began to squeeze his palmyra to extract its sweet juice. Suddenly his body began to tremble; the fruit began to glow and emit the sound of *Om*. As he watched—understandably transfixed—it transformed into a black Shivalingam, split in two, and released a handsome yogi, who tapped Sathyaraju between the eyebrows. Sathyaraju promptly dropped into a deep samadhi—which would continue virtually uninterrupted for the next twelve years.

For eight years, the Balayogi (boy yogi), as he came to be known, meditated twenty-three hours a day, only returning to ordinary consciousness to bathe, drink a glass of milk, or eat a little fruit. For another four years, he meditated twelve hours a day. His body was emaciated and gnawed by insects and rodents; but he emanated a spiritual bliss so intense that thousands of people began coming to sit in his presence. In 1961, on the twelve-year anniversary of his entry into samadhi, a crowd of 300,000 people assembled to witness his long-anticipated reemergence.

Since Shivabalayogi completed his austerities over thirty years ago, bhava samadhi—an esoteric aspect of the Indian spiritual tradition—has been a common experience during his programs in India. In bhava samadhi, it is said, a person is temporarily controlled by the astral body of a divine being. At evening bhajans at the ashram, you can witness the remarkable spectacle of men and women—many of them conservatively dressed Indian housewives and businesspeople—dancing and flailing around the room in sacred trance. Devotees say that bhava cures diseases and cultivates faith in God. But the main purpose is to get a taste of the divine, so that you're motivated to experience it again and again through meditation. "If the bhajan is good, I get perfectly immeasurable bliss. The better the bhajan, the better the trance," testified one devotee. "The bliss I experience cannot be described. I have never seen any other pleasure which can be compared with this."

Facilities and Food

The Shivabalayogi ashram is set in a four-acre garden in a residential, suburban district of Bangalore. The neighborhood is quiet with many trees; the grounds are thick with mango and banana trees, coffee beans, and a multitude of other vegetables and flowers. There's a large meditation hall with an arched concrete roof, where the bhajans and darshans are held; there's also a thousand-person auditorium with an attached dining hall and kitchen for marriages, plays and musicals, and other festive events. There's also a temple dedicated to Brahma, Vishnu, and Shiva—one of only two temples in India where Brahma is worshipped—where pujas are held three times a day.

The ashram can accommodate 150 to 200 people in shared rooms (four-person maximum) with attached baths. Flats are available for families.

Schedule

Meditation can be done on your own or in the temple or meditation hall when open. Guests of the ashram are expected to attend the meditation in the Dhyan Mandir at 5 A.M. every day for half an hour.

When present at the ashram, guests are also asked to attend the "naivedyam"—offering of food to the gods—at the temple at 8 A.M., 12 noon, and 8:15 P.M. and to attend the bhajans every evening at 6:30. From 7:30 to 8 P.M., Shivabalayogi's spirit gives darshan (through one of his disciples, who goes into a trance).

Fees

There is no charge for visiting the ashram, but guests who would like to stay for longer periods are expected to contribute three hours of service (such as gardening) each day. Donations are accepted.

Contact Information

SHRI SHIVABALAYOGI MAHARAJ TRUST
1/A, III PHASE
J. P. NAGAR, BANGALORE 560 078
TEL: 91-80-648-242
FAX: 91-812-648-822

U.S. Contacts
SHRI SHIVABALAYOGI MAHARAJ CHARITABLE TRUST
P.O. BOX 10595
PORTLAND, OR 97210-0595
TEL: (503) 285-6756

SHRI SHIVABALAYOGI MAHARAJ CHARITABLE TRUST
P.O. BOX 99703
SEATTLE, WA 98199
TEL: (206) 284-2885

SHRI SHIVABALAYOGI MAHARAJ CHARITABLE TRUST,
A NORTH CAROLINA TRUST
25 WEDGEWOOD ROAD
CHAPEL HILL, NC 27514
TEL: (919) 967-2361

The ashram is in J. P. Nagar, about 20 to 30 minutes by taxi or autorickshaw (or 45 minutes by bus) from the city center. Once you're in the area, the driver can ask local people for directions. Call the ashram for directions and bus numbers.

Other Services

All services are available in Bangalore, which has a population of approximately 4 million.

Books and Tapes

Books and photographs are available at the center in India. Books, tapes, photographs, and videotapes are also available through the U.S. centers (see Contact Information).

I tried to open my eyes but found that they remained forcibly closed. A soothing feeling began to take hold of me and I began to reel with the music, without even the slightest effort on my part. I heard my friends laughing, but I was past caring. I made a final effort to control myself and to hold myself still; just then I got a big shock on my right toe, as if it had been inserted into an electric plug. I was unable to move; my body became rigid. The force came right up into my stomach, accumulated there, and began to rise higher. I began to black out; a suffocating feeling engulfed me; a tremendous force started shaking me from within. I rose clutching my stomach. People around me were alarmed; they thought that I had got an attack of colic. My eyes were still closed but a force began to impel me forward. My limbs were no longer under my control. I believe I trampled over a few people as I moved forward . . . My eyes opened and I found myself standing near the Yogi. I was shivering involuntarily. His powerful eyes looked at me as if penetrating into my very being. He motioned to me to sit down and gave me some consecrated vibhuti to drink, mixed in

water. Immediately the force within me subsided and I began to sway with the music, enjoying the peaceful calm that once again enveloped me. In the mind's eye came visions of many gods and goddesses and of many ancient sages. This was my first experience of Bhava Samadhi.

> —A DEVOTEE'S ACCOUNT
> (from *Shri Shri Shri Shivabalayogi Maharaj: Life and Spiritual Ministration*)

Vivekananda Kendra Yoga Research Foundation
Bangalore, Karnataka

 Dr. H. R. Nagendra, Ph.D. (Founder/Secretary) (1943–   )

Located in the countryside thirty-two kilometers outside of Bangalore, the Vivekananda Kendra Yoga Research Foundation feels more like a corporate conference center than an ashram, complete with a cinema-size auditorium and an administration building in the shape of a giant *Om*. This is yoga gone mainstream—a large-scale experiment in fusing yoga with science, medicine, and organizational development.

Teachers and Teachings

VK Yogas, as the foundation is called for short, is the research and education wing of the Vivekananda Kendra, a spiritual service mission (headquartered in Kanyakumari, Tamil Nadu) dedicated to realizing the vision of the world-renowned teacher Swami Vivekananda. VK Yogas aims to bring together science and spirituality, so science can benefit from the ancient wisdom of yoga and yoga can be made more useful and accessible to the modern world.

If you're looking for mystical experiences, you may be in the wrong place. You'll meet more M.D.s than sadhus at the thirty-five-acre Prashanti Kuteeram campus (although you're welcome to book a private cell in the 84-chamber "Patanjali Block" meditation complex). What you will find are comprehensive, scientifically oriented courses in the fundamentals of yoga practice, including a teacher training course, a diploma program in yoga and naturopathy, and dozens of "personality development camps" based on yogic principles. The center also boasts a 160-bed holistic hospital; a yoga research laboratory; a stress-reduction program for corporate executives; an annual yoga and science conference; and an annual All-India yoga Olympiad.

The founder and director of VK Yogas is Dr. H. R. Nagendra, a Ph.D. in mechanical engineering who worked with NASA in the early years of the space program. Deciding that he was "more interested in human engineering than mechanical engineering," he returned to India and became the director of training at the Vivekanandra Kendra service mission. Under the auspices of the Vivekananda Kendra, he traveled all over the country studying with different yoga masters. By founding VK Yogas in 1979, he hoped to combine the most effective techniques of all the different schools and ground them solidly in a scientific context.

Today, VK Yogas has swelled to a massive complex serving patients, students, and scholars from all over the world. Over a thousand patients a year visit the yoga-based "health home" for holistic relief from ailments ranging from depression, asthma, migraine, and ulcers to cancer, mental retardation, and cerebral palsy. ("Yogasanas, pranayama, meditation, lectures, devotional meditation, and counseling are the 'pills' offered to the therapy participants for curing their ailments," says the Center's annual report.) The health home aims to wean patients from conventional medicine, with impressive results: For example, in 1995, 80 percent of anxiety patients were able to stop their medication, along with 90 percent of back pain patients, 70 percent of asthma patients, and 50 percent of diabetes patients.

The health home works closely with the neurophysiology and biochemistry research laboratories, which are engaged in ongoing scientific studies on the effect of yoga practices on illnesses such as asthma, allergy, cancer, arthritis, paralysis, hypertension, and even infectious diseases such as tuberculosis. The research lab's findings also bolster the two-day corporate intensives in "self-management of excessive tension" (SMET). A regular conference on yoga research (which draws nearly eight hundred international participants) features lectures on topics such as "Can science explain consciousness?"; "The psychophysiology of prana"; and "Quantum physics and the Upanishads."

Most of the foreign visitors, though, come for the educational offerings, which include a government-recognized teacher's training diploma program and a therapy course to train students in the art of using yoga to cure ailments. Residential programs range from a few weeks to a year in length, and the orientation, not surprisingly, is therapeutic and scientific. Advanced asanas are not encouraged; rather, gentle yoga poses are taught with an emphasis on relaxing the muscles, quieting the mind, and slowing down the breath, so that the life force energy can flow unimpeded. The goal is to learn to carry that relaxed attitude into everyday life—to be able to execute any task, regardless of its difficulty, without striving or stress. (The asana instructors are all themselves graduates of VK Yogas—some of them quite recent—and some students complain that they are not sufficiently experienced to be conducting teacher's trainings. There's no complaint, though, about the therapeutic and philosophical content, which is taught by scholar-practitioners and medical doctors.)

The program is intensive, with regular oral and written examinations on yoga philosophy, therapy, anatomy, and physiology. The emphasis is on developing the whole person, so the program contains some highly non-traditional elements—for example, participants are all required to give regular creative performances—such as story-telling, singing, dance, etc.—to help them overcome fears and inhibitions.

Facilities and Food

In addition to the 160-bed hospital, the thirty-five-acre Prashanti Kuteeram campus has beds for 154 guests in dormitories, small cottages, and single, double, and triple rooms. Rooms are fairly new and quite clean; bedding is provided. Be sure to bring a flashlight, as the electricity is unreliable. In the dormitories, earplugs are indispensable.

Other facilities include a meditation dome; a block of eighty-four individual meditation cells; a 1,300-person auditorium; and multiple classrooms and lecture halls.

The dining hall serves good south Indian vegetarian food.

The Vivekananda Kendra also has a coordinating center in Bangalore proper. The Vivekananda Kendra has over seventy branches all over India. For a complete listing, contact the Bangalore center.

Schedule

Schedule varies from program to program.

Rates for foreigners are given in $ U.S. and average about $250 to $300 per month.

VIVEKANANDA KENDRA YOGA RESEARCH FOUNDATION
PRASHANTI KUTEERAM RESIDENTIAL CAMPUS
JIGANI, ANEKAL TALUK
BANGALORE
TEL: 91-80-425-535
FAX: 91-80-425-385

CITY COORDINATING CENTER
EKNATH BHAVAN
19, GAVIPURAM CIRCLE
BANGALORE 560 019
TEL: 91-80-6608645

The Prashanti Kuteeram campus is 32 kilometers outside of Bangalore. To arrange a van or taxi from Bangalore, contact the Vivekananda Kendra city coordinating center in Bangalore.

There is a pay phone and fax available at Prashanti Kuteeram, but the line to use them is often long. All services are available in Bangalore, but that's a good hour away.

Books are available at the Center.

Spiritual personality is not something other worldly; in simple words, it means less and less selfishness, holistic perspective, act-

ing in tune with cosmic laws, life of simplicity and bliss, and higher powers used for good of the society and the country. These are the qualities given in abundance to Indians since ancient times; this is the personality of India itself.

—from *Yoga in Education* brochure of VK Yogas

Art of Living Foundation
Bangalore, Karnataka

 Sri Sri Ravi Shankar (1956–   )

With hundreds of teachers and centers in over forty countries, Sri Sri Ravi Shankar's Art of Living course—whose main base is in the countryside about 21 kilometers south of Bangalore—seems poised to become the Transcendental Meditation of the next generation. Like TM, the Art of Living neatly repackages traditional yogic techniques and Vedic philosophy into a simple, nonsectarian system that appeals to mainstreamers who might be uncomfortable in a traditional ashram. Its primary method is the "sudarshan kriya," a rhythmic breathing technique claimed to wipe out stress, eliminate toxins, increase vitality, and bring about profound physical and spiritual healing—all in as little as ten minutes of practice a day.

Teachers and Teachings

To stay at the country ashram, you must be enrolled in one of the Art of Living courses—either the introductory weekend or one of the four-to ten-day advanced courses. The program is billed as "fun and relaxing"—organizers stress that it doesn't conflict with any other religion or spiritual practice. "The course gives people a chance to dive deep into the joy hidden inside every man and woman, and come out smiling," claims a glossy promotional brochure. "The knowledge received is so simple and natural that there is no need for further instruction."

The Art of Living course aims to give you a direct experience of the silent, joyful core of your being, by cutting through the mental dust and debris that cover it up. Since body, breath, and mind are connected, you'll be taught to work with simple asanas, breathing exercises, and meditation techniques. The main method, though, will be the breathing technique called sudarshan ("right vision") kriya ("purifying action"), which is designed to "blow away all thoughts" and put you in touch with the natural rhythm of your body, breath, and soul.

According to Ravi Shankar's mother (who, admittedly, might be biased), he started meditating at the age of three and by the time he was four could recite the entire Bhagavad Gita. He's reticent about discussing the details of his spiritual training; however, it did include a number of years with Maharishi Mahesh Yogi, the founder of TM. Since what followers describe as his enlightenment experience in the early 1980s, he has been traveling worldwide, teaching the timeless message of staying in the present and opening the heart. "We think that at some time in the future when we are dead and gone, then we will meet God," he says. "No. God has to be realized in one's heart."

Today, Punditji, as his students call him, is a striking, charismatic man in his early forties, with long, wavy hair and beard and swirling white robes. His commanding presence is softened by his warmth and his playful, almost childlike charm—he has a quick wit and a easy, mischievous laugh. Of course, there's no guarantee you'll actually find him at his ashram, since he's often on tour worldwide—courses are generally led (according to a standardized curriculum) by his trained teachers. (To find out his schedule, contact the Bangalore city center or the office in Santa Barbara, California.)

The ashram draws people from all over India—most of them young, modern, middle-class professionals—as well as an increasing number of foreign visitors. A graduate student in psychology from California recently visited the ashram to compile psychophysiological data on seventy Art of Living course participants from twenty countries. When they arrived at the ashram, she reported, they suffered from symptoms that included rheumatism, asthma, arthritis, bronchitis, hay fever, migraines, high blood pressure, and anemia, as well as a full range of emotional problems. By the end of their retreat, all but two with physical problems felt that they were substantially improved; 95 percent of those with emotional problems reported marked breakthroughs.

Unlike TM, the Art of Living has a minimal organizational structure

("Sometimes the picture frame can start eating the picture," Ravi Shankar points out) and a strong orientation toward service projects. The ashram is very engaged in community service, including free primary education for rural children, vocational training for women, environmental protection projects, and nutritional and medical programs.

Facilities and Food

Located in the green, rolling farm country south of Bangalore, this ashram is clearly a growing concern—in addition to the hundred acres already developed, there's additional property awaiting further expansion. It can accommodate about four hundred people in shared rooms with attached baths and ten-bed dormitories. Vegetarian food is served.

The ashram has a banana plantation, vegetable gardens, and a lake. Their milk is produced by their own cows; the cow dung is used for a biogas plant that provides energy for the kitchen. A large meditation hall seats about one thousand people; a smaller hall is for ceremonies, meditation, and smaller programs. Volleyball courts are available. Construction is underway for numerous other facilities, adding to the air of growth and dynamism (though detracting somewhat from the tranquillity).

Other facilities include an ayurvedic clinic and a Vedic school.

Schedule

A typical introductory course begins with a puja at 5:30 A.M., followed by hatha-yoga asanas, pranayama, sudarshan kriya, and meditation. There are several hours of instruction and practice in the morning and afternoon, followed by a nature walk. In the evening is satsang with the teacher. The advanced course is largely conducted in silence. Special pujas are celebrated on Monday mornings.

Fees

In India, the fees for the introductory course (two evenings and one day) is Rs 500. The advanced course (five to ten days) is approximately Rs 1000. When staying at the ashram, donations are accepted to cover meals and accommodations.

City Center:
VYAKTI VIKAS KENDRA
19, 39TH A CROSS
11TH MAIN, IV T BLOCK
JAYANAGAR
BANGALORE 560 041
KARNATAKA
TEL: 91-80-6645106
FAX: 91-80-6635175

Ashram location:
VED VIGNAN MAHAVIDYAPEETH
UDAYAGIRI, 21ST KM.
KANAKAPURA ROAD
BANGALORE SOUTH TALUQ 560 062

U.S. Contact:
ART OF LIVING FOUNDATION
P.O. BOX 50003
SANTA BARBARA, CA 93108
TEL: (805) 565-3603

How to Get There

The ashram is located 21 kilometers south of Bangalore and is accessible by taxi or bus. Buses from Bangalore go about every 10 to 15 minutes on Kanakapura Road to the village of Hdipalya, which is next door to the ashram. Advance registration is essential.

Other Services

The nearby village of Hdipalya has a population of about 250 people, and services are basically nonexistent. Bangalore, 21 kilometers away, has all services.

Books and Tapes

Books and tapes are available at the Bangalore center and in the United States through the Art of Living Foundation Mail Order, P.O. Box 80068, Portland, OR 97280.

When God created man, man went to him for every small little thing, asking him for favors, complaining to him about everything. Man would pray for God to come. If God came, he would say, "Don't come now. Come later. You have come too soon." If God didn't come, he would complain, "I have called you so many times and you have come so late." God grew really tired of this. He wanted to go and hide somewhere, but that was not easily done. He knew man would go to the moon to find him.

At this point God met a wise man. The wise man whispered in God's ear, "Hide in the heart of man. That is where he never goes." Since that day, God has hidden in the heart of man. Anyone who goes there will not be able to complain. All complaints will drop away. One person here and there among a million goes to his own heart and finds God. And when a person finds God in his own heart, he has no complaints.

—Sri Sri Ravi Shankar
(from *The Language of the Heart*)

Ashtanga Yoga Research Institute
Mysore, Karnataka

K. Pattabhi Jois (1915–)

The octogenarian hatha-yoga master K. Pattabhi Jois has become increasingly sought-after in recent years, as his fiery brand of Ashtanga yoga—a bruising hatha-yoga workout—surges in popularity in the United

No-Frills Ashtanga Yoga

If you want to study Ashtanga vinyasa yoga in Mysore but can't afford Pattabhi Jois's rates, the same system is also taught by B. N. S. Iyengar, a seventy-year-old teacher who learned Ashtanga from Krishnamacharya (Pattabhi Jois's guru) in the 1940s and 50s. (He's no relation to the famous B. K. S. Iyengar of Pune—Iyengar is a common brahmin name in south India.) For $70 a month, foreigners can join the daily classes (mostly composed of local Indian students) in the traditional Ashtanga series. Unlike Pattabhi Jois, Iyengar is fluent in English and eager to teach the theory behind the practice—he'll give you specific information about the physiological, psychological, and spiritual effects of each asana, as well as theories about yoga philosophy, kundalini, and the subtle energetic effects of the Ashtanga practice. Men and women practice separately. You won't be part of the tight-knit Western Ashtanga club that practices with Pattabhi Jois—but you will have the chance to meet lots of Indian practitioners (something you won't get at Pattabhi Jois's center), who are very friendly to the handful of Westerners who practice here. Classes are held daily from 5 to 7 A.M. and 5 to 7 P.M. at Sri Patanjala Yogashala, Sri Brahmatantra Swatantra Parakaal Mutt, Jaganmohan Palace Circle, Mysore.

States and Europe. Seemingly unaffected by his sudden fame, Jois continues to teach classes six mornings a week—assisted by his grandson Sharat—in a tiny, concrete-floored room in his modest Mysore home.

Teacher and Teachings

Sweat is the salient characteristic of a session with Jois. This is not the place to go if you're looking for lectures on yoga philosophy. ("A lot of questions shows busy mind," he's fond of telling students. "Just do your practice and all will follow.") Nor should you expect much in the way of seated meditation. ("Sit still and you get monkeys in the head.") Instead, the daily routine consists of two to three hours of strenuous asana practice, in which increasingly challenging postures are synchronized with the breath in an unbroken, mesmerizing flow.

Known in Sansrit as *vinyasa,* this combination of deep breathing and vigorous movement is designed to stoke the internal fires, generating intense *tapas*—or heat—that purifies and energizes the body. Profuse perspiration washes out toxins, while increased circulation enables the muscles to melt more easily into the postures. ("Even iron will bend with heat," Jois says.) On a more subtle level, vinyasa practice is said to vastly increase the flow of *prana,* or life-force energy. And sustained concentration on the breath quiets the mind, creating meditation in movement.

According to Jois, the six standard routines that he teaches—which range from an already quite challenging "introductory series" to a culminating sequence that no one but he has ever mastered—derive from an ancient text called the *Yoga Korunta.* Jois was an early disciple of the great hatha yogi and Sanskrit scholar Krishnamacharya, whose other well-known students include B. K. S. Iyengar (p. 221) and T. K. V. Desikachar (p. 247). As Jois tells it, in the early 1930s he and Krishnamacharya were perusing obscure Sanskrit texts in the musty archives of a Calcutta library when they stumbled across a collection of verses on hatha yoga written on a bundle of crumbling leaves. The manuscript itself appeared to be about 500 years old; the verses were in an archaic form of Sanskrit that indicated they might reflect an even older tradition. Krishnamacharya handed the manuscript to Jois and said, "This is your life work."

Some suspect this story of being apocryphal. No one now alive has seen a copy of the *Yoga Korunta*—or even a complete translation of it—and Jois claims that the original manuscript has been "eaten by ants." But whatever their origin, the series are undeniably potent. The primary series is said to detoxify the physical body. The intermediate series purifies and strengthens the *nadis,* the subtle energy channels that link the seven chakras. The four advanced series draw the prana up the *sushumna nadi*— the central energy channel in the spine—to the crown chakra, where it produces radical changes in consciousness that culminate in the ecstatic state called *samadhi.*

Students of all ages and abilities practice together—from rank beginners who can barely see their toes, let alone touch them, to adepts who think nothing of back flips and five-minute handstands. Jois does not lead the class in a common practice—rather, each student progresses through an assigned series at her own level, while Jois and his assistant (his twenty-something grandson, Sharat, who is the heir to the Ashtanga throne) roam the studio coaching and making vigorous adjustments. As each student finishes, a new one takes her place, until the room finally empties out at about 10 A.M.

At first glance, the steamy, cramped studio with its concrete floor seems far from ideal for yoga—in fact, it's challenging just to avoid colliding with the sweaty bodies of fellow practitioners. But students invariably claim that their practice has never been better, a phenomenon they attribute to the powerful presence of Pattabhi Jois.

At eighty-one years old, Jois is a short, barrel-chested man with mischievous eyes and a radiant smile, who looks a good twenty years younger than he actually is. After completing his studies with Krishnamacharya, Jois went on to study yoga philosophy at the Sanskrit Collee in Mysore, where he taught from 1937 to 1973. He can push a student along as fiercely as an Army drill sergeant—using the full weight of his body, if necessary, to drag an uncooperative limb into positions its owner never dreamed of—but his scoldings are always good-humored: "Bad lady. Why so fat? Twenty-five-dollar fine!" Be prepared to cope with minor injuries—"Ashtanga casualties" are common. Jois will invariably dismiss your aching back, sore neck, or throbbing hamstring as "some little pain—one week, all over. Keep practicing!"

After asana class is over, students are on their own. No rules govern extracurricular activities, and celibacy is definitely not the norm. Some students use their free time to study Sanskrit and yoga philosophy at the nearby Sanskrit College of India. Others spend it shopping, swimming at a local hotel pool, sightseeing, or socializing.

Be sure to bring workout clothes—tights and leotards for women, shorts for men. Bring several sets, as they'll get soaked with sweat every day. Woven rugs are provided to cover the concrete floor, but a yoga "sticky mat" is also useful to prevent slipping. In addition to your standard first-aid kit, you'll probably want to bring something to rub on sore muscles.

Schedule

A minimum one-month stay is required. It's best to write ahead and let Jois or his grandson Sharath know when you are coming; drop-in visitors may be turned away at busy times of the year. Since only twelve students at once can squeeze into Jois's tiny studio, asana practice takes place in shifts, with the first round beginning at 4 A.M. Practice sessions are held every day except Saturdays, full moons, and new moons. Women are asked to take three days off during menstruation.

Fees

$250 (U.S.) a month for yoga classes, plus a $100 "initiation fee" for the first month.

Facilities and Food

The Ashtanga Yoga Research Institute does not provide accommodations, but rooms can be rented at local hotels for Rs 30 to 100 per night. A popular choice among yoga students is the Kaveri Lodge at 369 Cheluvamba Road. Many students also team up to rent houses together.

Within walking distance of the Ashtanga studio are several good vegetarian restaurants.

Contact Information

ASHTANGA YOGA RESEARCH INSTITUTE
876/1, 1 CROSS
LAKSHMIPURAM
MYSORE 570 004
TEL: 91-821-25558
FAX: 91-821-520357

Other Services

Mysore is a city of about 650,000, and all services are available.

How to Get There

Trains and buses run regularly to and from Bangalore (about three hours away).

For an introduction to the Ashtanga system, read *Power Yoga* by Beryl Bender Birch (HarperCollins). There's also a booklet on the Ashtanga series available from the office at Pattabhi Jois's house.

The dun-colored dust of India eddied about the bare feet of the villagers as they gathered in an open field to hear the yogi speak. It was the early 1930s, and Sri Krishnamacharya was touring the country with his young shishya (student), K. Pattabhi Jois, for the express purpose of reminding these people of their own great heritage. The science of yoga had been born among these very hills and plains.

Casting his eyes about for a suitable platform, Krishnamacharya had an idea. Why not use a practical demonstration of mental focus and strength to accompany the philosophical aspects of his talk? He summoned his eager disciple and pointed to a spot in the center of the growing crowd. Pattabhi Jois hurried over, drew some deep breaths, and prepared to execute the asana his teacher had chosen—Kapotasana. A thin cloth was spread over the lumpy ground to hold back the choking dust. The young yogi bent backward from a kneeling position, arching ever more tightly until he had an ankle grasped in each hand. With the exception of deep, regular breathing, he settled motionless into the completed posture. Krishnamacharya's face betrayed no trace of pride as he stepped onto the flat, hard stomach of his student to begin the lecture.

The story is made more memorable when Pattabhi Jois recalls with a wry smile that half an hour later, when Krishnamacharya at last ordered him up from the posture, a rusty metal spike came up with him. It had been embedded in his arm by the weight of the lecturer.

—CHRISTINE HETHER
(from *Yoga Journal*)

🌀 *Sri Ganapathi Sachchidananda Swamiji (1942–   )*

Devotees of Sri Ganapathi Sachchidananda Swamiji believe him to be an incarnation of the deity Dattatreya, an ancient yogi who was born with three heads representing the Hindu trinity of Brahma, Vishnu, and Shiva. As Dattatreya was both a great yogi and a great musician, Sri Ganapathi's teachings focus on these two elements. He's best known for his concerts of "healing music," which use classical ragas and his own improvisations to address emotional and physical imbalances. When he's not on tour, hundreds of devotees show up at his ashram on Chamundi Hill every Sunday morning for rollicking bhajan concerts with a ten-piece Indian band—"Sri Swamiji can easily handle harmonium, a Casio keyboard, or a most updated Roland keyboard," asserts a biographical pamphlet—followed by a discourse and an elaborate fire ceremony, or "homa."

Teachers and Teachings

"Mind must get healing. Music is the best way," according to an ashram publication. "Swamiji wants you to hear good music which indirectly acts as medicine for the injured mind." According to Sri Ganapathi, his music is designed to vibrate the 72,000 nadis (energy channels) in specific combinations, thus healing diseases ranging from depression and headaches to cancer and mental illness.

He has tens of thousands of Indian devotees, including many wealthy and influential politicians (the former prime minister of India used to visit him regularly); and increasing numbers of Westerners are coming to his ashram to witness his apparent miracles and learn his unique form of "kriya yoga."

Sri Ganapathi is, among other things, a consummate performer, drawing stadium-size crowds to his bhajan concerts in Indian cities, where his singing is often accompanied by some of India's top musicians. Bhajans, he believe, are a path to self-realization, as well as a means of bringing about physical healing: his compositions are crafted to address particular ailments, and he'll often preface a bhajan by saying "This one is to lower blood pressure" or "This one is for the back pain," and suggesting that the audience concentrate on that part of the body. You can order cassettes to treat specific diseases, ranging from "Nada Himalaya" for "body pains, sleeplessness, joint pains" to "Nada Prasara" for "skin problems, mental sick."

When he's at the ashram, his Sunday bhajans are often followed by a homa, or fire worship, a traditional purification ritual—passed down in his family for generations—in which he steps into a five-foot-deep pit filled with blazing coals. The fire, he says, serves as the messenger between human beings and the gods. In an annual Shivaratri extravaganza, thousands of devotees come to watch him perform a special homa, in which he dances in the pit for up to forty-five minutes, pouring ghee on the fire and making ritual offerings while the flames leap higher and higher around him. At this time, devotees say, he performs miracles and materializes objects, such as producing enormous stone lingams from his mouth; he then emerges from the flames and makes predictions on such matters as the future of the world. (A videotape of this event is available from the ashram or from his U.S. headquarters.) Depending on the audience, his satsangs are delivered in English, Kannada, Telugu, or one of several other Indian languages in which he is fluent.

Sri Ganapathi's only guru was his mother, whom he describes as a saint. (She was his father's second wife; as the story goes, his father went mad after the death of his first wife, and Sri Ganapathi's mother voluntarily married the madman, then restored him to sanity.) Before his spiritual awakening, Sri Ganapathi worked as a schoolmaster, a weaver, and a postman. Now, he says, "I am still a postman, in a sense—but now I carry the messages from the people to God."

Sri Ganapathi teaches a simple form of kriya yoga, which involves no asanas, but twenty-one pranayama techniques to raise the energy and purify the nadis, or nerve passageways. Most devotees are Indian, but when Swamiji is present, there will usually be several dozen foreigners there as well. Published (but unproven) charges of black market money laundering have not crimped the swami's swelling popularity. Since the ashram is very much centered on the personality of Sri Ganapathi, not much goes on there while he is on tour; you're welcome to visit, but the place will be virtually deserted. At festival times, when Swamiji is present, the ashram is very busy, so you're advised to write in advance for permission to stay; an initial short stay will probably be approved, but it can only be extended with Swamiji's permission.

The ashram has an increasing number of charitable works, including a hospital, an ayurvedic dispensary, and schools.

Facilities and Food

The ashram is set on twenty-two acres of landscaped grounds with flower gardens, coconut groves, and lotus ponds. The ashram facilities are startlingly grand, including an immense marble-floored prayer hall (hung with silkscreened banners bearing slogans like "No God No Peace— Know God Know Peace") that can accommodate several thousand people. You can descend a small staircase to visit the dark marble cave where Swamiji goes to sit in samadhi in style for up to ten days at a time. When he's not on tour or in samadhi, Swamiji dwells in a stately pale-yellow mansion built for him by devotees who, according to one follower, "want to see him live like a king."

The ashram can comfortably accommodate about five hundred guests in dormitories, private rooms with attached baths, and shared rooms. (For special festivals, though, as many as one thousand may be squeezed in.) Celibacy is required while staying at the ashram. An ayurvedic herb garden features 245 species of herbs—practitioners can do pranayama there to inhale the plant energy, and Swamiji plucks herbs every morning to prepare a sacred water to distribute to devotees. A music studio is used for music therapy, audio recording, and meditation. An ayurvedic clinic caters to devotees free of charge. The ashram has its own small dairy, featuring one special cow who, it is said, will fulfill your wishes if you propitiate her with bananas.

Vegetarian meals are served in the dining hall, which seats about five hundred people. A separate canteen serves dosas, coffee, and other snacks.

Schedule

When Swami is in residence, there is a concert every Sunday morning. The rest of the week, the day begins at 5 A.M. with meditation (on your own), followed by a puja and fire ceremony. Most of the schedule is taken up by seva (work in the hospital, kitchen, music studio, etc.). The day concludes with bhajans from 6 to 8 P.M.

There is a minimum charge of Rs 25 per night. A specific donation for daily meals is not stipulated.

Contact Information

GANAPATHI SACHCHIDANANDA ASHRAM
NANJANGUDA ROAD
DATTA NAGAR—OOTY ROAD
MYSORE 570 004
KARNATAKA
TEL: 91-821-22662

U.S. Contact:
DATTA YOGA CENTER, U.S.A.
139 CHINQUIPIN COVE
RIDGELAND, MS 39157
TEL: (601) 856-4783

How to Get There

Mysore can be reached from Bangalore by train, bus, or taxi. The ashram is on Chamundi Hill about 5 kilometers from the Mysore city center and can be reached by taxi or autorickshaw.

Other Services

Mysore has a population of about 650,000, and all services are available.

Books and Tapes

Books and tapes of healing music are available at the ashram or by contacting the U.S. center. The ashram has twenty-eight branches all over India: a list is available from the Mysore ashram office.

An interesting experience is that of Mr. H. V. Krishnaswamy, who was afflicted by the Guillain-Barre Syndrome (GBS), a rare viral disease which strikes one in a million, with the survival factor being one in two billion. When doctors had given up hope of his survival, Mr. Krishnaswamy was on a diet of exclusive bhajans and music rendered by the Swami. His condition slowly improved and subsequent tests proved he was completely cured. He says his surgeon is of the opinion that hearing the bhajans continuously had had a soothing effect on his brain, which paved the way slowly to ease the tension on the tiny nerves emanating from the brain to the eyes, throat, and other parts of his body, helping his recovery.

—from *The Hindu*, "The Concept of Music Therapy,"
November 29, 1991

Anjali Ashram

At the base of Chamundi Hill on the outskirts of Mysore is the Anjali Ashram, a tranquil multireligious retreat center directed by an Indian Roman Catholic priest who is also a Hindu swami. Every month the ashram offers an organized one-week program in "Indian Christian spirituality," presenting traditional Indian philosophy and practice in a Christian context. (This is "not a seminar but a lived-experience in wholeness at the ground of being. It takes place in an atmosphere of total silence, interior and exterior." Register in advance, as the programs tend to fill up.) You can also come for a personal retreat—of anywhere from a few hours to several months—and stay in one of the private cottages tucked in a grove of date and ashoka trees. A day at the ashram is a welcome respite from the bustle of Mysore. Contact Anjali Ashram, Chamundi Hill Road, Mysore 570 011. Tel: 30226.

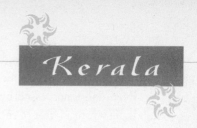

Anandashram
Kanhangad, Kerala

※ *Swami Ramdas (1884–1963)*
※ *Mother Krishnabai (1903–1989)*
※ *Swami Satchidananda (1919–ˋ)*

All day long you'll hear the singing, blending with the bellowing of the cows and the shrieks of the parakeets: "Om Sri Ram Jai Ram Jai Jai Ram," accompanied by the bright chime of silver hand bells. Because the mystic known as Papa Ramdas and his spiritual partner, Mother Krishnabai, both attained God-realization simply by chanting this mantra in praise of Ram—defined by Ramdas as the "subtle and mysterious power that pervades and sustains the whole universe"—that's the only formal practice that's done at the ashram they founded on this jungly Kerala hillside. "Devotees are advised to keep chanting the Holy Name as much as possible," explains an ashram brochure. "In due course, see God in everything and submit to his will in all matters."

Teachers and Teachings

At the Anandashram, every guest is welcomed as Ram in disguise. Arrive late at night, and they'll open the kitchen for you. Catch a train before dawn, and someone will come to your room to offer you tea before you go.

Seeing Ram in everything was the attitude that transformed Ramdas from a floundering and ineffectual textile mill manager into an ecstatic mystic revered as a saint by devotees all over India. In the early 1920s, Ramdas—then named Vittal Rao—began chanting the name of Ram to help him through his personal miseries (which included debt, unemployment, and a failed business venture). Calling on Ram, he found, brought not just relief, but bliss. To his wife's consternation, he began crying out

"Ram, Ram," as he walked down the street, and sleeping only one or two hours to leave more time for devotional singing.

Eventually, possessed by the longing to put his whole life in Ram's hands, he wrote a letter of renunciation to his wife, wrapped himself in two pieces of ochre cloth, and took the name Ramdas, or "servant of Ram." He then set out to wander all over India, with three weapons to protect him from all fear: the constant chanting of Ram Nam, the name of God; looking on everyone and everything as forms of his beloved Ram; and accepting everything and all situations as happening by Ram's will.

He spent two years wandering in ecstasy from holy site to holy site— getting onto whatever train Ram happened to place at the train station; getting off when Ram, in the form of an angry ticket taker, told him it was time. His travels included an encounter with Ramana Maharshi, the advaita vedanta master of Tiruvannamai (p. 286), who plunged him even deeper into bliss. Finally devotees built him an ashram in Kerala, where, in 1928, he was joined by a young woman named Krishnabai, who was to become his most ardent devotee. (He, likewise, addressed her as Mother and spoke of her as his guru.) After Ramdas's death in 1963, she took over the spiritual guidance of the devotees who, like Ramdas, referred to her as Mother.

Today, the ashram is headed by Swami Satchidananda, a taciturn but kind teacher who has been a devotee of Ramdas since 1947. From 5 A.M. to 10 P.M., small groups of devotees—both residents and guests—circumambulate the samadhi shrines of Ramdas and Krishnabai, singing the official mantra and clanging handbells. Visitors are welcome but not required to participate—you can sign up for a particular half-hour shift, or just join in whenever you want. Meanwhile, in the bhajan hall, there's an all-day program of devotional singing, with special periods for children. Meals are served to the accompaniment of chanting, and even the cows are sung to every morning as they are being fed.

None of this is mandatory, however—"We want you to be able to do your own sadhana," explained one swami. Meals are optional; you're not expected to work around the ashram, because "Mother prefers that you work on yourself." This low-key but heartful approach makes this an ideal place to do a personal retreat.

The only formal teaching is an optional afternoon gathering with Swami Satchidananda, in which he and other disciples read aloud from

Ramdas's books and respond to questions. (Warning: in the afternoon heat people tend to doze off during this session, including Swami Satchidananda himself.)

The ashram has a strong tradition of service, including starting a local grade school and medical clinic (which it later turned over to the community) and training villagers in work skills. Every day free food is offered to village children.

Facilities and Food

The ashram is lush, with hills on three sides and the Arabian Sea on the other. It offers over seventy comfortable private and semiprivate rooms, in addition to two dormitory halls with twenty to twenty-five beds each. Bedding is provided, but you'll need your own mosquito net.

The bhajan hall seats approximately 100 to 150 people. There is also a library with about 5,000 spiritual and religious books. The ashram has its own cowshed, housing some of the happiest cows you'll see anywhere in India. (Cows were beloved by Mother Krishnabai, and caring for them is viewed as a spiritual practice. Some cows, it's said, used to refuse to give milk unless Krishnabai sang to them.)

The food (served on banana leaves on the floor) is excellent, including superb milk and buttermilk from the ashram cows—nonspicy food is available for Westerners. The ashram water comes from its own spring and is safe to drink.

Schedule

The day begins with chanting to Vishnu at 5 A.M. in the bhajan hall. For the rest of the day, Ram Nam (chanting of the Om Sri Ram mantra) alternates with other sorts of devotional chanting. The final round of Ram Nam is at 10 P.M.

Fees

Donation.

Contact Information

ANANDASHRAM
ANANDASHRAM P.O. 671 531
KANHANGAD
DIST. KASARAGOD
KERALA, SOUTH INDIA
TEL: 91-499-703036

How to Get There

The ashram is located in north Kerala, 69 kilometers by train and 80 kilometers by road south of Mangalore (in Karnataka). You can take a train, bus, or taxi to Kanhangad. The *Trains at a Glance* schedule doesn't show a train stop at Kanhangad but the train does have a brief stop here. From the railway or bus terminal you can take an autorickshaw the 5 kilometers to the ashram. Air service is available into Mangalore from Bombay and Bangalore.

Other Services

Kanhangad is a town of about 100,000 and has most services available, although lodging selection is fairly limited. Mangalore has all services available.

Books and Tapes

Books by and about Swami Ramdas, Mother Krishnabai, and Swami Satchidananda are available at the ashram bookstore or by mail. *In Quest of God* and *Hints to Aspirants* are good introductions. Also available are cassettes of Ram Nam sung by Swami Ramdas and Mother Krishnabai.

One early morning at about 4 A.M., descending from the mountain, Ramdas walked straight to the railway station, and finding a train waiting, got on the platform without being obstructed, and

entered a compartment. A few minutes later the train moved. Where was the train taking him? It was none of his concern to try to know this. Ram never errs and a complete trust in him means full security and the best guidance . . .

A ticket inspector, a Christian, dressed in European fashion, stepped into the carriage at a small station, and coming up to the sadhus asked for tickets.

"Sadhus carry no tickets, brother, for they neither possess nor care to possess any money," said Ramdas in English.

The ticket inspector replied: "You can speak English. Educated as you are, you cannot travel without a ticket. I have to ask you both to get down."

The sadhu-Ram and he accordingly got down at the bidding of the inspector. "It is all Ram's will," assured Ramdas to his guide.

They were now on the platform and there was still some time for the train to start. The ticket inspector, meanwhile, felt an inclination to hold conversation with Ramdas who, with the sadhu-Ram, was waiting for the train to depart.

"Well," broke in the inspector, looking at Ramdas, "may I know with what purpose you are traveling in this manner?"

"In quest of God," was his simple reply.

"They say God is everywhere," persisted the inspector. "Then, where is the fun of your knocking about in search of Him, while He is at the very place from which you started on this quest, as you say?"

"Right, brother," replied Ramdas. "God is everywhere but he wants to have this fact actually proved by going to all places and realizing His presence everywhere."

"Well then," continued the inspector, "if you are discovering God wherever you go, you must be seeing him here, on this spot, where you stand."

"Certainly, brother," rejoined Ramdas. "He is here at the very place where we stand."

"Can you tell me where he is?" asked the inspector.

"Behold, he is here, standing in front of me!" exclaimed Ramdas enthusiastically.

"Where, where?" cried the inspector impatiently.

"Here, here!" pointed Ramdas, smiling, and patted on the broad chest of the inspector himself. "In the tall figure standing in front, that is, in yourself, Ramdas clearly sees God who is every-where."

For a time, the inspector looked confused. Then he broke into a hearty fit of laughter. Opening the door of the compartment from which he had asked the sadhus to get down, he requested them to get in again, and they did so, followed by him. He sat in the train with the sadhus for some time.

"I cannot disturb you, friends, I wish you all success in your quest of God." With these words he left the carriage and the train rolled onwards.

—SWAMI RAMDAS,
from *In Quest of God*

Isalayam
Thiruvananthapuram (Trivandrum), Kerala

 Swami Isa (1956–   )

Young, articulate, and confident, Swami Isa appears to be an up-and-coming guru who hasn't yet been discovered by many Western spiritual seekers. An ashram is under construction next door, but for now, he lives and teaches in the modest suburban home that he shares with his parents, sister, and brother on the outskirts of Trivandrum. About a hundred devotees—most of them local residents—visit the house each day for spiritual guidance, sacred gifts (said to be "materialized" out of the air), and initiation into traditional Vedic mantras and rituals, which Swami Isa believes are the gateway to God.

Teachers and Teachings

You'll probably be received by Swami Isa in person—a bearded, bright-eyed man in a plain white dhoti, who speaks persuasively (in excellent but heavily accented English) of the transformative power of Vedic practices. "When the individual performs the rituals knowing the fact that God is within himself, or realizes the presence of God within himself by performing the rituals, the rare treasure house of sublime experience, pulsating, beyond words, is laid open before him," says an article in *Om Gayatree*, Isalayam's monthly magazine. The spiritual values of ancient India are being annihilated by modernization, Swami Isa laments. To revive them, he prescribes the systems developed by the ancient rishis—an equal combination of devotion (bhakti) and knowledge (jnana).

Swami Isa refers to his budding ashram—named simply Isalayam, or "Isa's home"—as a "man-making center." His daily satsangs focus on the practical application of classic Hindu philosophy in the modern world. His central teaching is to surrender to and worship God, through the practice of rituals, mantras, and other forms of traditional vedic sadhana. Breaking with tradition, he initiates both men and women—of all castes, ages, and religions—into practices like Upanayana (the brahman sacred thread ceremony) and the Gayatri mantra.

Music is central to his approach—in Sunday morning music sessions, sitars and other instruments are used to open the energy of the chakras. "Through meditating on mantra, one can cross the ocean of materialistic life," he says. "Turn mantra into song. That song will become the rhythm of the mind. And that rhythm of the mind will become the pulsation of the prana or life force. Ultimately that enables the individual to reach the timeless existence of the soul."

Facilities and Food

As long as the ashram remains in Swami Isa's family home, there are no residential accommodations for guests. However, the ashram under construction will have several single rooms and dormitory space for about twenty people.

Schedule

Satsang is held from 6:30 to 7:30 P.M. daily. On Sunday, satsang begins at 9 A.M. with music and singing; from 2:30 to 3:30 P.M. there is a Sanskrit class, and from 3:30 to 5:30 P.M. a discourse by Swami Isa. On second Saturdays Swami Isa leads meditation instruction from 7 to 9 A.M.

In addition to formal satsang, Swami Isa is available for personal satsang throughout the day, beginning at 9:30 A.M.

Fees

Donation.

Contact Information

ISALAYAM
KADAKAMPALLI LANE
ANAYARA
THIRUVANANTHAPURAM (TRIVANDRUM) 695 029
KERALA
TEL: NONE

How to Get There

The ashram is about 5 kilometers from the center of Trivandrum (Thiruvananthapuram). By taxi or autorickshaw, go north from Pettah Junction in Trivandrum along the road to Anayara. Turn left on Kadakampalli Lane. Inquire for the exact house once you are in the area.

Other Services

Trivandrum has a population of about 900,000. A wide range of accommodations, restaurants, and other facilities is available.

Books and Tapes

Om Gayatree: The Man Making Magazine, an ashram publication, is available by writing the ashram.

"Do you have a favorite deity?" Swami Isa asked me as my friend Kristayani and I sat talking with him in his living room.

"No, I really don't have one," I said.

"How about you?" he asked Kristayani.

"Gayatri," she responded.

He waved his right hand in the air, then opened his fingers. There in his palm was a small silver Gayatri for Kristayani. He waved his other hand and opened it up, revealing a beautiful silver and sandalwood mala for me.

He couldn't have taken them out of his sleeve, because his arms were bare; his only clothing was a simple white lunghi wrapped around his waist. Granted, any high school magician can fool me. But it's hard to imagine how that could have been a trick.

On our way out the door he smiled and reached out his hands to us again. Suddenly his palms were full of vibhuti, sacred ashes, which he offered to us as a blessing.

—JERRY JONES

Sree Rama Dasa Madhom Ashram
Thiruvananthapuram (Trivandrum), Kerala

Swami Sathyananda Saraswathy (1935–   )

Located in a small village about 20 kilometers outside of Trivandrum, the Sree Rama Dasa Madhom Ashram is a quiet, low-key establishment headed by Swami Sathyananda Saraswathy, who has been living and teaching there for over thirty years. A commanding man in his sixties, with floor-length hair wrapped around his head, Swami Sathyananda does not particularly encourage Western visitors, feeling that they tend not to be serious. "Only a mature person can receive shaktipat from a sadguru," he says. However, if you do show up, you probably won't be denied the opportunity to receive the blessings, healings, and spiritual advice he bestows on the devotees who come and go throughout the day.

Teachers and Teachings

Because Swami Sathyananda—unlike many gurus—exhibits virtually no interest in being included in a spiritual guidebook, it was difficult to collect any concrete information about his life and teachings. Although he seems both knowledgeable and charismatic, he doesn't give formal satsang; he distributes no books or publicity brochures. Instead, he spends every day tending to the needs of the constant stream of people that come to consult with him. Like an old-fashioned country doctor, he patiently listens to their problems—whether physical, emotional, financial, or spiritual—and dispenses encouragement, prayers, and practical advice (such as prescribing yoga postures for a bad back). Occasionally, he will interrupt the darshan line to receive a call on his cellular phone.

Although he doesn't particularly cater to foreign devotees, Swami Sathyananda speaks excellent English and has traveled in America, so communication is not a problem. While the ashram is generally fairly quiet, devotees claim that huge crowds may visit during festival times.

Facilities and Food

The ashram consists of several rather old buildings—with two new ones under construction—that are not clearly separated from the surrounding village. Most devotees come during the day and do not stay overnight. The ashram has sleeping facilities, but they may be too spartan for most foreign guests.

Schedule

There is no regular daily schedule. Swami Sathyananda is available to receive visitors from 9:30 A.M. to 2 P.M. There are two daily poojas— one in the early morning, one around 9 P.M.

Fees

Donation.

Sree Rama Dasa Madhom Ashram
Chankottukonam, Alinera P.O.
Thiruvananthapuram (Trivandrum) 695 581
Tel: 91-471-418809

How to Get There

The ashram is about 15 kilometers from the center of Trivandrum in Chankottukonam village. Take a taxi, bus, or autorickshaw to Chankottukonam. Once you're there, inquire as to the exact location of the ashram.

Other Services

Thiruvananthapuram (Trivandrum) is a city with a population of about 850,000. A wide range of accommodations, restaurants, and other facilities is available.

Books and Tapes

None.

Sivananda Yoga Vedanta Dhanwanthari Ashram
P.O. Neyyardam, Trivandrum, Kerala

🍃 Swami Vishnudevananda (1927–1993)
🍃 Swami Mahadevananda (1942?–   )

This ashram is best known for its two-week "yoga vacations," and the setting couldn't be better for a tropical resort—a twelve-acre Eden on the banks of a silver lake, in the foothills of Kerala's Sahyadri Mountains, in a lush jungle of jackfruit, tapioca, rubber, banana, mango, and coffee beans. But don't expect to spend a lot of time lounging by the lake in your bathing suit or sipping cold pineapple juice in the shade of a mango tree. Instead, you'll get a dose of of fairly strict training in the five basic principles of yoga: proper exercise, proper breathing, proper relaxation, proper diet, and positive thinking and meditation.

Teacher and Teachings

Less a traditional ashram than an ongoing "yoga camp," the center was founded by Swami Vishnudevananda, a senior disciple of Swami Sivananda of Rishikesh (p. 343), for whom the ashram is named. One of the most influential figures in the transmission of yoga to the West, Vishnudevananda began his yoga career at seventeen, when, as an engineer in the Indian army, he found one of Sivananda's pamphlets stuffed in his office garbage can. Within three years, he had left the Army and taken vows of sannyasi in Sivananda's ashram in Rishikesh.

Recognizing his young disciple's talent for hatha yoga, Sivananda encouraged him to concentrate on this practice, and appointed him "hatha-yoga professor" at the Yoga Vedanta Forest Academy. Eventually Swami Vishnu went to the West, and over the next four decades his teaching spawned over thirty International Sivananda Yoga Vedanta Centers worldwide, serving hundreds of thousands of students. His "Complete Illustrated Book of Yoga" introduced a generation of flower children to hatha yoga.

Since his death in 1993, this ashram in his Kerala homeland—like other Sivananda centers worldwide—continues under the guidance of his senior disciples. The current director is an Italian man named Swami Mahadevananda, one of Vishnudevananda's first Western students, who has been at the Kerala ashram since it was founded.

The teachings at this ashram follow the formula that you'll find at Sivananda centers all over the world. You'll get asana and pranayama to strengthen your body and deepen your breath; meditation to focus your mind; lectures on yoga philosophy to deepen your understanding; and plenty of devotional chanting to open your heart to God.

Two-week "yoga vacations" are offered year-round, beginning on the first and fifteenth of every month. You can join at any time and do not necessarily have to stay for the full two weeks. "A Yoga vacation is a disciplined adventure. It brings out the happiness from within yourself which you once sought in typical vacations, but failed to find," wrote Swami Vishnu.

The typical vacation schedule includes early morning and evening meditations; morning and evening sessions of pranayama and asanas; karma yoga (cleaning, gardening, and other ashram work); a lecture by one of the swamis; and a screening of an episode from the popular TV serialization of the classic spiritual epic the Mahabarata. All events are compulsory, and the schedule leaves little time for yourself—so you may wish to schedule some quiet time after your program finishes, to relax and digest what you have learned.

Prices and programs seem to be geared for a Western clientele. Most of the people who come for "yoga vacations" are Westerners, and you're just as likely to get a Western yoga teacher as an Indian—in that sense, it's much like going to a Sivananda center in your hometown.

The hatha yoga training—held in an airy outdoor courtyard covered with a tile roof—revolves around the twelve basic postures of the Sivananda system: Headstand, Shoulderstand, Plow, Fish, Seated Forward Bend, Cobra, Locust, Bow, Seated Twist, Standing Forward Bend, Triangle, and Crow or Peacock; plus six repetitions of the Sun Salutation. (Some teachers throw in additional poses; however, these are not viewed as essential.) After each posture, you lie down to relax and absorb its benefits. You won't get precise anatomical instructions; if you've never done hatha yoga, be careful, as teachers may not know how to modify poses for beginners to avoid injury. (Teachers are drawn from Sivananda's own four-week teacher-training program, so levels of experience vary widely—some may have been practicing less than a year, others may have twenty years of sadhana behind them.)

If you want more in-depth study, try the four-week teacher's training course—you don't need to be an advanced practitioner or wish to become a teacher to enroll. Other special programs include a Sanskrit camp; an ayurveda camp; and a two-week ayurveda and culture program, which features in-depth classes on Keralan ayurveda and workshops on south Indian arts and dance (with performances almost every evening).

Facilities and Food

The twelve-acre ashram is located at the edge of a national park and wildlife preserve—at night you can hear the coughlike roars of lions from across the lake. Looming nearby is Mt. Agasteya, named for the ancient sage of medicine—who was sent here by Shiva, legend has it, so that his weight would keep the continent from tilting when all the other gods assembled in the Himalayas for Shiva and Parvati's wedding.

There are two types of accommodations: the Kailash building, with twelve spacious double and triple rooms with attached private baths and balconies; and twelve double and triple stone huts with common baths. Bedding and mosquito nets are provided. The annual teachers' training camp draws about two hundred people who must be housed in makeshift dormitories.

Swim at the ashram's private beach at your own risk—signs warn to beware of crocodiles, but residents will assure you that they only come out at dawn and twilight. There's a small library and a bookshop selling Sivananda writings.

Food is simple, non-spicy Indian vegetarian. If you're craving a treat, you can buy chai, ginger-lemon tea, fruit salad, and assorted sweets at the ashram chai shop.

Schedule

Two-week yoga vacations begin on the first and fifteenth of every month; because of the oppressive summer heat, the peak season is December through April. The four-week teacher's training course is generally held from the mid-November to mid-December and mid-January to mid-February every year. Preregistration is required. Every other year there's an advanced teacher's course (you must have taken the regular teacher's course to join).

Each February, the ashram sponsors a pilgrimage to temples and holy sites of south India; in the fall, there is often a guided pilgrimage to Badrinath and Gangotri in the Himalayas.

Write for details of individual training camps.

Fees

In the high season, daily rates (including room and food) are Rs 250 if you're staying in Kailash; Rs 200 if you're in a hut. (They're about Rs 50 less from May through November.) For the teacher's training course, the rates are $1,000 for a campsite; $1,200 for a room with shared bath; $1,400 for a room with private bath.

Sivananda Yoga Vedanta Dhanwanthari Ashram
P.O. Neyyardam, Trivandrum DT 695 576
Kerala
Tel and fax: 91-471-290493

Headquarters:
Sivananda Ashram Yoga Camp
8th Avenue
Val Morin, Quebec JOT-2RO
Canada
Tel: (819) 322-3226
Fax: (819) 322-5876

How to Get There

The ashram is in Neyyar Dam, 28 kilometers from Trivandrum. You can take the bus or train to Trivandrum; there are also daily flights from Bombay, New Delhi, and Madras. From the Trivandrum central bus station, there is a regular bus to Neyyar Dam; or you can take a rickshaw or taxi. If you have any difficulties once you have reached Trivandrum, contact the Sivananda center in Trivandrum on Airport Road (Tel: 0471-450942).

Other Services

Neyyar Dam is quite isolated—to change money or send faxes, you'll have to go to Trivandrum. Trivandrum is a major city, and all services are available.

Books and Tapes

The Sivananda Boutique sells books, videos, and cassettes by and about Swamis Sivananda and Vishnudevananda, including the famous *Complete Illustrated Book of Yoga.*

Health is wealth; peace of mind is happiness. Yoga shows the way through proper exercise, proper breathing, proper relaxation, proper diet, positive thinking, and meditation.

—Swami Vishnudevananda

Mata Amritanandamayi Math
Vallickavu, Kerala

 Mata Amritanandamayi (1953–   )

If the Divine Mother should choose to incarnate somewhere, it seems not unlikely that it would be here: in these fecund backwater islands, thick with coconut groves and rice paddies, where the very soil—rich and dark—seems bursting with life. For devotees of Mata Amritanandamayi—known to millions worldwide as "Ammachi," or "darling Mother"—that's exactly what has happened. Ammachi, they say, is the embodiment of Devi, the Divine Mother of the Universe. At her ashram in this small fishing village by the Arabian Sea—built on the site of her birthplace and childhood home—thousands of people from around the world come to experience her unique darshan, in which she holds each devotee in her arms like a mother embracing a child.

Teachers and Teachings

Ammachi's principal teaching is not her words, but the experience of being with her. Earthy, vital, and archetypically maternal, she personally receives every person who comes to her—laughing, scolding, consoling, and finally wrapping the devotee in a mammoth hug (usually accompanied by a chocolate kiss or some other sweet as prasad). She's been known to embrace over 15,000 devotees in one night, greeting each one with the same radiant, unforced smile. Her disciples estimate that to date she has hugged about twenty million people.

Mata Amritanandamayi was born in 1953 into a poor fisherman's family. By the age of five, young Sudhamani, as she was named, was completely devoted to Krishna. She carried a picture of him tucked within her shirt and began composing songs of devotion and longing, which she sang all over the village. Then, as a teenager, Sudhamani became possessed by the yearning for the Divine Mother. Ablaze with love for the Mother, she would kiss the earth, embrace the trees, weep at the touch of the breeze. She lapsed into trance for days at a time. Finally, she says, the Divine Mother appeared and merged with her. From that day on, she states, "nothing was different from my own formless Self, in which the entire Universe exists as a tiny bubble."

Local people began to acclaim the young woman as a saint and visit her to seek her blessings and miraculous healings. (In one often-repeated story—witnessed by both Indian and Western devotees—Ammachi cured the oozing sores of a leper by licking them with her tongue.) In the late 1970s, the first Western disciple appeared. Today, her devotees worldwide number in the millions; and her ashram attracts hundreds of visitors every day.

"The path of devotion is the best for Westerners," Ammachi says. "In the West, society is such that people, even from early childhood, take an intellectual approach to everything. Their analytical minds are well developed, but their hearts are dry."

For most disciples, devotion takes the form of devotion to Ammachi herself—a frenzy of love and longing that can approach hysteria. (Just see what happens if you accidentally cut in front of someone in the darshan line.) Some devotees even purchase small Ammachi dolls, which they hold in their arms and talk to, weeping, when Amma herself is not available. Those not attuned to the bhakti path may find such activities disconcerting.

Every morning and evening there's devotional chanting in the main hall, accomanied by tabla and harmonium and amplified through loudspeakers. When Ammachi is here, she leads it herself, with infectious passion and abandon—flinging her arms in the air as she cries out, rapturously, the names of the gods and goddeses. The audience shares in the passion, with devotees sometimes rolling on the floor, sobbing out Krishna's name.

The ecstasy reaches peak levels on Thursday and Sunday nights, during Devi Bhava, a ritual in which Ammachi dresses in a spectacular costume and crown, enters a trance, and assumes the form of the Divine Mother. On these days, the queues for darshan can be staggering—so many thousands of Indians come that they must be given tickets to get their hugs. (Foreigners, though, don't have to wait in the main line: you can enter through the side doors of the inner temple, where Amma is sitting.) Whole families camp out all night in the courtyard and corridors, sleeping sprawled in corners and stair landings until their time for darshan approaches. (Amma, remarkably, shows no signs of fatigue; she'll stay up most of the night greeting devotees, then show up at sunrise to lead more bhajans and supervise morning work.)

All visitors are required to sign up for daily karma yoga (cleaning, food preparation, etc.). The sheer volume of people here—combined with the constant activity and the frequent singing of bhajans—means that this is not a particularly quiet place (except when Ammachi goes on tour, when it's virtually deserted). If you're looking for a contemplative or meditative retreat, it's probably not for you.

The ashram runs a number of charitable, medical, and educational programs, including an orphanage, a free housing program for poor widows, and a hostel for tribal children; a hospice for cancer patients; a five-hundred-bed hospital; an ayurvedic clinic; a computer technology institute; and a technical school.

Facilities and Food

Hidden in a grove of coconut palms about a hundred yards from the ocean, the ashram physically consists of one six-story building (a combination temple and dormitory), one seven-story apartment complex that is still under construction, and a number of smaller residential buildings—all packed onto a relatively small amount of land. It can accommodate up to five hundred people at any one time, most of them in spartan dormitories designed to sleep about twelve people to a room (although at peak season, as many as forty may be squeezed in). There are some semi-private rooms with attached bath for married couples—families with children have priority. Thin mattresses are available for rent but you must provide your own bedding and mosquito net.

A small library is available for reading and study. The land area of the ashram is somewhat limited, but there is a spectacular black-sand beach nearby for quiet contemplation. (Watch out for fecal land mines: the beach also serves as the local toilet.) Snacks, books, pictures, clothing, soaps, and other items are available for purchase at a small store. You can make phone calls (booked in advance) in the cloak room. The fax works only intermittently.

The food is rather nondescript Indian vegetarian fare—rice and vegetables, but no chappatti. Much better is the non-spicy, more Western food that can be purchased for breakfast and dinner at a separate canteen. (This includes excellent homebaked bread from a wood-fired brick oven constructed by the resident German baker.) Filtered and boiled water is available.

Schedule

The daily routine begins at 4:30 A.M. with Archana (chanting the 1,000 names of the Divine Mother). When Ammachi is in residence, there's darshan every morning, starting around 11 A.M. In the evening, she leads bhajans.

Devi Bhava is held every Thursday and Sunday evening in the temple. On these days, the evening bhajan, which is led by Mother, starts at 5 P.M. Ammachi is generally out of the country from mid-May until mid-August, as well as from early November until early December.

Other Services

Vallickavu is a relatively small village. It has some fruit stalls and other small shops but has very limited (if any) suitable lodging. The city of Kollam (Quilon) (approximately 35 kilometers) is the closest city with all services and a good range of accommodations.

Fees

Rs 50 per day (including food and accommodations).

Contact Information

MATA AMRITANANDAMAYI MATH
AMRITAPURI P.O., KOLLAM DISTRICT

KERALA 690 525
TEL: 91-4756-21279, 897578

U.S. Contact:
M.A. CENTER
P.O. BOX 613
SAN RAMON, CA 94583-0613
TEL: (510) 537-9417 OR 9427
FAX: (510) 889-8585

How to Get There

Ammachi's ashram is located in the tiny village of Vallickavu in south
Kerala between the backwater canal and the Arabian Sea. The closest
major cities with airports are Kochi (Cochin) and Thiruvananthapuram
(Trivandrum).

A scenic and fairly simple way to visit this ashram is to take one of the
backwater boats that go from Kollam (Quilon) to Alappuzha (Alleppey).
From Thiruvananthapuram go north (by train, bus, or taxi) to Kollam (77
km), then by autorickshaw or taxi to the backwater boat docks. Boats leave
Kollam at about 10:30 A.M. and arrive at the ashram pier across from Vallickavu at about 1:30 P.M. Small boats will take you across the river to the
ashram for a few rupees (depending on the amount of luggage you have).
The ashram is approximately 100 meters down the path from the pier. Following a stay at the ashram, you can continue north by boat to Alappuzha
or return by boat to Kollam.

From the north, you can also take one of the backwater boats (from
Alappuzha) to the ashram pier. Trains and buses also go to Kayam Kulam
where you can take a bus or taxi to Vallickavu (10 kilometers).

Books and Tapes

Books, pictures, and tapes are available at the ashram or the centers in
the United States and France. The *Awaken Children!* series makes a
good introduction to Ammachi's teachings. A small brochure is available,
giving additional information regarding ashram conduct, dress, and other
practical information for the ashram.

*N*ot long after two in the morning everyone who got a numbered card has had a chance to sit at the feet of the guru. It looks like the darshan is over, but it isn't. One last supplicant enters from the darkness outside. As he does, there is a sudden and terrified silence. The man's affliction is horrifying beyond belief. It looks as though the skin from the top of his head to the tops of his feet is covered with thousands of hanging caterpillars, clinging to him, weaving their cocoons on his skin. But the disgusting encrusted things are not external creatures clinging to his skin. They are a part of his skin; dangling, shriveled, wormlike appendages to his skin. . . .

Only one person doesn't recoil. Amma. She reaches out, beckons him to come forward, and the afflicted man moves to her. He kneels, but doesn't dare reach out to touch her.

Now, for the first time since the darshan began seven hours ago, Amma rises from her throne. She reaches down, takes his hand, and pulls him to her feet. He stands before her, his eyes filled with tears. She stands before him, her eyes filled with love. Projecting that love directly into his eyes, Amma opens her arms, steps forward, and embraces him. . . .

He starts to pull away, but she holds him in her embrace, kissing each encrusted growth on his face. She overflows with compassion, she bursts with love, and he in turn dissolves in love and gratitude. . . .

As she ends the embrace, one of her attendants approaches with a small straw basket. Amma reaches into it, clenches her fist, turns back to the afflicted man, and holds her hand over his head. Then, just as everyone in the room is experiencing what must be an orgasm of compassion, Amma opens her hand and releases hundreds of pink flower petals, which cascade down on the disfigured object of her love.

—HART SPRAGER
(from *The Sound of the Earth*)

❧ **Kaladi.** Kaladi is the birthplace of the great ninth-century philosopher and religious reformer Shankaracharya, one of Hinduism's most influential figures. He was devoted to the god Shiva, and because of his extraordinary abilities was considered by some to be an incarnation of the god. Kaladi features a small temple complex and the Sringeri Math, which is said to mark the site of Shankaracharya's house. Kaladi is about 50 kilometers northeast of Cochin (Kochi), a day trip by road. Cochin has air and rail links and lots of hotels. You can also stay in guest houses and lodges in Kaladi.

❧ **Ayappan Temple.** Millions of pilgrims a year—over twenty-five million, by some counts—make the arduous barefoot trek up a mountain to the Ayyappan Temple in Sabarimalai, about 190 kilometers north of Trivandrum. The god Ayappa is one of the sons of Shiva. His devotees—mainly male, since women of menstruating age are not allowed in the temple—can be spotted on the roads and buses all over south India, barefoot and dressed in black, blue, or ochre for the duration of their pilgrimage. For the forty-one days preceding the visit to the temple, pilgrims must be celibate and vegetarian.

There are no major roads leading all the way to the temple, which must be reached on foot; the easiest trek is from Pampa (reachable by bus from Trivandrum), which is about 5 kilometers from the temple. Plenty of basic accommodations are available for pilgrims.

—LEA TERHUNE

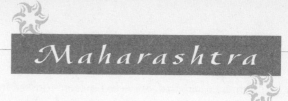

Maharashtra

Meherabad
Ahmadnagar, Maharashtra

Meher Baba (1894–1969)

If you've ever sung along to the popular song "Don't Worry, Be Happy," then you've already had a taste of Meher Baba's teachings—that was the slogan he distributed on cards to his Western devotees back in the 1960s. Followers of Meher Baba consider him not just a guru, saint, or teacher, but "the Avatar": a manifestation of God in human form who is born again and again to awaken living beings to divine love. For "Baba lovers," as devotees call themselves, Meher Baba is identical with Zoroaster, Rama, Krishna, Jesus, and other divine incarnations. Meher Baba died in 1969; but Baba lovers still congretate at his Meherabad community near Ahmadnagar to visit his samadhi shrine, study and discuss his teachings, and celebrate his life through music, poetry, dance, and drama.

Teachers and Teachings

Love was Meher Baba's primary message. For the last forty-four years of his life, he lived and taught without speaking, communicating only through gestures and letters pointed on an alphabet board: "Things that are real are given and received in silence," he said. He told his devotees, "I have come to sow the seed of love in your hearts so that, in spite of all superficial diversity which your life in illusion must experience and endure, the feeling of oneness, through love, is brought about amongst all the nations, creeds, sects, and castes of the world."

This love—more than any specific verbal teachings—is what people come to the pilgrim center to experience. You won't find much in the way of structured programs here. What you will find is a warm and peaceful environment with plenty of time to pursue your own practice and connect with other Baba lovers.

Born as Merwan Sheriar Irani into a Zoroastrian family in south India,

Meher Baba began his spiritual journey in his college years, when an ancient woman named Hazrat Babajan—herself widely revered as a fully enlightened sadguru, or perfect master—kissed him on the forehead as he sat with her under a neem tree. With that kiss, an inner veil was lifted from Merwan's consciousness, and he realized that he was "the Ancient One." "Many consider it blasphemy for one to say he is God," he was to say. "But in truth it would be blasphemous for me to say I am not God."

Over the next seven years, Merwan sought out several other masters, including Sai Baba of Shirdi (a Moslem saint) and Upasani Maharaj, a Hindu teacher who, it's said, guided him to full Self-realization. By the early 1920s, a band of disciples had gathered around him, who gave him the title Meher Baba—"Compassionate Father"—and established the colony of Meherabad. Meher Baba began traveling all over India, feeding the poor and bathing lepers with his own hands. In 1925 he entered into silence, but his work continued unabated. He quickly gained an enormous following, sometimes attracting crowds of up to 100,000 people. In 1953, he publicly announced what his inner circle already believed—that he was a God-man, the "Avatar of the Age."

Meher Baba was especially devoted to his work with "masts" (pronounced musts)—a term he coined from the Sufi word "mast-allah," meaning "God-intoxicated." He crisscrossed India to search out and work with over 20,000 of these ragged and apparently deranged street-people—indistinguishable, to most observers, from madmen—whom he felt were actually highly evolved souls who simply lacked adequate spiritual guidance. Many of them he brought to special ashrams, where he fed and tended them. He claimed that the masts he worked with—while outwardly changing little—became channels of divine love, assisting Meher Baba with his invisible, esoteric work in the service of the world.

Meher Baba made thirteen trips to the West and attracted the attention of counterculture icons such as Timothy Leary and Ram Dass with his lucid writings on mystical states of consciousness. However, he subsequently surprised the psychedelic community with his denunciation of drugs such as LSD, which, he said, "give only a semblance of 'spiritual experience,' a glimpse of a false reality." Today, most of the pilgrims who visit Meherabad are upper middle-class Westerners, primarily Americans, who come for anywhere from a few days to several months. Because Meher Baba was adamantly opposed to ritualistic religion, there are no prescribed ceremonies or practices at Meherabad. Instead, pilgrims pour out their love through spontaneous gatherings of guitar-playing, song, and storytelling at Meher Baba's samadhi shrine.

If you're not a Baba lover, you may feel out of place in this environment. Baba lovers believe that devotion to Meher Baba is devotion to God; the real "Baba," Meher Baba used to tell his devotees, would be awakened within the hearts of everyone who loved him, whether or not they had ever met him physically. "I want you to make me your constant companion," Meher Baba told his devotees. "Think of me more than you think of yourself. Your duty is to keep me constantly with you in your thoughts, speech, and action. . . . Surrender to the God-Man, in whom God reveals Himself in His full glory."

Facilities and Food

The Meherabad Pilgrim Centre can accommodate about fifty-six guests in clean, attractive rooms for one to eight people each. Men and women are housed separately. Writing ahead for reservations at least six weeks in advance is recommended. Initial bookings are made for up to two weeks; space permitting, your stay may be extended.

The dining hall serves wholesome vegetarian food—more Western than Indian—on Western-style tables and chairs. You can visit Meher Baba's stone samadhi shrine, whose inner walls are painted with murals of his life; you can also visit his tiny "table house," a low, cavelike structure in which he wrote. If the Pilgrim Centre is full, you can stay in Ahmadnagar, 9 kilometers away; recommended hotels include the Chanakya, the Sanket, and the Amar.

Fourteen kilometers from Ahmadnagar, in the opposite direction from the Pilgrim Centre, is Meherazad, the site of Meher Baba's former home. Visitors can't stay there; however, you can attend informal satsangs with Meher Baba's resident disciples. There you can also see the famous "blue bus" in which Meher Baba and his devotees toured all over India.

Schedule

The Pilgrim Centre is open from June 15 to March 15. During the summer months (from March 16 to June 14) it is closed; the Meherabad property is closed an additional four weeks, closing March 1 and reopening July 1. During the open season, arati is held from 7 to 8 A.M. and from

7 to 8 P.M. at Meher Baba's samadhi shrine. It includes singing by devotees, often to the accompaniment of guitars. Meals are 8 A.M., 1 P.M., and 8 P.M. Other than that, Meherabad is fairly unstructured; you are encouraged to pursue your personal development in whatever way is best for you. Drugs and alcohol are prohibited.

Visiting hours at Meher Baba's home in Meherabad are 11:30 A.M. to 2 P.M. on Tuesdays, Thursdays, and Saturdays; 11:00 A.M. to 12:30 P.M. on Sundays.

Fees

About Rs 100 for lodging and three meals a day.

Contact Information

THE MEHER PILGRIM CENTRE
PILGRIM RESERVATIONS
AVATAR MEHER BABA TRUST OFFICE
KING'S ROAD, POST BAG 31
AHMADNAGAR 414 001
MAHARASHTRA
TEL: 91-241-341821 OR 91-241-323666
FAX: 91-241-341967 (AT POST OFFICE)
EMAIL (FOR RESERVATIONS):
PIMCO.OFFICE@AMBPPCT.SPRINTRPG.SPRINT.COM

U.S. Contact:
MEHER BABA INFORMATION
P.O. BOX 1101
BERKELEY, CA 94701
TEL: (510) 562-1101

How to Get There

The Pilgrim Centre is in Meherabad, 9 kilometers from Ahmadnagar. However, it's important to register first at the Pilgrim Registration Office in Ahmadnagar (three passport-sized photos required. The office is located in the Avatar Meher Baba Trust Compound, also known as the Meher Nazar compound, off of King's Road.

To get to Ahmadnagar, take a bus, taxi, or train from Pune. (You can also get there from Aurangabad or Nasik.) State Transport buses leave Pune every 15 minutes for the three-hour ride to Ahmadnagar; or you can catch the daily Goa Express or Jhelum Express trains.

Other Services

Ahmadnagar has a population of about 155,000 and has most services.

Books and Tapes

For a catalogue of books and tapes by and about Meher Baba, write to the U.S. contact. A good introduction to Meher Baba's teachings is *Meher Baba: The Compassionate One* by Rick M. Chapman (Berkeley: White Horse).

Today the urgent need of mankind is not sects or organized religions, but Love. Divine love will conquer hate and fear. It will not depend upon other justifications, but will justify itself.

I have come to awaken in man this divine love. It will restore to him the unfathomable richness of his own eternal being and will solve all of his problems.

—MEHER BABA

(from *Meher Baba the Awakener*)

Divine Knowledge Society
Bombay, Maharashtra

Gurudev Shree Chitrabhanu (1922–)

In the early 1970s—after walking 30,000 miles barefoot around India—Gurudev Shree Chitrabhanu put on rubber-soled shoes and flew by airplane to the Spiritual Summit Conference in Geneva, Switzerland, thus becoming the first Jain monk to renounce the ancient rules prohibiting footwear and traveling by vehicle. Since then, he has journeyed all over the world—from Kenya to the Harvard Divinity School—to spread the Jain message of nonviolence and compassion. But he still spends half of each year living in his Bombay apartment overlooking the ocean, where students and devotees can seek him out.

Teachers and Teachings

Absolute nonviolence and reverence for life are the key pillars of the Jain religion. Jains are strict vegetarians. Jain monks wear masks to avoid inhaling small insects and limit their bathing to minimize the death of microorganisms in the water. Some sects go naked ("sky-clad") to eschew all attachments. Chitrabhanu's teachings translate these principles—often viewed as ascetic and extreme—into terms that are practical for the average seeker.

"The need for propagating Ahimsa [nonviolence] and focusing on this ideal is not a result of otherworldly or unrealistic considerations. It is the result of concern for a world torn by conflict," he insists. "Unless we live with nonviolence and reverence for all living beings in our hearts, all our humaneness and our acts of goodness, all our vows, virtues, and knowledge, all our practices remain meaningless and useless."

The Jain religion was founded in the 6th century B.C. by a teacher named Mahavira, a contemporary of the Buddha. Jains believe that Mahavira was the last of twenty-four great teachers known as "thirthankaras," or "ford-makers"—realized beings who show the way across the sea of ignorance. There is no external Supreme Being in Jainism. Rather, Jains believe in liberating the jiva—the radiant energy of the soul—through individual effort, including ethical vows, ascetic practices, and meditation.

Born into a highly religious Jain family that had been vegetarian for seventeen generations, Chitrabhanu was initiated as a Jain monk at age twenty. For twenty-nine years, he lived as a wandering monk, walking barefoot through the villages of India. He rapidly won a large and devoted following, which included increasing numbers of Western students. In 1965, he founded the Divine Knowledge Society in Bombay, which operated medical and famine relief stations and educational programs throughout India. After first breaking with tradition to travel to the West (a decision that almost provoked a riot as mobs of hardline Jains tried to block his entry to the airport), he renounced the monastic life so that he could accept the many invitations he had received to teach in America. Since then, he has led retreats, seminars, and workshops at many major universities, including Princeton, Cornell, and Harvard. He has written over thirty books and inspired fifty-seven Jain meditation centers in the United States, England, Europe, Africa, and Brazil.

A vigorous man in his mid-seventies, Chitrabhanu emphasizes the importance of a disciplined and ethical life. (In India, Jains in general are trusted businesspeople, because of their strict prohibitions against lying and stealing. And you can set your watch based on the punctuality with which Chitrabhanu begins his talks and meditation sessions.) In particular, Chitrabhanu stresses the power of our actions—and even our thoughts—to create karmic vibrations that shape every aspect of our lives.

"From the time of our birth we are 'on the air.' But no one turns the red light on to warn us!" he writes. "It is not only what we say that is heard, but whatever we *think* goes out into the universe and returns to us like an echo or a boomerang. If we want to receive beautiful vibrations from the universe, we have to send out vibrations of a like nature. If we send out negative thoughts, we cannot expect to receive otherwise."

Facilities and Food

When in India, Chitrabhanu receives students—by appointment only—at his spacious apartment overlooking the ocean in an upscale Bombay neighborhood. No residential facilities are available at his apartment. A complete range of accommodations is available in Bombay, though hotels here tend to be expensive compared to elsewhere in India.

Schedule

Chitrabhanu is generally based in Bombay from October through March, although he also travels within India and other Asian countries and sometimes accompanies Western students on pilgrimages to temples and sacred sites not generally known to tourists. He is based in New York City from April through September. (Asked about his choice of home cities—about as far from a Himalayan cave as it's possible to get—he responds, "The outer conditions need not affect one's inner peace. In these places there are a lot of people to serve.")

Fees

Donations are accepted to help fund the Divine Knowledge Society's medical and famine relief stations and educational programs.

Contact Information

DIVINE KNOWLEDGE SOCIETY
E-1, QUEEN'S VIEW
28/30, WALKESHWAR RD.
BOMBAY 400 006
TEL: 91-22-362-0887 OR 6958

U.S. Contact:
JAIN MEDITATION INTERNATIONAL CENTER
244 ANSONIA STATION
NEW YORK, NY 10023-0244
TEL AND FAX: (212) 362-6483

How to Get There

Chitrabhanu's residence is on Walkeshwar Road in Bombay. This is a major road and a taxi should find it without difficulty.

Other Services

Bombay is a city of about ten million people, and all services are available.

Books and Tapes

Books by or about Gurudev Shree Chitrabhanu are available in the United States through the Jain Meditation International Center (see Contact Information). Good introductory books are Dynamics of Jain Med-

itation, Psychology of Enlightenment, and *The Jain Path to Freedom* (all by Dodd, Mead & Company).

No one stops us from being happy, creative, secure, and enlightened; yet we are afraid to leave behind the familiar habits of negative thinking. Why? Why don't we realize that every problem has a solution just as every lock has a right key? Our difficulty is that our daily haste and confusion prevent us from discovering the key that is needed. If we have refined our energy, however, it will guide us in the right time to the right place.

—GURUDEV CHITRABHANU
(from *The Psychology of Enlightenment:*
Meditations on the Seven Energy Centers)

Ramesh Balsekar
Bombay, Maharashtra

Ramesh Balsekar (1917–)

If your idea of an enlightened master is an ash-covered ascetic in a mountain cave, Ramesh Balsekar may come as a bit of a surprise. A retired bank president and an avid golfer and badminton player, Balsekar lives in a comfortable Bombay flat—where he dispenses the radically nondual teachings of advaita vedanta to a steady stream of primarily Western students who view him as a Self-realized master.

Teachers and Teachings

A disciple of the famous advaita vedanta master Nisargadatta Maharaj, Ramesh Balsekar is best known in the West through his book *Consciousness Speaks,* a collection of dialogues on consciousness and enlightenment compiled by a Western student. "There is no solidity at all, either

Another Advaita Master

Now in his eighties, Ranjit Maharaj has just been discovered by Western seekers and made his first Western tour in 1996. A contemporary of the now-famous Nisargadatta Maharaj (both were disciples of the same guru), he is said to have achieved Self-realization at the age of twelve, but it wasn't until fifty-eight years later—in 1983—that he began giving satsang.

Ranjit Maharaj has no ashram, but he is available to receive students every day (from 12 to 1 P.M. and from 3 to 5:30 P.M.) at his tiny flat off a debris-filled lane in a busy commercial district in Bombay. His teachings are classic advaita vedanta; he uses Ramana Maharshi's method of self-inquiry (the constant question, "Who Am I?") as the path to Self-realization. His English is excellent, but sometimes difficult to understand due to his heavy accent (and possibly his lack of teeth). Western students—many of whom are also students of Ramesh Balsekar—say that they are drawn to him by "his softness, his transparency"—and by the opportunity to work with an advaita master in a small and intimate setting.

Ranjit Maharaj's home is at 45 Dubash Lane, Nairayan Bldg., Off V.P. Road, Bombay, 400 004. The telephone is 022-388-6906. Take a taxi to the area off V.P. Road near the C.P. tank. Dubash Lane is a small street off V.P. Road; the Nairayan Building entrance is actually on the street next to the one marked Dubash Lane. Ranjit Maharaj's apartment is on the second floor.

at the most sublime level of the body or at the heart of the universe," he teaches. "The human being is virtually empty space and utter illusion."

There are rarely more than twenty-odd students at his informal daily satsangs, which include no rituals, pujas, or devotional ceremonies of any kind. With wit and precision (and in perfect English), he fields questions on duality, predestination, enlightenment, karma, good and evil, the guru-disciple relationship, and the nature of God—all, apparently, without attachment to people's reactions, or even to whether the satsangs take place at all. Asked what he would do if his following grew too large for his apartment, he responded with enthusiasm, "I have absolutely no idea! Not my problem."

Born in India, Balsekar was educated at the London School of Economics and rose through the ranks of the Bank of India to become its general manager. During his ten years at the helm, he oversaw the opening of hundred of new branches in India and around the world. However, throughout his secular career—as well as his marriage and family life—Balsekar retained the spiritual intuition he had felt since childhood: that his true identity was not his body or his mind. He read the teachings of Ramana Maharshi and spent twenty years as a devotee of a guru—who, he later recounted, was not able to give him the insight he was looking for.

Shortly after his mandatory retirement at age sixty, Balsekar read an article in a Ramanashram publication about Nisargadatta Maharaj, who was then teaching advaita vedanta in a poor section of Bombay. When he heard Nisargadatta speak, he "knew at once that this was my ultimate guru." Within a few months, Balsekar began translating for his teacher at his daily morning talk; and about a year later, while translating one of those talks, his own Self-realization happened.

"I found that the translation began to come so spontaneously that in actual fact I was not translating, I was merely witnessing the translation taking place," he recounts. "It was as if Maharaj was translating and I was merely sitting there, a witness." Nisargadatta promptly confirmed his Self-realization. Two years after Nisargadatta died in 1981, Balsekar himself began giving satsang.

Ramesh Balsekar's teachings can be summed up in a single sentence: "All there is, is Consciousness." The idea of a separate self is an illusion: "You are only an instrument through which action is produced, impersonally. You are merely an instrument through which Consciousness is functioning." Each individual organism, he explains, "is conceived and created with certain characteristics, so that certain actions will take place through that organism."

"Then there's really nothing to do but relax and enjoy the ride?" a seeker asked. "Yes, that's exactly it!" he responded. "There is really no effort, nothing that worry or work can change." Even enlightenment, he says, is an impersonal event, not a personal achievement: "There is a flood, a fire, an earthquake; there is enlightenment, just one happening in the whole process, all part of the phenomenal process."

Facilities and Food

Satsangs are held in Ramesh Balsekar's home. No residential facilities or food are provided.

Schedule

Satsangs are held daily (except sunday) from 10 to 11:30 A.M.

Fees

In Ramesh Balsekar's words, "nothing is demanded, nothing is refused."

Contact Information

RAMESH BALSEKAR
NAURAJI GAMADIA RD.
SINDHULA BUILDING #10
BOMBAY 400 026
MAHARASHTRA
TEL: 91-22-492-7725

U.S. Contact:
ADVAITA PRESS
P.O. BOX 3479
REDONDO BEACH, CA 90277
TEL: (310) 540-9197
FAX: (213) 876-0708

How to Get There

The apartment is located in the Cumballa Hill area of Bombay, near the Maha Laxmi Temple. From Pedder Road go past the hospital; turn left at the first light on Nauraji Gamadia Road. The Sindhula Building is next to last on the right. The name of the building is clearly marked. A doorman is at the front door to take you up in the elevator.

Other Services

Bombay has a population of ten million; all services are available.

A good introduction is *Consciousness Speaks: Conversations with Ramesh S. Balsekar* (Advaita Press). This and other books are available at his apartment or in the United States from Advaita Press (see Contact Information). In India they are published by Zen Publications, 9 Raja Bahadur Bldg, 156 Dadajee Rd Tordeo, Mumbai 400 034; telephone/fax 022-492-3446.

If there's one thing which I've always been anxious for participants in my seminars or retreats to be sure of it's that I'm not selling anybody, anything. Then it suddenly dawned on me that that is not true. I am selling something, which is nothing on behalf of the Divine Entity, which is really no entity and therefore nothing either. And the biggest joke is, I'm selling this nothing to you who are all nothing! This is really the joke. But until the joke is realized as a joke, it can be a terribly tragic joke.

—RAMESH BALSEKAR

(from *Consciousness Speaks*)

The Yoga Institute of Santa Cruz
Santa Cruz, Bombay, Maharashtra

❧ *Shri Yogendra (1897–1989)*
❧ *Smt. Sitadev Yogendra (1912–)*
❧ *Dr. Jayadeva Yogendra, Director (1929–)*
❧ *Hansaji Jayadeva Yogendra, Dean (1947–)*

W elcome to the Heart of the Modern Yoga Renaissance," reads the plaque at the gate to the Yoga Institute of Santa Cruz. Don't come here for a sylvan retreat—once a remote jungle outpost, the center now lies in a busy suburb directly under the flight path of Bombay's Sahar International Airport. But the round-the-clock roar of jets somehow seems a fitting backdrop for an institution that since its inception nearly eighty years ago has been dedicated to "yoga for householders." The Yoga Institute was the first to make available to the general public the specific techniques of hatha-yogic practice, which for centuries had been the closely guarded secrets of sannyasins. Today, it emphasizes a practical, scientific approach to asana, pranayama, meditation, hygiene, diet, and ethics—packaged to address the health and lifestyle concerns of the urban Indians who are its primary clientele.

Teachers and Teachings

Asana junkies beware: You won't learn any dramatic gymnastics at the Yoga Institute of Santa Cruz. Although students are taught basic, gentle postures for health and stress reduction, the Institute teachers deplore the current trend toward yoga as a form of physical fitness. Little mention is made of tantric teachings about chakras, kundalini, and shaktipat. Long hours of meditation are viewed as unproductive and even dangerous. What's stressed instead is the slow transformation of a person's life through a combination of personal willpower and surrender to God.

"Do not pamper the weaknesses in your personality! You must use willpower to forcibly throw them out!" urges the Institute's dean, Hansaji Yogendra, slapping the back of her hand into her other palm with a emphatic thwack. "Anyone can attain the balanced, peaceful state of yoga—it just requires faith and effort. But your effort alone is not going to take you anywhere. Also present must be God's grace."

The Institute was launched in 1918 by Shri Yogendra, an iconoclastic young Gujarati—he was only twenty-one when he founded the Institute—who dropped out of the prestigious St. Xavier's College in Bombay to enter the ashram of Paramahamsa Madhavadasaji, a 118-year-old bhakti yogi from Malsar. However, the young man entered the ashram with one stipulation: After his studies were completed, he would return to society, marry, and live a householder's life. "I am interested in spirituality in order to live life more fully and not to seek an escape from life," he told his teacher. After three years of intensive study, Mani left the ashram and founded the Yoga Institute in Bombay, where he began using yoga to help local people with their medical problems.

In a radical departure from tradition, Mani made classical yoga teachings available in public classes for the first time ever. When necessary, he modified traditional asanas, pranayamas, and kriyas (cleansing techniques) to make them safe, hygienic, and accessible to the average person. In another move that shocked his contemporaries, he offered yoga classes to women, who had traditionally been barred from such studies. He invited doctors and scientists to study the effects of yoga on his students, and recorded their findings in pamphlets and leaflets that he disseminated to the public.

After Shri Yogendra's death, direction of the Institute fell to his eldest son, Dr. Jayadeva Yogendra. While his father's emphasis was on science and health, Dr. Jayadeva—a tall, shy man with a sweet, clench-jawed smile—is interested in the more spiritual dimensions of yoga, as expressed in the householder's life. "Techniques can only take you so far," he says. "Yoga should be a way of life, a kind of culture."

Dr. Jayadeva is assisted by his wife, Hansaji, whose lively, down-to-earth style and pragmatic approach to yoga philosophy make her a popular teacher. The "Lilias" of India, Hansaji starred in a fifty-episode program called "Yoga for Better Living" that has been rerun five times on Indian national television.

About eight hundred students pass through the center each day, most of them local Bombay residents who have turned to yoga to help them cope with back pain, asthma, stress, and other mind-body ailments. In addition to ongoing daily asana classes, the Institute offers regular weekend residential "health camps" (on topics such as "Cardiac and Hypertension"; "Stress Management and Abdominal Disorder"; "Pregnancy: Antenatal and Postnatal") and "educational camps" ("Concentration"; "Relaxation"; "Memory and Mind Training"). Every month, it conducts a twenty-one-day "Better Living Course," with an hour-long class every day introducing students to the basics of yoga practice. Every Saturday, anyone can stop by for an individual consultation on health, nutrition, diet, and yogic lifestyle (bring your medical reports).

For more serious practitioners, there's a comprehensive seven-month teacher-training course, certified by the government of India—it's divided by topic into month-long modules, so a student may start the program at the beginning of any month.

The best way to get a taste of the Institute, though, is the week-long residential "introduction to yoga" camp, which begins on the second Saturday of every month. In seven packed days—the first lecture starts at

6 A.M., and the last one doesn't end until 9 at night—this program covers the fundamentals of the yogic life, tailored to suit modern times (or, at least, modern India). Lectures cover everything from personal hygiene to positive thinking, and in guided discussion groups students discuss how yoga principles could help them get through their own life challenges. (You may be surprised at how often "mothers-in-law" crop up in these conversations.)

Since the students are primarily Indian—unlike many centers in India, where you'll meet the same sort of people you would in a yoga class in your hometown—one of the side benefits of the program is the chance to make local friends and learn firsthand about contemporary Indian life.

Schedule

Ongoing yoga classes (separate for men and women) are held daily. The Health Checkup is Saturday at 1:30 P.M. Satsang is Sunday, 9:30 to 10:30 A.M. Two-day health and education camps are held on a regular basis.

The week-long residential yoga camp begins on the second Saturday of every month and consists of lectures and classes 6 A.M. to 9 P.M., with breaks for breakfast, lunch, and dinner.

Fees

Seven-Day Introductory Yoga Camp: Rs 1000 (including food and lodging)
Two-day Health Camps: Rs 300 (including food and snacks)
Two-day Educational Camps: Rs 100 (including food and snacks)
21-day Better Living Course: Rs 100
Teachers Training Course: Rs 1500—residential; Rs 2000—nonresidential
Daily Yoga Classes: Rs 150 per month for first month; Rs 100 per month thereafter

Facilities and Food

The Institute—nested on two acres of land, with trees and flower gardens surrounding its three large concrete buildings—is the only place within miles that you can hear birds. The sweet, spicy smell of a blossoming Kailash tree drifts through the smoggy air; chalked signboards offer messages like "Gratitude to God should be as regular as our heartbeat."

Shared accommodations are available for about thirty visitors, in dormitories—four to a room—with shared bath. Men and women are required to stay in separate buildings. Mosquito nets and bedding are provided; be sure to bring earplugs, as the roar of jets overhead can make sleeping difficult. Additional facilities include a small yoga library (about 2,500 volumes); a "museum of classical yoga," with exhibits ranging from antique eye-wash cups to photos of sadhus from different sects; and several spacious halls for lectures and asana classes.

Food is strictly sattvic, with no spices and little salt; it's also heart-healthy, with little oil and only diluted milk. No chai or other caffeinated beverages are served. During the residential programs, no outside food or drink is permitted, other than fruits. Smoking is prohibited. Filtered water is always available.

Contact Information

The Yoga Institute of Santa Cruz
Santa Cruz East
Bombay 400 055
Tel: 91-22-612 2185; 611 0506

How to Get There

From Bombay, take the train or bus to Santa Cruz East; the center is a short walk or rickshaw ride from the train and bus stations. If you are flying into Bombay's domestic or international airports, the center is about 15 minutes away by taxi.

Other Services

Santa Cruz is a large suburb of Bombay. Fax, STD/ISD, and other amenities are easily available.

Books and Tapes

The Institute has over two dozen books available on yoga therapy, philosophy, and asana practice, including a three-volume "Yoga Cyclopedia." Write for a complete list and order form.

Suppose you do asanas. You have developed flexibility of body:
Now whether you do one asana or twenty asanas does not make
a difference. Society needs you! Don't be so selfish that you just
do your asanas, eat your good food, develop your strong body,
that's all! What is the purpose of your strong body and strong
mind? Society needs you—but you don't have time to help, be-
cause every day you must do two hours of asana, one hour of
pranayama, one hour of meditation . . . To us, this is looking very
funny. Yogis should see that their students become better people,
and do something useful for the world."

—HANSAJI YOGENDRA

I just spent fifteen minutes in the ashram bathroom, trying to
snort warm salt water up out of the palm of my hand with one
nostril, then blow it out the other, as I was taught in my kriyas
class this morning. I know I'm supposed to start with a particular
nostril, but in my jet-lagged stupor I can't remember which one,
or whether I'm supposed to invoke a particular deity as I snuffle.
The real question in my mind, though, is this: Why would anyone
design a bathroom with the shower head directly over the
Western-style toilet, with no shower curtain, so that the seat is always slimy and wet? And why does the shower drain through a
hole in the wall into my bedroom? And is there a law that all
bathroom shelves, in India, must slope gently downward, so that
your toothbrush rolls inexorably onto the wet, gritty floor? My
pants legs trail in the puddle; I've left wet footprints in the dust of
my dormitory floor, and gritty black streaks on my sheets. So
why am I so happy to be here?

    At dinner tonight, I talked to a 60-year-old woman from Cal-
ifornia, with close-cropped hair, a dingy white sari, and a Sanskrit
name that means Daughter of Bliss. This is her sixth time in India,
she told me, but it never gets easier.

    "Why do you keep coming back?" I asked her, scooping my
fingers through a thick slop of relentlessly sattvic rice.

    "Because it's my destiny," she says. She takes a sip of the
milky lemon-grass tea, painfully sweet with jaggery. "It trashes

my body, it warps my mind, it wrecks my nerves. But I have to keep coming. Because I believe that the land of India, the actual earth itself, soaked up some knowledge from the gods thousands of years ago—absorbed it into her very soil—that's the secret I've been looking for my whole life."

—ANNE CUSHMAN
(from India journal)

Gurudev Siddha Peeth Ashram
Ganeshpuri, Maharashtra

Swami Muktananda Paramahansa (1908–1982)
Gurumayi Chidvilasananda (1955–)

Located in a tiny village about two hours from Bombay, Gurudev Siddha Peeth is the "advanced university" of Siddha yoga and the original ashram of Swami Muktananda, one of the most prominent Eastern teachers to come to the West during the spiritual explosion of the sixties and seventies. Today, tens of thousands of people are students of Muktananda's America-based successor, Swami Chidvilasananda, known to devotees as Gurumayi. Be forewarned—this isn't a place where you can just drop in. Visitors are welcome to pay their respects at Muktananda's peacock feather–lined samadhi shrine and the temple to his guru, Swami Nityananda. But the ashram itself is reserved for serious students of Siddha yoga, who must apply at least three months in advance to be vetted for a one-month minimum stay.

Teachers and Teachings

Because the popular and charismatic Gurumayi is headquartered in New York State, this isn't the place to come to seek her darshan, unless she's here on one of her periodic Indian tours. However, if you're drawn to Siddha yoga, it's an opportunity to tap into the spiritual energy of three generations of Siddhas ("perfected ones"). "The atmosphere of a Siddha's abode is charged with enormous force," wrote Muktananda. "The Ashram may appear to be an ordinary place to our physical eyes, but its every leaf, flower, fruit, tree, and creeper is pervaded by the Kundalini Shakti."

Siddha yoga is derived from Kashmir Shaivism, a school of Hindu thought centered on devotion to the god Shiva. Shiva—known as the greatest meditator and ascetic—is one of the three most important gods of the Hindu pantheon. In Shaivite practice, Shiva represents pure divine consciousness. His inseparable counterpart is Shakti, divine power. The individual practitioner strives to unify with the divine consciousness and harness divine power through yoga, mantra recitation, and meditation.

In Siddha yoga, Self-realization is achieved through the awakening of the intense spiritual energy called kundalini shakti, which lies coiled and dormant at the base of the spine. In an initiation called shaktipat, the Siddha guru transmits a blast of his or her own shakti to the disciple, thereby jump-starting the disciple's dormant energy. The activated kundalini rises through the six psychic energy centers, or chakras, ultimately reaching the crown chakra, where it manifests as intoxicating bliss. "In shaktipat, one's inner energy is kindled by the fully unfolded energy of the Guru, just as a lit candle lights an unlit one," Swami Muktananda wrote. "Then, one no longer has to make an effort to meditate. Meditation comes spontaneously on its own."

In the 1970s, Swami Muktananda brought these teachings to the West, planning to start a "meditation revolution." He jetted around the world giving teachings; published more than thirty books; gave shaktipat to tens of thousands of devotees; and founded ashrams and meditation centers across the United States and Europe. His SYDA (Siddha Yoga Dham of America) Foundation became one of the wealthiest and most popular of the West's blossoming Eastern spiritual groups. (Before his death, however, he was dogged by widely publicized accusations of sexual activities with female disciples, which most devotees vigorously deny.)

After Muktananda's death in 1982, the organization's spiritual leadership passed into the hands of Swami Chidvilasananda, one of the two successors he had named. A glamorous woman with a radiant smile, Gurumayi continues the work that Muktananda began, presiding over five hundred fifty meditation centers and ten ashrams around the world and giving shaktipat to tens of thousands of devotees every year. Like Muktananda, Gurumayi stresses the primacy of the guru-disciple relationship.

However, there are spiritual techniques that can facilitate the rising of the awakened kundalini, and these are what is taught in the Ganeshpuri ashram.

The yoga study program offers in-depth training in meditation, hatha yoga, and mantra and courses in Indian philosophy and scripture—all in a highly Westernized setting ("At least you know you're not going to get bedbugs in this place," commented one weary seeker) characterized by a very un-Indian degree of organization and efficiency (at what other ashram are you likely to be given a computerized nametag?). The schedule includes plenty of meditation and devotional chanting, and you'll be kept busy with long hours of seva (voluntary work as a spiritual practice).

The ashram's charitable activities include the Muktananda Mobile Hospital, which treats more than 40,000 patients each year in over 150 villages; and four eye camps, which perform free or low-cost cataract surgery.

Facilities and Food

Built on the site of the tiny hut that Nityananda gave to Muktananda, the Ganeshpuri ashram has grown to a fenced-off campus whose locked gates are monitored by uniformed guards. Once inside, it's green and peaceful, with meditation flower gardens adorned with statues of Indian deities. The buildings are spotlessly clean; in tranquil, dimly lit meditation halls, Sanskrit chanting croons from speakers.

The ashram itself provides accommodations only for enrolled students. High-quality vegetarian food is available for the residents. Visitors to the temple and the samadhi shrine can get basic Indian food at the Samadan Restaurant across from the temple, which is reputed to be clean. The village of Ganeshpuri has only very limited hotel accommodations.

Schedule

The schedule includes daily meditation, yoga, lectures, and courses. The Nityananda temple and Muktananda's samadhi shrine are open to the public from 7 A.M. to 12 P.M. and from 3 to 6:30 P.M. October to March is the best time to visit; summer and monsoon season in this region are apt to be uncomfortable.

Fees

Donation.

Contact Information

GURUDEV SIDDHA PEETH ASHRAM
P.O. GANESHPURI 401 206
DIST. THANA
MAHARASHTRA
TEL: 91-2522-61-221

U.S. Contact:
SYDA FOUNDATION
P.O. BOX 600
SOUTH FALLSBURG, NY 12779
TEL: (914) 434-2000

How to Get There

Getting to Ganeshpuri can be done expensively by taxi from Bombay, or less expensively by taking the train from Bombay to Vasai, and then taking a bus or autorickshaw for the 36-kilometer ride to the ashram. Taxis are not readily available in Vasai.

Other Services

Ganeshpuri is a tiny village; for most services, you'll have to go to Vasai.

Books and Tapes

A full line of books and tapes on Siddha yoga is available at the ashram, as well as through affilitated centers in the West. A recommended introductory book by Swami Muktananda is *In the Company of a Siddha*. A recommended collection of talks by Gurumayi is *My Lord Loves a Pure Heart*.

When the Truth comes, it does not always come in a mild way. There is an explosion, an absolute explosion. Even though you may think it is subtle, it shatters your brain and shatters your heart. That's not to say that your brain, heart, and mind won't be intact; but their limited existence explodes. Everything inside explodes.

For this reason, when you look at the sages, they may look no different from other human beings: they eat, they drink, they sleep; they talk and they observe silence. On the other hand, they are absolutely different, because the Truth has exploded within their beings; whereas in us, the Truth is dormant.

—SWAMI CHIDVILASANANDA
(from *Darshan* magazine)

Vipassana International Academy
Igatpuri, Maharashtra

S. N. Goenka (1924–)

To newcomers, they may seem like meditation bootcamps: ten days of near-total silence, with up to eleven hours of seated meditation every day. Founded by Burmese-born meditation teacher S. N. Goenka, the Vipassana International Academy in Igatpuri—like its sister centers in Europe, the United States, and elsewhere in India—offers intensive ten-day courses in vipassana, or "insight meditation," a technique taught by the Buddha in India 2,500 years ago.

Teachers and Teachings

Beginners, be prepared: these courses are rigorous, and you are required to commit to the full ten days. If you can stick it out, though, there's no better introduction to this ancient practice, which Goenka defines as "seeing things as they really are."

An Indian born into a Hindu family in Burma, Goenka discovered vipassana meditation while searching for a cure for his severe migraine headaches. For fourteen years he studied closely with a Burmese meditation master, while continuing with his life as a successful industrialist and head of a large family. In 1969, he settled in India and began teaching vipassana courses in Bombay, thereby fulfilling his teacher's dream that the teachings of the Buddha—which had died out in India centuries ago—would one day return to the country where they had been born. Today, the headquarters in Igatpuri is just one of about thirty centers he has established all over Asia, Europe, and the United States.

The nonsectarian training consists of three steps. The first step is sila, or morality. For the ten days of the course, you'll be asked to abide by the five traditional Buddhist precepts: abstaining from killing, stealing, sexual activity, lying, and intoxicants. "One cannot work to liberate oneself from defilements of the mind while at the same time continuing to perform deeds of body and speech which only multiply these defilements," says Goenka. "By abstaining from such actions, one allows the mind to quiet down sufficiently in order to proceed with the task at hand."

The next step is to develop concentration by focusing the mind on the breath (a technique known as "anapana"). For the first three and a half days of meditation, you'll be instructed to keep your attention focused on the sensation of the breath entering and leaving the nostrils. This quiets the mind in preparation for the third step, vipassana—"purifying the mind of defilements by developing insights into one's own nature."

In Goenka's system, vipassana is a body-based practice. "In order to develop experiential wisdom, we must become aware of what we actually experience; that is, we must develop awareness of sensations," he says. "Sensation is indispensable in order to explore truth to the depths." Starting on the fourth day of the retreat, you'll be told to spend your meditation sessions sweeping your attention systematically through your body, from head to toe and from toe to head. Whatever sensations you encounter, neither cling to them nor push them away. As you sense these feelings ebb and flow, you will gradually come to experience directly what may previously have been just abstract concepts: that the world is impermanent; that every particle of the body and every process of the mind is in flux; that there is nothing that can be labeled "I" or "mine"; and that attempting to cling to anything is bound to bring unhappiness. From these realizations, says Goenka, springs the equanimity that is the source of true freedom from suffering.

There are eight meditation periods throughout the day, totaling about eleven hours of sitting—however, some of these can be conducted in the privacy of your own room, so it's possible to take a break if you absolutely have to (although monitors—dubbed the "thought police" by one disgruntled meditator—do come around to make sure you're sitting upright). Goenka is generally not physically present at these courses; his instructions—practical, insightful, and often humorous—are given via videotape. (After hours of sense-deprivation, these taped discourses prove as entertaining as a Hollywood summer blockbuster.) Assistant teachers are there in the flesh to answer questions and give additional instructions. "Noble Silence" is observed and any form of communication with fellow students is strictly prohibited. However, you may speak with the teachers when necessary.

Men and women are separated, including married couples. You are asked not to practice yoga and other physical exercises and to discontinue any other spiritual practices such as chanting, burning incense, praying, or reciting mantras. People with serious mental disorders are advised not to come.

Facilities and Food

Accommodations are spartan, with options of dormitories, individual cement cells, or individual rooms with shared bathrooms. Cots and blankets are provided, but you may want to bring your own bedding. Hot water for bathing is provided.

Food is simple Indian vegetarian, served in small but adequate quantities (every morsel tastes unusually good due to the sensory deprivation). There are no full meals after noon. (During an afternoon tea break, new students or those with health problems may eat a little fruit or even a light meal; experienced students have only herbal tea or fruit juice.) Safe drinking water is provided.

Other Goenka centers are located all over India: a list is available through the Igatpuri ashram or the United States contact.

Schedule

The usual Vipassana meditation course is ten days in length. Days start at 4 A.M. There is about ten to twelve hours of meditation daily—usually in one-hour or one-and-a-half-hour segments, with short breaks between sessions. There is about one and a half hours of videotaped instruction daily from S. N. Goenka. Assistant teachers are available for specific questions.

Fees

Courses are free and participants are not allowed to pay for the teaching, meals, or lodging. After you have successfully completed a course, you can make a donation to benefit future students, but such donations are not solicited.

Contact Information

VIPASSANA INTERNATIONAL ACADEMY
DHAMMAGIRI
P.O. BOX 6
IGATPURI (DIST. NASIK)
MAHARASHTRA 422 403
TEL: 91-2533-4076, 4086, 4032
FAX: 91-2533-4176

U.S. Contact:
VIPASSANA MEDITATION CENTER
DHAMMA DHARA
P.O. BOX 24
SHELBURNE FALLS, MA 01370
TEL: (413) 625-2160
FAX: (413) 625-2170

How to Get There

Igatpuri is approximately 130 kilometers (3½ hours by train) from Bombay on the Bombay-Nasik railway line. You can go by train, bus, or taxi.

Dhammagiri is located about 1 kilometer from the railway station. Autorickshaw drivers or porters will know the way to the center. If you walk (which takes about 15 minutes), porters are available to help you with your luggage, but be sure to set the price in advance or be prepared to carry your luggage if the porter wants to renegotiate part way to the center.

Other Services

Igatpuri is a relatively small town with restaurants, shops, food stalls, and very limited accommodations. Accommodations generally are not an issue if you plan to arrive on the same day as the course begins. If you plan on staying overnight in Igatpuri, Manas Hotel has been recommended by the Vipassana Center in Massachusetts. Reservations are highly recommended. Budget accommodations are available at Satkar Lodge, opposite the railway station.

Books and Tapes

A pamphlet by S. N. Goenka explaining the vipassana meditation training entitled *The Art of Living: Vipassana Meditation* is available by writing to any vipassana meditation center. For more in-depth instruction, read *Vipassana Meditation as Taught by S. N. Goenka*, by William Hart (Harper & Row). Books and tapes are available at the Vipassana International Academy Dhammagiri. In the United States, contact:

For Books:
PARIYATTI BOOK SERVICE
P.O. BOX 151
HAYFORK, CA 96041
TEL: (916) 628-5094

For Audio & Videotapes:
AUDIO PRODUCTIONS
8806 SOUTH LAKE STEVENS ROAD
EVERETT, WA 98205-2912
TEL: (206) 335-5223
FAX: (206) 334-7866

Observing reality as it is by observing the truth inside—this is knowing oneself directly and experientially. . . . From the gross, external, apparent truth, one penetrates to the ultimate truth of

mind and matter. Then one transcends that, and experiences a truth which is beyond mind and matter, beyond time and space, beyond the conditioned field of relativity: the truth of total liberation from all defilements, all impurities, all suffering. Whatever name one gives this ultimate truth is irrelevant; it is the final goal of everyone.

—S. N. GOENKA
(from *The Art of Living: Vipassana Meditation*)

Kaivalyadhama Yoga Institute
Lonavla, Maharashstra

 Swami Kuvalyananda (1883–1966)

Kaivalyadhama is the place to come if you're interested in knowing, for sure, whether it's better for your psychomotor performance to chant "om" in a high pitch or a low pitch; how "breath of fire" practice affects blood sugar and hemoglobin counts; exactly how long a yogi can stay in an airtight "samadhi pit." Sprawled on one hundred sixty rural acres in the popular hill station of Lonavla, it's a yoga institute with a three-pronged mission. Its educational wing offers a six-week yoga certificate course and a nine-month, government-certified diploma program. Its research branch conducts scientific studies on yoga's physiological and psychological effects, with the students from the diploma program as the principal guinea pigs. And its yogic hospital provides residential treatment programs for patients suffering from high blood pressure, back pain, asthma, diabetes, constipation, chronic headaches, and other ailments on which their research shows that yogic techniques can have a significant effect.

Teachers and Teachings

Kaivalyadhama is a good place for a relaxing week of yoga and naturopathic treatments in the company of twenty to thirty primarily Indian patients (many of whom seem to view it as a sort of yogic prison camp, in

Atmasantulana Village

If you're passing through Lonavala, you might want to check out the Atmasantulana Village, an ayurvedic healing center a few kilometers from Kaivalyadhama. Founded by an Indian ayurvedic physician—but staffed mainly by expatriate Germans—the center offers panchakarma (an ayurvedic healing regime), yoga, and meditation. The general course of treatment consists of a special vegetarian diet; massage and steam bath; ingestion of medicated ghee to release toxins; purgatives to cleanse the gastrointestinal tract and bowels; and enemas with medicated oil and herbs. Specialized treatments are available for heart, brain, muscles, joints, sinuses, back pain, arthritis, and other ailments.

The facilities are immaculate, including an ayurvedic pharmacy that manufactures its own line of medicines and cosmetics; a meditation pavilion surrounded by a small lake; a temple dedicated to Om as the symbol of the Absolute; and a small tea-shop. Evening meditation (6:45) is open to the public (except on Thursdays, when the center is closed). Foreigners can stay for about one thousand dollars per month, including food, accommodations, classes, and treatments (medicines extra). Indian guests must find lodging elsewhere (like at the adjacent MTDC holiday resort). It's advisable to book several months in advance. For information, contact Atmasantulana Village, Bombay-Pune Road, near MTDC Holiday Resort, Karla 410 405. Tel: 91-2114-82232. Fax: 91-2114-82203.

which they've been incarcerated on doctor's orders). It's also worth visiting just for a tour of the research lab, which bristles with aging but still functional equipment—looking like something you'd see in footage from the 1960s space program—including such custom-built treasures as a "nostril dominance apparatus" (for studying the effects of alternate nostril breathing) and a "trataka box" (for measuring the effects of the meditation practice of gazing steadily at a single point).

Kaivalyadhama was founded in 1924 by Swami Kuvalyananda, a self-taught scientist and yoga practitioner whose lifelong obsession was bringing together science and spirituality. Astounded by the mysterious potency of yoga techniques—which challenged his strict rationalist beliefs—he set out to ferret out their secrets with medical equipment. In his very first experiment, for example, he used X-rays and a manometer to examine the effects of nauli and uddiyana bandha, two techniques that involve drawing in and manipulating the muscles of the abdomen. The power of these practices, he concluded, stemmed from the fact that they reduce the air pressure inside the large intestines, creating a temporary vacuum.

This experiment set the tone for the next seventy years at Kaivalyadhama, which has continued to flourish after the founder's death in 1966. Kuvalyananda's quarterly journal *Yoga Mimamsa*—still in existence today—has published the results of hundreds of studies, charting such things as the improvement in diabetes patients after six weeks of practicing simple relaxation postures and the effect of Savasana (the classic relaxation posture) on neural network resource management in the human brain. At the yoga hospital, these findings are put into practice on a steady stream of clients. (One of Kuvalyananda's first patients, in 1927, was Mahatma Gandhi, for whom he prescribed a program to treat what he diagnosed as a "nervous breakdown.")

In addition to scientific research, Kaivalyadhama scholars conduct what they term "philosophico-literary research"—collecting and critically editing ancient texts from all over India, many of which were destroyed or hidden during the Moslem invasions. For example, their new edition of the classic Hatha Yoga Pradipika contains an added fifth chapter, reconstructed from previously lost fragments.

Obviously, Kaivalyadhama lies on the rational, scientific end of the yoga spectrum; you won't find much here in the way of devotional or mystical practices, although these topics are covered, in an academic way, in the nine-month diploma program. (However, there is a resident swami tucked in a cottage next to the cowshed.) What you are taught largely depends on which program you enter. If you're just passing through for a short time, your only option is to check into the yogic hospital (minimum stay, eight days—at least fifteen days recommended for optimum benefits). Don't be scared off by the intimidating list of disorders treated here (which range from "piles" to "mild schizophrenia")—it's also possible to stay here just to relax and renew. You'll do kriyas (cleansing practices) and very gentle asanas in the early morning, and another hour of asanas in the late afternoon; throughout the day naturopathic treatments such as mud baths and massage are available in the hospital clinic. Other than that, you'll be on your own to browse in the library or sight-see in the surrounding area.

If you want more serious instruction, you'll have to enroll in either the six-week or nine-month course—both of which are offered annually and require that you apply in advance. Topics covered in the six-week course include yoga and physical education; anatomy and physiology of yogic practices; traditional yoga philosophy (the main text being *Astangayoga of Charandas,* with supplementary readings in the *Hathayogapradipika, Yoga Sutras of Patanjali, Gerenda Samhita,* and other classics); and yoga and mental health. Curiously, only students age thirty-five and under are permitted in the program. Rules of conduct are strict: men and women may not visit each other's rooms; failing to attend any class is "a gross breach of discipline"; and "routine of the course must be strictly followed and *a happy manner adopted.*" The course concludes with written, practical, and oral exams.

For the nine-month course, most of the students are Indians seeking a government-certified diploma, but there are usually one or two foreigners as well. The intensive program is divided into five main subjects: Patanjali Yoga Sutra; Yogic Texts (including *Hathayogapradipika, Shiva Samhita,* and other classics); Yoga and Cultural Synthesis (which examines Vedic culture, the Upanishads, the Mahabarata, and other Indian classics, as well as looking at the spiritual traditions of other cultures); anatomy and physiology of yogic practices; and yoga and mental health. As a student, you'll automatically be a source of raw data for the research department—be prepared to have your vital statistics (weight, blood pressure, etc.) monitored daily throughout the course.

Facilities and Food

The Kaivalyadhama campus is vast, grassy, and quiet, with only a distant hum of traffic from the highway. The yoga hospital offers clean and comfortable single and double rooms and family suites, with bedding and mosquito nets provided; shared bathrooms are down the hall. For the yoga courses, you also have a choice of single and double rooms (dorms are only for Indian students)—however, you'll have to bring your own bedding, blanket, mosquito net, yoga mat, glass, thali, spoon, and drinking cup. The food is excellent—only mildly spiced, with milk and curd from the ashram cows, and salads from vegetables grown in Kaivalyadhama's own garden.

A research laboratory bristles with equipment. There's also an excellent 25,000-volume library, tranquil and well-organized—if you're interested in yoga history and philosophy, it's worth coming to Kaivalyadhama just to spend a few days browsing among texts you won't find anywhere else.

Schedule

The six-week course is offered annually, starting at the beginning of May—application deadline is the end of March. (Unfortunately, May is the hot season in India—however, since Lonavla is a hill station, the temperature remains bearable.) The nine-month program starts in the middle of August and lasts for two terms, with two midterm vacations (one of which must be used for an "educational tour"). Application deadline is the end of June.

Every January there is a ten-day "spiritual camp" featuring intensive pranayama and meditation practice.

Fees

Fees for foreigners are considerably more than those for Indians. For foreigners, the rates are:

Yogic hospital (including food, room, treatments, yoga lessons; minimum stay eight days): double room—$6 (U.S.) per day; single room—$10 (U.S.) per day.

Six-week course: registration fee—Rs 20; board and lodging—double room $450 (U.S.), single room $750 (U.S.); tuition—$20 (U.S.); refundable deposit—Rs 150.

Nine-month course: registration fee—Rs 20; board and lodging—$3,000 (U.S.); tuition—$150 (U.S.); college uniform—Rs 1,200; refundable deposit—Rs 150; educational tour—Rs 300; final examination fee—Rs 25.

KAIVALYADHAMA
SHRIMAN MADHAVA YOGA MANDIR SAMITI
LONAVLA 410403
TEL: 91-2114-73001; 73039
FAX: 91-2114-71983

U.S. Contact:
KAIVALYADHAMA
104 UNION AVE
PHILADELPHIA, PA 19004
TEL: (610) 617-8548

How to Get There

Lonavla is between Bombay and Pune and can be reached by bus or train.

Other Services

Lonavla is a small hill station. STD and fax are available; however, there is *nowhere to change foreign currency.* Make sure you bring all you need.

Books and Tapes

Kaivalyadhama offers over forty books on various aspects of yoga practice, including both modern works and critically edited editions of classic texts. Write for a catalogue.

The project on "pit burial samadhi" revealed that the adept yogis could stay in the underground pit for eighteen hours in comparison to a normal person (with no yoga exposure), who could stay for only twelve hours. The tolerance to increasing concentrations

of CO_2 in the pit was found to be of vital importance for prolonging the stay inside such airtight pit.

 —brochure of Scientific Research Department, Kaivalyadhama

International Meditation Center
Matheran, Maharashtra

Dr. Bhagwan D. Awatramani (1941–)

Located in a picturesque hill station about ninety kilometers from Bombay, the International Meditation Center (not to be confused with the center by the same name in Bodh Gaya) is both a resort hotel and a meditation school. The resort caters to affluent Indian families on holiday, while Westerners (primarily Swiss) come to study with resort owner and meditation teacher Dr. Bhagwan D. Awatramani.

Teachers and Teachings

As meditation centers go, this is a very Westernized, businesslike operation—it may be off-putting to those expecting a traditional Indian ashram (or traditional Indian prices). As a resort, however, it's a pleasant place to relax, and Dr. Awatramani offers a user-friendly introduction to the teachings of advaita vedanta master Ramana Maharshi (p. 286).

There's no rigorous meditation regime—instead, you can enjoy long, vista-studded hikes through the forested mountains, play a bit of ping-pong in the resort game hall, and still get back in time for informal meditation instruction in the afternoons. The town of Matheran has a bit of a "wild West" feeling, with a wide, red-earth main street lined with shops. As no vehicles are allowed in this area, there's a constant procession of pedestrians, horseback riders, porters carrying boxes and suitcases on their heads, and pack horses or mules laden with saddlebags.

A medical doctor, Dr. Awatramani became interested in meditation in his early twenties as a way to alleviate the stresses of medical school life in Bombay. According to his brochure, "his roots are in the tradition of Ramana Maharshi"; he teaches Ramana's method of self-inquiry, in which the meditator is told to ask, again and again, "Who am I?"

"Fundamental changes would take place in our lives if we would shift our awareness away from the periphery, from the observed toward the observer, toward the source of our being," he says. "We would find out that there is no world apart from us, that we are the center of the universe."

There are generally fewer than five students at the center, although sometimes groups of ten to twenty visit together. Most are previous students who have taken one of his seminars or retreats in Europe, where he has been teaching regularly for many years. Dr. Awatramani recommends that people come for two weeks or longer: "We don't want walk-ins and curiosity seekers."

Facilities and Food

The center has twelve rooms, each with attached bath with shower and Western-style toilet. It's currently set up as a resort, with a badminton area, ping-pong, swings, hammock, and a television room as well as a meditation room. Food is buffet style and includes both vegetarian and non-vegetarian selections.

Schedule

The schedule is relaxed. New arrivals have private sessions with Dr. Awatramani in the morning. At around 4 or 5 P.M. there's a discussion or question-and-answer session, followed by a period of silent sitting.

Dr. Awatramani plans to establish a permanent center in Switzerland, where he will spend six months a year. Most meditators come to the Matheran center in December, January, and February—if you come at another time, there's no guarantee Dr. Awatramani will be there.

Fees

The cost of food, lodging, and meditation instruction is about 1200 rupees a day (although payment in dollars or Swiss francs is preferred). A tip of Rs 50 to Rs 100 per day is suggested for the staff. If you have reservations and are delayed, you must give two days' notice or you are expected to pay from the date of your reservations.

Contact Information

INTERNATIONAL MEDITATION CENTER—MATHERAN
MALDOONGA RESORT
MATHERAN A10102
MAHARASHTRA

Mailing address in Bombay:
204 RAJ MANDIR, YARI ROAD
VERSOVA, BOMBAY 400 061
MAHARASHTRA
TEL: 91-21-483-0204, 91-21-483-0399
Telephone in Bombay: 91-22-626-9981
Fax in Bombay: C/O WEST END HOTEL, 91-22-205-7506

How to Get There

Take a train or bus from Bombay to Neral Junction (about 90 kilometers). From there, you can take a taxi or a narrow-gauge "toy train" that winds its way slowly up the steep mountainside to the 2,500-foot elevation of Matheran. You can then complete the journey by foot, horseback, or human-drawn rickshaw. Porters are available to carry your bags.

Other Services

This is a tourist town and restaurants, lodging, and shops abound. There is a phone booth in town, but no fax.

Books and Tapes

None.

*A*sk yourself, 'Who am I and what is the world?' There is no answer, and in pursuing this inquiry the mind finally disappears."
—DR. BHAGWAN D. AWATRAMANI

Christa Prema Seva Ashram
Pune, Maharashtra

✤ *Sister Brigitte, Acharya*

The Christa Prema Seva Ashram is run like a traditional ashram in every respect but one: "Our guru," explains its spiritual head, an 81-year-old German nun, "is the Lord Jesus Christ." Founded by an Anglican priest and now in the hands of a small group of Anglican and Roman Catholic nuns, this tiny ashram—a tranquil garden in the smoggy heart of Pune—seeks to foster a truly Indian Christianity, which embraces and learns from India's rich spiritual heritage, rather than trying to supplant it. Today, it attracts spiritual seekers from all over the world who are interested in the dialogue between Christianity, Hinduism, and yoga.

Teachers and Teachings

The ashram was founded in 1927 by Father Jack Winslow, the head of a small group of Indian and English Christians who were interested in living the teachings of Jesus within the context of Indian society. (An early supporter of this project was Mahatma Gandhi, who was a frequent visitor.) That community eventually disbanded, but the ashram was relaunched in 1972 by a community of Anglican sisters from Pune and Catholic sisters from Bombay, under the leadership of an Indian nun named Sister Vandana (p. 337).

From the beginning, the ashram was intended to be, in the words of Sister Sarah Grant, "above all a place of prayer, where all who came should be helped to enter into the Mystery of God by whatever name they called him." Guided by a local pundit, the nuns began studying the Upanishads, the Gita, and traditional Indian methods of meditation and prayer, while continuing to celebrate the Christian Eucharist daily.

"When Christians came to India, they tried to plant Christianity like a full-grown tree. If you became a Christian you had to become alienated from your culture, your roots, your own spirituality," explains Sister Sarah. To counter this tendency, the community tried to conform to Indian ashram customs, in small ways and large, from vegetarian food—served from thalis on the floor—to a twice-daily arati (offering of fire). Gradually,

Neo-Buddhist Headquarters

On the outskirts of Pune, in an area called Dapodi, is the headquarters and temple of the Trailokya Bauddha Mahasangha Sahayaka Gana—an order founded by British Buddhist monks as a spiritual center for India's "neo-Buddhists."

In October 1956, almost a half million of India's Dalits (outcasts) came together on a vast field in the Maharashtran town of Nagpur, where they converted en masse to Buddhism under the leadership of an outcaste politician named Dr. B. R. Ambedkar. In converting to Buddhism, these people—most of them part of the Mahar caste, part of the lowest stratum of Hindu society—were proclaiming their freedom from the Hindu religion and its rigid caste system. However, at that time Buddhism was virtually nonexistent in India—there were no schools, monasteries, temple, or teachers—and for twenty years Maharashtra's "neo-Buddhists," as they were called, existed more as a fragmented political movement than a spiritual one.

The first teachers to come—in a curious reversal of Buddhism's gradual spread from East to West—were a handful of British Buddhist monks from a group called the Friends of the Western Buddhist Order. They began teaching classes in Buddha dharma—in venues ranging from a police station to an abandoned railway—to eager crowds of Indian Buddhists. Today, the order they started has about 180 ordained monks and nuns and offers ongoing classes at the center in Dapoti.

The TBMSG also runs a retreat center near the Bhaja caves in Lonavla. For information, contact TBMSG Pune, Dhammachakra Pravartan Mahavihar, Raja Harishchandra Road, Dapodi, Pune 411012. Tel: 91-212-58403.

nuns discarded their habits in favor of saris and loose, comfortable Punjabi suits.

Today, the community's leader—known as the "acharya," a Sanskrit word meaning "teacher"—is Sister Brigitte, a German-born Anglican nun who began practicing yoga and Zen Buddhism in her fifties and spent four years as a hermit in Wales before coming to India. The core community consists of a handful of nuns, about half Indian and half European.

Although the original intention had been to reach out to Indian Christians, most of the current visitors are Europeans interested in exploring Indian spirituality without abandoning their Christian roots. You'll usually find one or two Iyengar yoga students staying here, since it's only about a fifteen-minute walk to the Ramani Iyengar Memorial Yoga Institute.

As with any Christian community, the central spiritual celebration at the CPS ashram is the daily celebration of the Eucharist—but with several key modifications. Instead of hymns, you'll get bhajans in Sanskrit, Hindi, and Marathi. Along with readings from the Old and New Testament, you'll get excerpts from the Gita, the Upanishads, the Mahabharata, and other Indian classics.

Guests at the ashram are not required to attend the daily Eucharist—or anything else, for that matter, although you're encouraged to come to the morning, noon, and evening arati (which includes offering the flame to Jesus, Mohammed, and Buddha as well as the traditional Hindu deities). Instead, you're left on your own most of the time to do your own practice, sit in the flower garden by the lotus fishpond, or browse in the library. Depending on the wishes of the guests, the nuns will organize interfaith discussion groups.

The ashram has just been granted "Indian Heritage" status by the government, a move that guarantees that its land and buildings will be preserved as they are (thereby fighting off a land grab by a powerful group of real estate developers). However, it continues to face opposition from other Christian groups that disapprove of its blend of traditions, and its future is somewhat uncertain. But the nuns remain optimistic. As Sister Sarah has written, "We are never quite sure how long we shall be able to go on, who will be in the community next year, what we shall be asked to do next. All we know is that in spite of all our shortcomings, the Lord seems to be doing something marvellous in this place, and that as long as he wants to go on doing it, we are happy to be here."

Facilities and Food

The ashram consists of a cluster of low stone buildings, painted pale yellow and cream and overgrown with a riot of bougainvillea, clustered around a lotus pond and a tranquil, deliciously untidy garden (roamed by the nun's dogs, Maya and Lila). Over a hundred different species of trees provide shade, freshen the air, and offer homes to more than forty types of birds. About twenty visitors can stay in small shared rooms, with common bath and toilet. Bedding is provided.

Food is Indian vegetarian, non-spicy, served Indian style (on thalis on the floor, without utensils). Guests are encouraged to help with food preparation and serving; however, this is not required.

The ashram has an excellent library (which resident yoga students can use as a practice room—there's even a collection of sticky mats and other Iyengar props); a meditation dome; and a chapel that is open for prayer and meditation at all times.

Schedule

Daily arati at 5:50 A.M., followed by Eucharist at 7 A.M. (full Mass on Sunday). Evening arati at 8 P.M.

Fees

Rs 250 per day covers food and lodging. No one will be turned away based on inability to pay.

Contact Information

THE ACHARYA
CHRISTA PREMA SEVA ASHRAM
SHIVAJINAGAR
PUNE
MAHARASHTRA 411 005
TEL: NONE

How to Get There

This ashram is located in Pune, approximately 192 kilometers from Bombay, three and a half to five hours on the train. Trains and buses travel frequently to Pune; you can also fly directly there from many cities in India. When you arrive in Pune, ask the taxi or rickshaw driver to take you to Shivaji Nagar, S.T. bus stand. (Do not mention the word "ashram" or the driver may insist on taking you to the Osho Commune.) A short distance past the S.T. bus stand, you will see a gate on your left with a large notice saying "CPS Hostel and Ashram." Go through the hostel compound to the next gate, which is the ashram.

Other Services

Pune has a population of about 2 million, and all services are available.

Books and Tapes

The Lord of the Dance, by Sister Sarah Grant, gives some of the background and philosophy of the ashram.

"*We feel that love is a greater value than rigid insistence on conformity.*"

—SISTER SARAH GRANT

Osho Commune International
Pune, Maharashtra

Osho (formerly Bhagwan Shree Rajneesh) (1931–1990)

Some people call it the "buddhafield" of an enlightened master. Others say it's the world's largest spiritual singles' club. One thing is certain: the Osho Commune International—founded nearly twenty-five years ago by Osho, the controversial guru formerly known as Bhagwan Shree Rajneesh—is not your typical Indian ashram. A New Age Xanadu that attracts thousands of visitors every day, the commune is a self-contained personal growth conglomerate, offering an astonishing variety of classes and workshops in everything from organizational development to tantric sex. And, if the courses don't interest you, you can spend your days romping in the swimming pool, sauna, "Zennis" courts, and bistro of the commune's "Club Meditation."

Teachers and Teachings

"For tantra everything is holy, nothing is unholy," Osho wrote in *The Book of the Secrets*. For Osho, world and spirit were not separate, the body was sacred, and sex was a valid path to enlightenment. His community—still flourishing nearly a decade after his death—is designed to celebrate his vision of the new human being: "Zorba the Buddha."

Dubbed the "sex guru" by the Indian press, Osho insisted that he did not advocate sex as an end in itself. Rather, he wanted his followers to liberate their raw, creative life force energy and use it as a tool for transformation—ultimately dropping sex altogether, without repression. "Sex can be just animalistic—that is possible—but it need not be. It can rise higher. It can become love, it can become prayer," he wrote. "That is the vision of Tantra: sex can become samadhi, through sex the ultimate ecstasy can enter in you."

Osho's career as a spiritual teacher began in the mid-1960s, when he left his post as a philosophy professor at the University of Jabalpur and began traveling around India, electrifying and outraging audiences with his radical vision of personal transformation. By the early 1970s, Western visitors were flooding into his newly formed Pune commune, attracted by his bold critique of cultural and religious traditions, his fusion of Eastern teachings with Western cathartic and body-based psychotherapies, and his no-holds-barred celebration of life in the present moment.

In 1981 Osho moved to the United States, where he and his followers established a small city called Rajneeshpuram on a 64,000-acre ranch in Oregon. However, Rajneeshpuram foundered amid internal intrigue and escalating conflicts with the surrounding community; and in 1985 Osho was convicted of immigration fraud (on what his followers insist were specious charges) and deported from the United States. After brief sojourns in various countries, he returned to his ashram in Pune, where he died in early 1990.

Today, the Osho Commune International rivals the Taj Mahal as one of India's largest tourist attractions, with thousands of visitors every day—almost entirely foreigners, with Germans forming the largest contingent—

roaming its green, exquisitely landscaped thirty-one-acre campus. The commune has been proclaimed an "AIDS-free zone"—to get an entry pass, you'll need a current clean AIDS test done by the commune's own testing center (located right at the main gates). You'll also need to buy a maroon robe—mandated to create a "unified field of energy" in the commune—from one of the dozens of entreprising robe-wallahs lining the street outside. ("Robe" is something of a misnomer—color is prescribed, but style is not, and women's outfits range from skimpy knee-length nighties to slit-thighed, spaghetti-strapped evening gowns, while most men favor elongated tee shirts.) If you want to use the Club Meditation facilities, you'll also need a maroon bathing suit and exercise wear.

Once inside, you can participate for no additional charge in a full schedule of various kinds of meditation, beginning at 6 A.M. with "dynamic," Osho's most famous technique. Dynamic meditation is based on the premise that modern people are too agitated, stressed, and overstimulated to benefit from plunging straight into seated, silent practice. Instead, a dynamic meditation session consists of five stages: ten minutes of deep, fast, chaotic breathing through the nose; ten minutes of wild, free-form catharsis; ten minutes of jumping up and down and shouting the Sufi mantra "hoo!"; ten minutes of absolute silence; and, finally, fifteen minutes of celebratory dancing.

Other forms of meditation are offered throughout the day, including vipassana and kundalini. The day concludes with the meeting of the White Robe Brotherhood, billed as the community's core spiritual event, for which you'll have to purchase—you guessed it. (An entrepreneur could make a fortune here selling maroon robes with a reversible white lining.) At the Brotherhood assembly, you'll dance to live music while Osho's image conducts from a giant video screen, climaxing with thunderous shouts of "Osho! Osho! Osho!" Then you'll watch one of Osho's classic videotaped discourses on topics ranging from the Buddha to Ronald Reagan.

For an additional charge, you can take courses at the Osho Multiversity, whose nine departments include a Meditation Academy, an Institute for Love and Consciousness, a School for Creative Arts, and a School for Centering and Zen Martial Arts. While course offerings seem more rooted in the spiritual traditions of California than those of India, their intent is emphatically transpersonal. One of the classics is a three-week course in the "mystic rose" meditation, in which you laugh for three hours a day for seven days; then cry for three hours a day for seven days; then sit in silence for three hours a day for seven days.

If you're inspired to do so, you can take Osho's nontraditional version of sannyas vows at a weekly ceremony on Saturday night. You'll be given a Sanskrit name to break your attachment to your old identity; your only vows consist of a internal pledge to your own spiritual growth. The ceremony is followed by a celebratory, free-form dance party.

Facilities and Food

There are no guest accommodations within the commune; you'll have to stay in one of the numerous hotels and guest houses in the surrounding area (which range from luxurious to spartan). The welcome desk at the commune's main gate has a list of local hotels.

The commune itself is verdant and impeccably clean, with stone pathways winding through a maze of gardens, trees strung with twinkling lights, and black marble buildings with name like "Osho Lao Tzu" and "Osho Jesus." A variety of restaurants serve delicious vegetarian food—both Indian and Western—made with produce grown on the commune's organic farm. You can purchase alcohol at the Meera Bistro if you obtain a "zen pass" from the front gate.

"Club Meditation" includes a beauty salon, massage rooms, sauna, lagoon-shaped swimming pool, and badminton, volleyball, and "Zennis" courts. (Warning: during Zennis matches, the referee is likely to halt the game and play points over if she feels the players need to look at their competitiveness issues.)

Osho's marble-and-glass samadhi shrine is a great place to meditate; white socks are required to walk inside it.

One of the commune's highlights is the twelve-acre garden called Osho Teerth, an eco-paradise reclaimed from a stinking refuse dump. A once-contaminated stream runs through it, turned sparkling clean through a natural biological filtration process.

Schedule

One-hour guided tours are offered in the morning and afternoon for a cost of ten rupees. The daily meditation schedule is posted at the entrance to Gautama the Buddha Auditorium. A three-day Intensive Meditation Camp begins on the second Friday of each month, and no Multiversity groups are scheduled for that time. Special celebrations are held on January 19 (Osho's death), March 21 (Osho's enlightenment), the July full moon, September 8, and December 11 (Osho's birthday). These are preceded by five-day festivals of music, dance, and other entertainment.

Osho Multiversity courses vary in length from a couple of hours to several months. Schedules are available from Osho Commune International.

Fees

Entrance fee: Rs 50 per day
AIDS test: Rs 125 (next-day result); Rs 350 (same-day result)
Food: available at commune restaurants for prices ranging from Rs 50 to 100 per meal
Club Meditation: Rs 70 for each use
Osho Multiversity courses: varies from course to course; prices start from Rs 1250 for a typical one-day introduction to meditation

Contact Information

OSHO COMMUNE INTERNATIONAL
17 KOREGAON PARK
PUNE 411 001
MAHARASHTRA
TEL: 91-212-660963
FAX: 91-212-644181
TELEX: 81-0145-7474 LOV IN
E-MAIL: CC.OSHO@OCI.SPRINTRPG.EMS.VSNL.NET.IN

U.S. Contact:
VIHA MEDITATION CENTER
P.O. BOX 352
MILL VALLEY, CA 94942
TEL: (415) 381-9861
E-MAIL:OSHOAVI@AOL.COM

How to Get There

Pune is approximately 192 kilometers from Bombay, 3½ to 5 hours by train (easy) or bus (less easy). You can also fly directly to Pune. The commune is in Koregaon Park, a suburb less than two miles from the bus and railway stations and approximately five miles from the airport. All taxis or autorickshaws know the Osho Ashram.

Other Services

Pune has a population of approximately 2 million, people and all services are available.

Books and Tapes

There are several hundred Rajneesh titles in print, many of which are available in bookstores in the psychology/religion section. A full range is available through the commune bookstore or through the U.S. contact. Recommended introductory titles include *My Way, the Way of the White Clouds; I Am the Gate; Dimensions Beyond the Known; The Book of the Secrets;* and *Meditation: The First and Last Freedom.* The commune offers a useful booklet entitled "Staying Healthy in India." Books can be ordered through the U.S. contact.

Registration at the Multiversity Plaza was as hectic and harried as any regular college registration. Dozens of us magenta-clad, overeager spiritual seekers stood in line to work out personalized enlightenment schedules with the frazzled swamis. My counselor was Swami Niven, and when I laid out my desires—to improve my tennis game, date beautiful women, and find the meaning of life—he recommended three courses: Opening to Feeling, Opening to Self-Love, and Opening to Intimacy. He also insisted that I attend dynamic meditation at seven every morning.

"I don't want to go overboard here," I confessed. "I just want enough Osho to, you know, get a little zip in my life."

Swami Niven shook his head. "You really need the Opening to Feeling seminar," he said.

—Karl Taro Greenfeld
(from *Condé Nast Traveller*, October 1996)

Ramamani Iyengar Memorial Yoga Institute
Pune, Maharashtra

B. K. S. Iyengar (1918–)

He's probably the most famous hatha yogi in the world. For thousands of students, the photographs of him in *Light on Yoga*—his illustrated Bible of yoga postures—are the ultimate standard for asana practice. And his precise, scientific approach to alignment and form have revolutionized the way yoga is taught in the West. Now in his early eighties, B. K. S. Iyengar—sometimes called the "Lion of Pune"—continues to roar in his lair at the Yoga Institute, where (with the help of his son and daughter, whom he's groomed as his successors) he's drilling a whole new generation in the fundamentals of practice.

Teachers and Teachings

Unless freedom is gained in the body, freedom of the mind is a far cry," says Iyengar. "It is through the body that you realize that you are a spark of Divinity." You won't do much seated meditation at the Iyengar Institute. Instead, you'll get rigorous classes in asana and pranayama, taught with an almost military precision and ferocity. The point, says Iyengar, is to awaken intelligence in every cell of the body, so that even the skin becomes conscious, alive, and alert. In the process, the mind becomes anchored in the present moment.

A weak and sickly child from a poor south Indian family, Iyengar was raised by his elder brother after the death of their father when Iyengar was nine. As a boy, he suffered from malnutrition, malaria, tuberculosis, and typhoid. Doctors predicted that he wouldn't live past the age of twenty.

At age sixteen, he was sent to Mysore to live with his sister, who was married to T. Krishnamacharya, a famous scholar and yoga teacher. (Krishnamacharya went on to teach many other influential yogis, including Pattabhi Jois (p. 142), Indra Devi, and his son T. K. V. Desikachar (p. 247). At first, Krishnamacharya refused to teach yoga to his feeble young brother-in-law, saying that such instruction required auspicious karma from previous births. But when Krishnamacharya's prize student ran away—just a week before a demonstration Krishnamacharya had scheduled for the Maharaja of Mysore—he quickly gave Iyengar a crash course in asana practice. "He almost broke my back," Iyengar recalls. But after a week of intense practice, Iyengar gave an impressive demonstration of backbends for the Maharaja—and Krishnamacharya accepted him as a student and assistant teacher at his yoga school.

After three years in Mysore, Iyengar left for Pune to teach yoga. For the next decade, he scraped out a meager living as a yoga teacher, while engaged in intense personal practice and experimentation. "I regarded the body as my temple and the asanas as my prayers," he writes in his autobiography. He began to explore yoga therapy; props (such as bricks and blankets) to make poses accessible to people who couldn't otherwise do them; meticulous and subtle adjustments of alignment.

In the early 1950s, Iyengar gave a session to celebrated violinist Yehudi Menuhin, who was in Bombay giving a concert to raise money for famine relief. Menuhin invited him to teach in Switzerland—a visit that proved to be the first of many trips to the West. Iyengar's largely self-taught system of yoga—with its emphasis on the physical body as the vehicle for enlightenment—was just what many Western students had been craving. By the mid-seventies, "Iyengar yoga"—exacting, scientific, and physically rigorous—had taken the yoga world by storm. Today, it's probably the most widely practiced hatha-yoga system in the West.

This practice involves strict attention to subtle anatomical details. Among other things, Iyengar is a master at physical therapy—stories abound about "miraculous" cures of everything from depression to near-paralysis through his meticulous routines. Even if you're basically healthy, it's not uncommon to spend a whole class working on one basic pose—with strict instructions on how to move the femurs, the kidneys, the skin on the inner front armpit. ("Self-realization must exist in every pore of the skin," he says.) Extensive use of props (such as straps, poles, and ropes suspended from the ceiling) helps you get the proper movement (although you might as well face it—you'll never *really* get it right. Breaking down the ego is an important element of this approach.) Those accustomed to a more flowers-and-incense style might be in for a rude awakening.

These days, the daily classes are taught not by Iyengar, but by his daughter, Geeta, and his son, Prashant. While remaining firmly rooted in their father's teachings, each brings a unique spin to the presentation: Geeta is reportedly a wizard with women's bodies, while Prashant specializes in integrating breath with movement. But Iyengar is usually hovering in the back of the room, doing his own practice; and he frequently interrupts, Zeus-like, to hurl a thunderbolt at a teacher or student. Two afternoons a week, he leads a medical class for people with health problems, which other students are welcome to watch. Stripped to his shorts, he storms about the room, guiding forty or fifty people through complex, completely personalized routines involving a staggering variety of ropes, weights, sandbags, and custom-built yoga furniture.

Space is limited at the Institute, and half the class is reserved for local Indian students. Consequently, there's a three-year waiting list for Westerners. If you want to study there, apply in writing and give your "yoga resumé," which must include at least a year of Iyengar-style classes. (It definitely helps your chances if you've been studying with a senior Iyengar teacher.) You can sign up for either one or two months; they will write back and tell you for what dates you've been scheduled. Once at the Institute, you'll be scheduled for six classes a week with Geeta and/or Prashant. In addition to classes, enrolled students are welcome to use the practice rooms and the library throughout the day—an opportunity, as one student eagerly put it, "to rub shoulders with the master."

Be sure to bring yoga wear that's appropriate for heat. Tee shirts and shorts (that won't be indecent when you turn upside down) are recommended. Leotards and tights will probably be too hot.

Facilities and Food

Named in honor of Iyengar's wife Ramamani (who died in 1973, just after the foundation was laid), the Institute consists of a semicircular cone of a building on a quiet residential street. The main practice room is a bright, airy room, furnished with a small department store's worth of yoga furniture—benches, horses, boxes, stools, weights, bars, footrests, and enough ropes for an S&M dungeon. There's a yoga library of close to eight thousand volumes.

The Institute has no residential facilities—students must stay in nearby hotels. It's also possible to rent flats in the vicinity.

Schedule

You'll be assigned to six classes a week (the Institute is closed on Sunday) with Geeta and/or Prashant. Iyengar supervises a medical class on Tuesday and Wednesday afternoons, which other students can watch with advance permission. Once a month, Geeta leads a discussion on yoga philosophy, interpreting classic texts from an Iyengar yoga perspective.

There are also several classes a week taught by senior students, including ones for women, children, and beginners. These are rarely attended by Westerners.

Each December 14, the Institute celebrates Iyengar's birthday. The Institute is closed during May.

Fees

Tuition: $150 per month for Westerners (Indians pay far less).

Contact Information

RAMAMANI IYENGAR MEMORIAL YOGA INSTITUTE
1107-B1
SHIVAJI NAGAR
PUNE 411 016
TEL: 91-212-356134

U.S. Contact:
IYENGAR YOGA NATIONAL ASSOCIATION OF THE UNITED STATES
1676 HILTON HEAD COURT, #2288
EL CAJON, CA 92019
TEL: (800) 889-9642

The Institute is on Hare Krishna Road in Shivajinagar, not far from the College of Agriculture. Pune is approximately 192 kilometers from Bombay (3½ to 5 hours by train). Trains and buses travel frequently to Pune; you can also fly directly there from many cities in India.

Other Services

Pune is a city of 2 million, and all services are available.

Books and Tapes

Books by and about Iyengar are available in over a dozen languages. Good introductory texts are *The Tree of Yoga* (Shambhala), *Light on Yoga* (Schocken), and *Iyengar: His Life and Work* (Timeless).

If you cannot see your little toe, how can you see the Self?
—B. K. S. IYENGAR
(from *Iyengar: His Life and Work*)

Stretch! Stretch! Stretch!" he yells. You are standing in a pose, stretching, you think, with every fiber in your body, when suddenly there is a slap on your shoulder and a harsh voice says, "Move the skin here!" You try to think of your skin moving and hope something is happening. Another slap on the back, "You did not move like I tell you. Armpits roll from back to top. Why are you so slow? Am I explaining correctly or incorrectly? Eh?" He stands in front of you, demonstrates, then pushing a seemingly angry face directly in front of yours, he yells, "You understand? You understand?" Bewildered, embarrassed, you shyly answer yes. "So see if you can love like that," he says and walks away, smiling his broad, white-toothed smile. "To show compassion," he explains to the class, "you must be merciless. Unless I shout she will not love." By "love," Iyengar means practice with devotion.

—Elizabeth Kent
(from "The Lion and the Lamb," *Yoga Journal*)

PILGRIMAGE SITES IN *Maharashtra*

Nasik. One of the four sites where the Kumbh Mela is held, Nasik is located on the train route from Bombay to Aurangabad, about 190 kilometers from Bombay. According to tradition, the gods Rama and Sita stayed here during their exile—pilgrimage highlights include a cave from which Sita is said to have been abducted by the demon Ravana. You can also visit the tank by the holy Godavari River where Rama and Sita used to bathe—bones dropped in here are said to dissolve, and famous bones that have been deposited here include Mahatma Gandhi's, Jawaharlal Nehru, and Indira Gandhi. About 30 kilometers from Nasik is the source of the Godavari River at Trimbak, said to be the spot where the nectar fell from the sacred pot in the famous story that the Kumbh Mela commemorates. Nasik has plenty of moderately priced hotels.

Ajanta and Ellora. The famous Ajanta and Ellora caves in Maharashtra are more accurately rock-hewn chambers, very well planned and executed, that housed Buddhist monks for about eight hundred years. The walls are ornamented with exquisite early Buddhist paintings, some of which date to the second century B.C.E. They are one of the few remaining examples of this sort of temple painting.

The easiest way to get to the Ajanta and Ellora caves is to fly or take the train to Aurangabad. From there Ajanta and Ellora may be reached by road. Ellora is only 30 kilometers from Aurangabad, and the city may be used as a base for day trips to the caves. Ajanta is somewhat farther, just off the road that leads from Aurangabad to Jalgaon, so it is more convenient to stay in the vicinity of the Ajanta caves—there is a travelers' lodge and a very small forestry rest house right next to the caves, but there are better options 5 kilometers down the road in Fardapur, which can be reached by bus.

Shirdi. Every day thousands of pilgrims visit the village of Shirdi, the former home of one of India's most beloved saints, Sai Baba of Shirdi, who died in 1918. (The contemporary superstar guru Satya Sai Baba [p. 69] is believed by his devotees to be a reincarnation of Shirdi Sai Baba.) You'll see Shirdi Sai Baba's picture on taxi dashboards all over India—a thin, grey-bearded man with a white scarf on his head, wrapped in a threadbare cloak. Some people believed him to be a Hindu sadhu, others a Moslem fakir; he was familiar with both Islamic and Vedic scriptures, and his teachings transcended creed. Devotional services—including arati and chanting—are held at his samadhi several times a day, starting at 5:15 A.M. and finishing around 10:30 P.M.

The closest railheads are at Manmad and Kopergaon, from which you can catch buses or taxis to Shirdi. Buses also run from Pune, Bombay, and Nasik. Plenty of food and lodging is available.

—LEA TERHUNE AND MURRAY FELDMAN

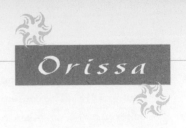

Karar Ashram
Puri, Orissa

🍂 *Swami Hariharananda Giri (1907–)*

His disciples call him the greatest living master of kriya yoga, the path popularized by Paramahansa Yogananda in his classic *Autobiography of a Yogi* (p. 390). Now over ninety, Swami Hariharananda Giri was a devotee of Yogananda's own guru, Sri Yukteswar, back in the 1930s. Nowadays, he divides his time between his disciples in the United States and this small, nonresidential ashram in the seaside pilgrimage and resort town of Puri.

Teachers and Teachings

If your only reason for going to Puri is to visit Hariharananda, be sure to call ahead and find out if he's there—these days, he spends most of his time in the United States, and there may not be much going on in his absence. The ashram's current president is Swami Yogeswarananda Giri, a taciturn man in his fifties who has been at the ashram for almost a quarter century. When Hariharananda passes away, Yogeswarananda will probably be the next guru.

For a place with such a strong lineage that's been around for so long, this ashram seems curiously lifeless, at least when Hariharananda is absent. The official schedule shows a variety of different classes, but you may want to check to make sure they are actually happening before you show up.

Daily meditations and kriya-yoga classes are only for initiates in Hariharinanda's system of kriya yoga, which—although similar in essence—has some distinct differences from the more widely known techniques taught by Yogananda's Self-Realization Fellowship. Anyone can receive the first level of initiation at the ashram, which normally takes a few days; after this, you're welcome to attend the daily sessions.

Like the SRF system, Hariharananda's yoga promises to vastly accelerate the process of spiritual evolution through a set of practices, or kriyas—divided into six sequential levels—that include simple postures, breathing exercises, visualizations, and concentration techniques. According to Hariharananda, kriya yoga incorporates the devotional elements of bhakti yoga, the energy-awakening techniques of hatha yoga, and the meditative concentration of raja yoga; however, kriya yoga eliminates the "meticulous austerities and painful processes" sometimes associated with these paths, making it accessible and useful to householders.

"During the practice of kriya, the entire spine is converted into a magnet which draws bodily currents away from the senses and the nerves," he writes. "A devotee becomes automatically introverted, experiences the divine sensation of sound vibration, touch of heaviness on the forehead, vision of glow of light in the midbrain, and becomes absorbed in meditation. Therefore, the kriya technique is the foundation of Self-realization."

Hariharananda was initiated into the first kriya by Sri Yukteswar, the second by Paramahansa Yogananda, and the third through sixth by a series of other masters, both within and outside Yogananda's organization. Medical doctors have verified his ability to stop his pulse at will; he has spent days at a time immersed in the deepest state of samadhi, oblivious to the external world. He's known for his knowledge of astrology, astronomy, and palmistry, as well as yogic philosophy, the Vedas, and the Upanishads.

He has frequently dismayed people in Yogananda's lineage by initiating some seekers immediately—sometimes within minutes of meeting them—into practices that, in the SRF system, require years of disciplined preparation. "Hariharananda can infuse the spiritual power in a person such that in two or three minutes you can hear the divine sound, you can feel the movement sensation in the brain, you can see the divine light," one of his disciples explained in an article in *Yoga Journal*. "When the desire comes in your mind to go for initiation, that is when you are fit. The voice within is telling you, so you don't have to wait years and years."

Facilities and Food

The ashram has no residential facilities for Westerners, but there are plenty of nearby hotels at all levels of luxury, since Puri is a major tourist town. It's on about half an acre, planted with flower and vegetable gardens, coconut palms, and papaya and banana trees. There's a meditation hall and the samadhi shrine of Sri Yukteswar, the guru of both Hariharananda Giri and Paramahansa Yogananda.

Schedule

Daily meditations are held from 5:30 to 6:30 A.M. in the summer (6 to 7 A.M. in the winter). On Sunday there's yoga instruction from 2 to 5 P.M. and a Bhagavad Gita or kriya yoga class from 5:30 to 8:00 P.M. (Classes may or may not be conducted in English, depending on who's there.) Classes in palmistry and astrology are also sometimes offered.

Fees

Donation.

Contact Information

KARAR ASHRAM
c/o SWAMI YOGESWARANANDA GIRI
PRESIDENT & ASHRAM-IN-CHARGE
SWARGADWAR
PURI 752 001
ORISSA
TEL: 91-6752-23004

How to Get There

The closest airport to Puri is at Bhubaneswar with flights from Calcutta, Delhi, Hyderabad, Madras, and Nagpur. Puri is 60 kilometers from Bhubaneswar and can be reached by train, bus, or taxi. There are also trains and buses into Puri from Madras, Calcutta, Delhi, and other major cities. From the railway station take an autorickshaw or bicycle rickshaw about 3 kilometers to the ashram, which is located one block up from the beach.

Puri has a population of about 125,000 people. As a major pilgrimage site and a seaside resort, it has most facilities available, including a wide range of lodging and food services.

Books and tapes are available at the ashram.

I have never met anyone so totally incapable of small talk as Hariharananda. "Hello! How was your trip?" And then, before we can reply, he launches into his one all-consuming passion. "Kriya yoga is a short cut to God realization. By the practice of this technique, within five or ten minutes' time, people can change their life force into a radiant, all-accomplishing divine force . . .

"This kriya yoga is a rare opportunity. Many people have taken initiation into other practices like mantra recitation or singing or dancing or reading books, but these are all extrovert. With kriya yoga, from the very beginning, you will not feel where is your body. You cannot feel where you have sat. You cannot imagine your own face. You cannot imagine that the whole world is there. You are offering your soul and your whole body in the fire, and the world is finished. You can only feel the omniscient."

—LINDA JOHNSEN
(from "Master of Kriya Yoga," *Yoga Journal*)

PILGRIMAGE SITES IN *Orissa*

Puri and Bhubaneshawar. The city of Puri is reknowned for its picturesque white-sand beaches—it's also a major pilgrimage center, known as the earthly abode of the god Vishnu. Pilgrims particularly flock here during the Rath Yatra at the Jagannath Temple, which takes place in June or July every year. In this festival, the raths, or chariots, of the Lord Jagganath (another form of Krishna—the name literally means "Lord of the Universe") and his brother and sister Balabhadra and Subhadra are dragged through the streets to the Gundicha Mandir, where the gods spend seven days. (Unfortunately, the Jagannath Temple—one of the most famous in India—does not admit non-Hindus.)

It's also worth a trip to Bhubaneshawar, 61 kilometers away, the capitol of Orissa and a famous pilgrimage center. It's one of the few remaining examples of the ancient Hindu temple cities that thrived during early medieval times, with ruins dating back to the second and third centuries B.C.E. Hundreds of temples remain in a city that at one time had thousands.

—LEA TERHUNE

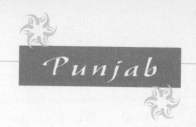

Radha Soami Satsang Beas
Beas, District Amritsar, Punjab

Maharaj Charan Singh (1916–1990)
Maharaj Gurinder Singh (1955–)

Over a million people worldwide belong to one of the sects of the Radha Soami movement, an offshoot of Sikhism whose primary teaching is "surat shabd yoga," a meditation on inner light and sound. The headquarters of one of the main Radha Soami sects, Radha Soami Satsang Beas is actually a self-contained colony—as squeaky-clean and orderly as a military base—inhabited by five to six thousand permanent residents. The community strongly discourages drop-in visitors. But foreign initiates are welcome to stay in the immaculate international guest-house compound and participate in the daily round of meditation, chanting, satsang, and work.

Teachers and Teachings

The Radha Soami movement was started in 1861 by a retired money-lender and mystic named Shiv Dayal Singh, who initiated his followers into a secret set of spiritual disciplines designed to help the practitioner connect with the blissful divine energy known as Radha Soami (literally, "the Lord of the Soul"). Although the movement has splintered into a number of sects with allegiances to different gurus, the basic teachings remain the same from group to group. The specific techniques are available only to initiates. However, the essence of the practice involves tuning in—through meditation on the third eye—to an inner current of sound and light, which is (in the words of the current guru, Maharaj Gurinder Singh) "so fascinating, so charming, so tempting, that once we are attached to it, we are automatically detached from the senses."

"A current of sound was the first activity of the Supreme Being at the beginning of creation. . . . When one of our members listens internally and expectantly for the divine sound, with controlled body, mind, and will, he will become lifted up towards the bliss and wisdom of the Supreme Being as soon as he hears the divine sound," an early Radha Soami guru explained to the British journalist Paul Brunton in the 1930s. "A sound carries the influence of the region whence it emanates and so, if you concentrate your attention inwardly in a certain way, you may one day hear the mystic words which sounded forth at the first upheaval in the primeval chaos and which form the true name of the Creator. The echoes of those words reverberate back into man's spiritual nature; to catch those echoes, by means of our secret Yoga practice, and to trace them up to their origin is literally to be carried up to paradise."

To learn the specific techniques for tuning in to this inner sound, you have to be initiated by an authorized representative of the Radha Soami Satsang Beas, which has branches in fifty-one countries. The RSSB will only initiate people who are over twenty-five years old; you must vow to maintain a strict vegetarian diet, abstain from alcohol and drugs, live a clean and moral lifestyle, and meditate for at least two and a half hours a day. These vows must be practiced for at least six months before initiation. If you're interested in being initiated, it's best to do so at a branch in your own country, rather than trying to do it at the headquarters in India.

Radha Soami members are forbidden to proselytize; you won't get a hard sell or be pressed to join the group (assuming you even get permission to visit without already being an initiate, which is somewhat unlikely). The current guru, Maharaj Gurinder Singh, keeps a deliberately low profile—he doesn't seek or even allow publicity about himself, preferring to draw appropriate students to himself through more subtle channels. Despite these restrictions—or perhaps because of them—the RSSB has grown to be a large international organization, with about a thousand centers in India and three hundred more worldwide. During the period when foreigners are allowed to visit (October 12 through January 15, and February 9 through April 10), there are usually about three hundred foreigners staying at the guest house (unless the guru is absent, in which case the number drops to just a handful). Children are not allowed, nor are people who are unable to care for themselves because of age, illness, or other conditions.

Discipline, hard work, and punctuality are stressed—you should plan to be about five minutes early for every scheduled event.

Facilities and Food

The main community encompasses about three hundred acres, plus additional land for a hospital complex and substantial farmland in the surrounding areas. Streets are well paved and the grounds are landscaped and immaculate; the whole place radiates tidiness, organization, and discipline. Facilities include a satsang hall, hospital, dispensary, bank, laundry, barber, communications center, and numerous shops and tea stalls.

Foreign guests are lodged in the International Guest House, a gated compound that can accommodate about three hundred guests in shared rooms with attached baths. The dining hall offers a choice of Indian and Western food.

Schedule

There is no group meditation, but all initiates are expected to meditate for two and a half hours daily on their own. The suggested time for meditation is between 3 and 6 A.M. Seva (service work) is permitted, but not required, in the morning from 9 A.M. to lunchtime and in the afternoon following lunch until satsang at 5:30 P.M.

Fees

There is no charge for food and lodging for foreign guests. Initiates may make a donation but this is not requested or encouraged. Guests who are not initiates are not allowed to make donations.

Contact Information

Radha Soami Satsang Beas
P.O. Dera Baba Jaimal Singh
Dist. Amritsar 143 204
Punjab
Tel: 91-1853-72345, 72346
Fax: None

U.S. Contact:
Normal L. Krause
General Secretary

RADHA SOAMI SOCIETY BEAS—AMERICA
18 COUNTRYSIDE DRIVE
HUTCHINSON, KS 67502
TEL: (316) 662-2242
FAX: (316) 663-6943

How to Get There

The closest airport is in Amritsar, Punjab. The community is about 40 kilometers east of Amritsar near Beas. You can take a train, bus, or taxi from Amritsar to Beas and an autorickshaw to the main gate of the ashram. From Delhi, trains or buses are available to Beas (approximately 410 kilometers).

The Radha Soami Satsang Beas secretary in New Delhi will make train reservations for accepted visitors, and they will be met at the train station in Beas by an ashram vehicle.

Other Services

The ashram is self-contained with all services that a visitor is likely to need. Foreign visitors are not permitted to stay outside the ashram (in the Beas area) and commute to the ashram.

Beas (population about 10,000) has food stalls and some services (but no foreigner accommodations). Amritsar (population 750,000) has all services available.

Books and Tapes

These are available from RSSB centers in India and worldwide. In the United States, contact:

R. S. BOOK SALES DEPT.
73-675 JUNIPER STREET
PALM DESERT, CA 92260

or

R. S. Audio Tape Sales
P.O. Box 611
Petaluma, CA 94953
(707) 762-5749

Contact the headquarters in India or the United States (see Contact Information) for a list of centers worldwide.

The Lord has provided both Sound and Light in each one of us to enable us to reach His mansion. With the sound we are to determine the direction and with the Light, complete our spiritual journey home.

—Maharaj Charan Singh

SIKH PILGRIMAGE SITES IN *the Punjab*

The Golden Temple. There are five sacred sites associated with the Sikh gurus, but by far the most sacred is the Golden Temple (Hari Mandir) in Amritsar, Punjab. The Golden Temple was begun by the fourth Sikh guru Ramdas in 1577 and completed by his son, the fifth guru Arjan, in 1601 to serve as a central place of worship for Sikhs. Its foundation stone was laid by the Muslim saint Mian Mir. From morning till night musicians sing devotional songs—prayers and selections from the holy book sung in classical raga style, beautiful and uplifting even if you don't understand the language. The environment is also an exquisite example of Sikh architecture, a devotional song in marble.

The daily routine at the temple begins at 2 or 3 A.M., depending on the time of year. It begins with prayers and offerings by the faithful, followed by kirtan and reading of the Granth Sahib, the Sikh holy book, which is brought each day from its place in the nearby Akal Tahkt. (The Akal Tahkt, or "eternal seat of authority," is the oldest of the five seats of Sikh religious authority, where decisions regarding Sikh religious practices are made.)

The priest opens the holy book and reads verses at random, explaining them to the congregation. After kirtan at noon, prasad (blessed food) is distributed and the temple is cleaned. Kirtan continues until 9:30 P.M. when the Granth Sahib is taken back to the Akal Takht and the main gate of the temple is closed.

In the temple is a sacred pool from which it is customary for pilgrims to take a handful of water. There is a first-floor balcony where people can sit to listen to kirtan and meditate. Connected to the temple are rooms where pilgrims can stay, a community kitchen where visitors are fed free of charge, and a museum of Sikh history.

Amritsar is a pleasant city in the heart of the Punjab, near the border with Pakistan. It is easily accessible by air or rail from Delhi. It is possible to stay at the temple, but only for a night or two.

Anandpur Sahib. Anandpur, the City of Bliss, is like a town of Sikh temples rising out of nowhere along an otherwise ordinary stretch of Punjabi highway. Founded by the ninth Sikh guru in 1644, it is important in Sikh history as the place where the tenth Guru Gobind Singh created the Khalsa Brotherhood by initiating the first five Sikhs in 1699.

There are more than sixty temples and numerous shrines at Anandpur, including a fort built by Guru Gobind Singh, his military training ground, his residence, and the cremation site of Guru Tej Bahadur's head, brought to Anandpur after he was killed in Delhi. There are plenty of places to stay.

Around the time of the Hindu feast Holi, which occurs in March, the Sikhs celebrate Hola Mohalla, a three-day fair first held in 1700. Thousands of people attend this fair, originally intended to instill martial spirit in Sikhs during the fight against Mughal tyranny.

Anandpur is located between Nangal and Ropar, about 80 kilometers from Chandigarh. The best way to get there is to fly or take the train to Chandigarh, then taxi or bus to Anandpur—unless you want to taxi all the way from Delhi, about a seven-hour trip.

—LEA TERHUNE

Brahma Kumaris World Spiritual University
Mt. Abu, Rajasthan

Brahma Baba, founder (1880–1969)
Dadi Prakash Mani, Chief Administrative Head (1922–)

It can take a whole day just to tour the facilities at the Brahma Kumaris World Spiritual University, a massive educational and spiritual complex set against the serene beauty of Mt. Abu. Founded to "establish Universal Peace through the impartation of spiritual knowledge and training in Easy Raja Yoga Meditation," the Brahma Kumaris—literally, the "daughters of Brahma"—are a booming organization, with 4,500 centers in sixty-six countries and about 400,000 members. The recipients of seven peace awards from the United Nations, the Brahma Kumaris emphasize morality, celibacy, peacework, and social action—all fueled by cultivating a relationship with God and the soul through the practice of meditation.

Teachers and Teachings

The Brahma Kumaris were founded in the 1930s by a former jewel merchant named Brahma Baba, who left his business and turned to the spiritual life after receiving a series of visions of God in the form of Shiva. According to these visions, the Kali Yuga—the present era of suffering—was soon to come to an end through a great catastrophe; it would be followed by the golden age of the Satyuga, "where man will be a veritable deity, where women will have equal rights with men, and where there will be no crime and no sin."

Brahma Baba devoted the rest of his life to trying to create a prototype of this new world order. Believing that women had been deprived of their due spiritual and social stature, he established a spiritual community primarily run by women. Although the students are composed of men and women about equally, the leadership is vested in a group of nine women known as "dadis," or sisters.

The central teachings of the Brahma Kumaris hold that there is only one God, the incorporeal, changeless, and eternal "Mother-Father of all souls," and that we can develop a "spiritual love-link" with God through the practice of "Raja Yoga Meditation." As taught by the Brahma Kumaris, this is not the classic raja yoga of Patanjali, but a simple, practical method of turning the mind inward and focusing on your true identity as a pure, peaceful soul. You are taught to see others as souls as well; to understand that all your actions have karmic consequences; to open your heart to the Supreme Being; and to cultivate the qualities of tolerance, courage, cooperation, accommodation, discrimination, judgment, and a quiet mind.

Virtue and morality are emphasized and symbolized by the white clothes of the brothers and sisters. Our true identity is said to be spirit, not flesh—celibacy is encouraged as a means of detaching from the body. Once we realize our true nature, the Brahma Kumaris say, we can rise above the limitations of gender, race, and nationality to create a harmonious global community.

Visitors can participate in a free meditation course (which takes a minimum of three days), which requires that you find your own accommodations and meals outside the ashram. You can also apply to stay at the ashram and follow the busy community schedule, which begins with a 4 A.M. meditation period and continues until 10 P.M. If the path appeals to you, you can become a "spiritual family member," a process in which you agree to follow certain practices that include celibacy and abstinence from alcohol and drugs. There's no formal initiation; participation is on the honor system. Family members are encouraged—but not obliged—to give a donation of one rupee per day to support the work of the Brahma Kumaris.

Facilities and Food

The extensive campus can house up to 15,000 guests and includes numerous conference centers, auditoriums (wired with individual headsets for simultaneous translation into sixteen languages), meditation halls, dining rooms, athletic areas, museums, a sewage treatment plant, and a free hospital. The International Spiritual Art Gallery is a combination educational center and museum with multimedia presentations and a laser-light show. Brahma Baba's former house and offices have been converted into meditation areas—especially charming is the garden house, surrounded by trellises of grapevines, where Baba did much of his writing.

Mt. Abu is a forested mountain oasis with huge rock outcroppings, palm and mango trees, beautiful lakes, clear air, and splendid stars at night. The buildings and grounds are beautifully constructed and maintained (with white being the dominant color, both inside and out); the food is among the best you'll have at any ashram in India.

Schedule

The free meditation course lasts a minimum of three days and consists of nine basic lessons. There's no particular schedule, but classes generally take about two hours a day, plus meditation periods and consultations with instructors. Course participants are responsible for their own meals and accommodations outside the ashram.

If you want to stay at the ashram, you can apply at any of the centers worldwide to stay for two weeks or more. If you stay at the ashram, you must follow the community schedule, which begins with meditation at 4 A.M., followed by a discourse from 6:30 to 7:30 A.M. You'll do community work in the morning and afternoon, then attend more classes in the late afternoon and evening.

Fees

All classes and activities are free. "Family members" are encouraged to give a donation of one rupee per day or more if they desire. Nonmembers are not allowed to give donations to the ashram, although if you wish you may give a contribution to the charitable hospital.

Contact Information

BRAHMA KUMARIS WORLD SPIRITUAL UNIVERSITY
POST BOX NO. 2
MT. ABU 307501
RAJASTHAN
TEL: 91-2974-38788 (OR 89, 90, 91)
FAX: 91-2974-22116

U.S. Contact:
GLOBAL HARMONY HOUSE
46 S. MIDDLE NECK RD
GREAT NECK, NY 11021
TEL: (516) 773-0971

How to Get There

Mt. Abu is about 195 kilometers from Udaipur, Rajasthan, and 224 kilometers from Ahmedabad, Gujarat. It's 27 kilometers from Abu Road, a major rail junction with trains from Delhi and Ahmedabad. You can also take a bus from Udaipur or Ahmedabad. The main Brahma Kumaris reception area is about 2 kilometers from the center of Mt. Abu on Subash Road.

Other Services

Mt. Abu is an active tourist area with a population of about 18,000. Most facilities are available.

Books, Tapes, and Affiliated Centers

The Brahma Kumaris publishes a booklet listing contact information for thousands of centers worldwide.

For the next few days just take up two or three simple themes or phrases, such as, "I am a peaceful soul," "I am a being of light and love spreading these feelings to others and the world" and "I am a subtle point of consciousness so different from the physical body." Repeat these thoughts gently to yourself, allowing them to sink more and more deeply, until your thoughts and your feelings match each other. When this happens, the tension between what you think you should be doing and what you actually are doing disappears, and the soul feels content and full. In addition, prac-

*tice seeing others as souls, seeing beyond the part to the actor
who is playing the part.*

—from *Practical Meditation*

$$\boxed{\text{PILGRIMAGE SITES IN } \textit{Rajasthan}}$$

Pushkar. Near Ajmer, about 140 kilometers from Jaipur, Pushkar is an important pilgrimage spot because it has the only temple dedicated exclusively to Brahma in all of India. Pilgrims bathe in Pushkar Lake, which Brahma decreed has the power to remove sins. A famous livestock fair is held here every year in November.

In season, hotels are often full. During the annual fair Rajasthan Tourism and private operators set up tent cities to accommodate the crowds. Pushkar may be reached by road from Ajmer.

Mt. Abu. The site of the Brahma Kumaris World Spiritual University (p. 239), Mt. Abu is also the home of the magnificent Dilwara Temples, one of the chief pilgrimage places of the Jain religion. There are several temples in the complex, but the two most enthralling for their intricate marble sculpture are the Vimal Vasahi and the Tejpal temples. The Vimal Vasahi temple is the oldest, built in 1031—it's said that it took fifteen hundred sculptors and twelve hundred laborers fourteen years to complete it. It is dedicated to Adinath, the first tirthankar (enlightened Jain teacher). The Tejpal temple was built in 1230 and dedicated to the twenty-second tirthankar, Neminath. In addition to representations of Mahavir and the other tirthankaras, the temples contain images of Hindu gods and goddesses, such as Krishna, Saraswati, Shitala, Narasingha, and others.

Mt. Abu is also full of Hindu sacred sites, including Nakki Lake. According to tradition, this lake was dug by a sage using only his fingernails—a dip in its waters is said to be as cleansing (spiritually, that is) as a bath in the Ganges. The lake is in the center of downtown Mt. Abu, next to the fourteenth-century Raghunathji Temple.

—LEA TERHUNE

Saccidananda Ashram, Shantivanam
Kulittalai, Tamil Nadu

Father Christudas (dates unkown)

The Benedictine monks at Saccidananda Ashram describe themselves as "Christian sannyasis"—they dress in the saffron robes of Hindu ascetics, walk barefoot and eat sitting on the floor, and study Vedanta and yoga as thoroughly as the *Rule of Saint Benedict*. Their rustic ashram— for many years the home of Father Bede Griffiths, a famous pioneer of Hindu-Christian dialogue—is meant to be "a place of meeting for Hindus and Christians and people of all religions or none, who are genuinely seeking God."

Teachers and Teachings

I had begun to realize that there was something missing in the Western Church; we only live out half of our soul; the conscious rational side," Father Griffiths wrote. "We still have to discover the other half, the unconscious, intuitive dimension." At the Saccidananda Ashram, Indian mysticism—with its emphasis on a direct experience of God—is embraced both philosophically and ritually. The church is built in the style of a south Indian temple. Two hours a day are set aside for meditation; prayer sessions include readings from the Vedas, the Upanishads, and the Bhagavad Gita; arati is performed before the Blessed Sacrament; sandal paste, kumkum, and vibhuti are placed at the third eye; "om" is chanted as part of the daily prayers. Even Christian teachings are often couched in Hindu terms (as when Father Griffiths referred to Christ as "the Atman, the true Self, of every being").

The ashram was founded in 1950 by two French priests who took Sanskrit names to show their identification with the Hindu quest for God. After one priest died and the other priest (Abhishiktananda, the author of several classic works on Hindu and Christian mysticism) became a hermit in the Himalayas, the ashram was taken over by the Benedictine monks of Father Bede Griffiths's order. Father Griffiths himself lived there until his death in 1993, and the place is still steeped in his spirit of simplicity, tolerance, and love.

According to one long-term resident, this ashram is for "silence, meditation, and new spiritual insights and interreligious dialogue and living. This is not a tourist center. The ashram is conducive to those who are seeking a deep spiritual interior life." Christmas, of course, is a particularly wonderful time to be there for Christmas rituals with an Indian twist.

Facilities and Food

Accommodations are spartan but adequate. The guest house has twelve private rooms, five semiprivate rooms, and thirty-two dormitory beds. Bedding and mattresses are provided.

Schedule

The day starts at 5 A.M. with prayers, meditation, and Eucharist. Midday and evening prayers and meditation are also held. Talks on yoga or Indian spirituality are often given in the afternoon. In the evening is satsang, which the monks define as "divine exchanges with friends and guests."

Fees

Donation.

Contact Information

SHANTIVANAM
TANNIRPALLI P.O. 639 107
KULITTALAI
DIST. TIRUCHIRAPALLI
TAMIL NADU
SOUTH INDIA
TEL AND FAX: 91-4323-22260

U.S. Contact:
BEDE GRIFFITHS TRUST
NEW CAMALDOLI HERMITAGE
BIG SUR, CA 93920
TEL: (408) 667-2456

How to Get There

The closest airports with scheduled air service are at Madras and Madurai. The nearest city is Tiruchirapalli (Tiruchy), which can be reached from Madras or Madurai by rail, bus, or taxi. Then proceed to Kulittalai (30 kilometers) by bus or taxi and then to the ashram (3 kilometers) by taxi or autorickshaw.

Other Services

About 3 kilometers from the ashram is the town of Kulittalai, which has a population of about 10,000. There are restaurants, food stalls, shops, and limited accommodations here. Tiruchirapalli, which is about 30 kilometers from the ashram, has all services available.

Books and Tapes

Books, ashram bhajans, and cassettes are available for sale in the office of the ashram.

It is the task of the Christian monk to try to enter into the whole tradition of Indian sannyasa, the renunciation of the world and all family ties in order to 'realize' God, to discover the in-dwelling presence of God both in nature and the soul. . . . This is the point at which Hindu and Christian spirituality have to meet. We have to make the discovery of Christ as the Atman, the true Self, of every being.

—FATHER BEDE GRIFFITHS

The Krishnamacharya Yoga Mandiram
Madras, Tamil Nadu

T. K. V. Desikachar (1939–)

The word "mandiram" comes from the Sanskrit verb "mandir," which means "to remove heavy burdens." That's the stated mission of the Krishnamacharya Yoga Mandiram, which was founded by T. K. V. Desikachar to perpetuate the teachings of his father, the world-renowned yoga master T. Krishnamacharya. At their small, unassuming headquarters on the edge of a slum neighborhood at the southern tip of Madras, the KYM offers one-on-one instruction in asana, pranayama, Vedic chanting, yoga therapy, meditation, and yoga philosophy to hundreds of primarily Indian students every week. KYM teachers are also establishing yoga programs in remote rural villages; offering yoga to inmates at mental institutions; researching the effects of yoga on asthma, schizophrenia, heart disease, and mental retardation. In the words of one staff teacher, "Yoga should be made available to everyone. We don't want yoga to be thought of as an elite activity."

Teachers and Teachings

The Institute's primary focus is public service to the local community, not yoga education for Western students, and they have been unable to keep up with the recent surge of foreign interest in Krishnamacharya's style of yoga. They can't accept drop-in foreign visitors—instead, they encourage you to study Krishnamacharya's method with a teacher from your own country. Occasionally, however, some of Desikachar's Western students lead groups to the Mandiram, so you can experience these teachings at their source.

Arguably no one has more profoundly influenced the transmission of yoga to the West than T. Krishnamacharya, a master of yoga, ayurveda, and Indian philosophy who died in 1989 at the age of 101. Born into a family of yoga teachers tracing its ancestry back to Nathamuni, a ninth-century south Indian sage, Krishnamacharya studied Sanskrit and philosophy at India's leading universities and lived for many years with a yoga master in the mountains of Tibet. He ran a yoga school at the royal palace of the Maharaja of Mysore which attracted students from all over India, including princes and government officials. Many of Krishnamacharya's students have gone on to be famous teachers in their own right, such as B. K. S. Iyengar (p. 221), K. Patthabhi Jois (p. 142), Indira Devi, and his own son T. K. V. Desikachar.

As Krishnamacharya's son, Desikachar grew up in an atmosphere steeped with the sage's encyclopedic knowledge of yoga, ayurveda, astrology, Sanskrit, and Vedanta. However, he pursued a degree in civil engineering, and didn't turn to yoga until his early twenties, when, with characteristic enthusiasm, he became his father's most avid pupil. Giving up his engineering career, he devoted the next three decades to intensive study and apprenticeship with Krishnamacharya.

At the core of Krishnamacharya's approach is the concept of *viniyoga*—the belief that yoga teaching must be individually tailored to suit an individual's age, cultural background, occupation, physical condition, mental ability, disposition, and other such factors. In keeping with viniyoga philosophy, there are no group yoga classes offered at the Krishnamacharya Yoga Mandiram. Instead, the twenty-five staff teachers—most of whom hold other jobs outside the Mandiram—volunteer an average of three to five hours each day to offer one-on-one sessions to the hundreds of clients that pass through the center's doors each week. Over the past two decades, KYM has served over 16,000 people—and an average of six to ten new ones sign in every day, most of them local residents seeking relief from asthma, back pain, headaches, stress, and other common ailments. (The KYM has developed an excellent track record with local doctors, who regularly refer clients.)

There are no quick fixes at the KYM. Each student is assigned to a teacher, who carefully observes everything about the client's demeanor during an initial interview. How does he sit on the backless stools in the interview room? Does she answer questions directly? Does he look the teacher in the eye? How wide does she open her mouth when she speaks, and how deep or shallow is her breathing?

The teacher then works with the student to develop an individually tailored regime—one that addresses not just the symptoms, but their source. For example, rather than prescribe a standard set of poses for back pain, the teacher will seek to ascertain its physical or emotional source. Is it a slipped disk? A critical mother-in-law? A sedentary job? A husband who works all the time? Incorrect lifting of heavy objects? Each of these situations will elicit a different recommendation. At the end of a session, stick-figure poses are scrawled on a ditto pad and handed to the student like a prescription, along with recommendations for dietary or other lifestyle changes. (Poses are precisely sequenced and synchronized with the breath, another key component of Krishnamacharya's teachings.) After several days or a week of practice, the student comes back to report on his progress, and a new set of practices is prescribed based on the student's feedback.

One of the Mandiram's specialties is teaching the chanting of the Vedas—ancient texts that Hindus believe are the direct words of God—both as a spiritual practice and a form of therapy. According to Krishnamacharya, chanting is a physical expression of the breath, which is the link between body and mind; the way you chant both reveals and influences your mental state. Chanting of classical Vedic texts—for centuries forbidden to anyone but Brahmin males—is taught as a form of meditation, which reveals instantly the student's level of concentration and presence.

Just as different asanas mold the body and nervous system in different ways, so each Sanskrit syllable has a precise effect on the consciousness. Chanting is used in combination with asanas for therapeutic purposes and to heighten the link between body and mind. Certain mantras are chanted for their stimulating effect; others for their soothing qualities. "The effect of sound depends on little details: the pitch, the phonetics, even the posture in which it is done," explains Sujaya, one of the senior teachers. "The same sound has a different effect done in a forward bend and a back arch."

Because the teachings are so subtle and precise, it is advised that you study with a viniyoga teacher in your own country before coming to the Mandiram. Desikachar's senior Western students often bring groups to the Mandiram for organized, intensive two- to three-week courses tailored to the group's specific interests (ranging from yoga therapy to Vedic chanting to Patanjali's Yoga Sutras).

The center also offers a two-year, nonresidential teacher-training program (covering all aspects of yoga philosophy, therapy, and practice) and a three-month certificate program (focusing primarily on asana practice). These courses are primarily geared toward local Indian students.

Facilities and Food

The KYM consists of one small concrete building in a poor neighborhood at the southern tip of Madras. There are no residential or kitchen facilities and no restaurants or hotels in the immediate neighborhood.

Some Western students stay at Woodlands, a hotel about ten minutes away by rickshaw. Others rent rooms in local houses—one favorite is at 38, 6th Main Road, a few blocks away.

Schedule

Schedules are worked out individually with your assigned teacher. Desikachar conducts a public class on the Yoga Sutras every week—check the current schedule.

Fees

Fees are determined on an individual basis. Local people with limited funds receive sessions at no charge. Westerners generally pay more—the typical donation is about 150 rupees for each private session.

Contact Information

THE KRISHNAMACHARYA YOGA MANDIRAM
13, 4TH CROSS STREET
RAMAKRISHNA NAGAR
MADRAS 600 028
TEL: 91-49-37998

U.S. Contact:
VINIYOGA NETWORK
1164 NORTH HIGHLAND AVENUE
ATLANTA, GA 30306

How to Get There

The Mandiram is located at the southern tip of Madras in the district called Ramakrishnanagar. If your driver doesn't know where it is, tell him it's adjacent to Raja Annamalaipuram. Once you're there, ask locals for directions to the Mandiram.

Other Services

Madras is a major city, and all services are available.

A good introduction to the teachings of Krishnamacharya is *The Heart of Yoga: Developing a Personal Practice* by T. K. V. Desikachar (Inner Traditions). Other books and the quarterly journal *Darsanam* are available through the KYM.

The way yoga is taught nowadays often gives the impression that there is one solution to everyone's problems and one treatment for every illness. But yoga affects the mind, primarily, and each person's mind is different. . . . It is not that the person needs to accommodate him or herself to yoga, but rather the yoga practice must be tailored to fit each person.

—T. K. V. DESIKACHAR
(from *The Heart of Yoga*)

A. G. Mohan
Madras, Tamil Nadu

A. G. Mohan (1945–)

Initially, A. G. Mohan wasn't sure he was willing to be listed in a spiritual guidebook at all. "I'm sorry, but that is so American!" he said when he finished laughing about the idea. "I don't encourage yoga shopping." For eighteen years a student of the master T. Krishnamacharya, Mohan was one of the founding teachers at the Krishnamacharya Yoga Mandiram (p. 247). He now has a substantial international following of his own and offers private instruction and group courses—with the assistance of his wife, Indira, and his daughter, Nitya—at his seaside home in a village just south of Madras.

Mohan's teachings are rooted firmly in Krishnamacharya's lineage: practices tailored for the individual, integration of breath and movement, use of sound and chanting as spiritual and therapeutic tools. More than just focusing on techniques, though, he's interested in imparting the vision of a stable and unified way of life firmly based on the principles of the Vedas, the texts that have governed all aspects of Hindu life for thousands of years. "People come to India looking either for a guru who will do all the work for them, or a few techniques that will change their lives," he says. "But you have to develop some kind of inner stability, or the techniques are useless."

A former engineer, Mohan stresses the importance of understanding the fundamental principles of breath, movement, mind, and prana that underlie all the different yoga techniques. He emphasizes that yoga is a complete, internally consistent system—developed in conjunction with ayurveda—that can be explained on its own terms, without reference to Western anatomy and physiology. Each practice, he says, has two parts: the technology and the spiritual attitude. If you do a forward bend, for instance, you should know the proper body mechanics; but you should also know the right attitude to take, which is that "you are placing your head and heart at the feet of the Divine."

Mohan's daughter, Nitya, is a classically trained musician—she recorded her first cassette of Vedic chanting at age nine—who teaches Vedic chanting, bhajans, voice exercises, and other musical explorations as therapy and spiritual practice. You can arrange private sessions with Mohan, Indira, or Nitya. Upon request, Mohan will conduct group courses on topics like ayurveda, therapeutic yoga, and yoga philosophy. (He's extremely knowledgeable but somewhat disorganized, so it's best to spell out clearly your area of interest, or you may get a brilliant series of lectures on Vedic family values when what you wanted was information on yoga techniques for lower back pain. On the other hand, you may find out that the two topics aren't so far apart as you might have thought.)

Mohan is especially good at teaching Westerners how to observe and learn from Indian culture—which, he says, is the only real reason to come to India to study yoga. "There are very few people here who can really teach asana and pranayama—and what most people are teaching here you can get in the West anyway," he says with characteristic bluntness. "So why come? Because India has something valuable to teach you, if you know how to look at her." He often arranges tours for groups of foreigners, giving them pointers beforehand on how to see the spiritual lessons that India has to offer. "If you just see the filth, you're missing it," he says. "You may feel sorry for the people you see living in the street. But if you look closer, you may see that they are happy—and you are not."

Facilities and Food

Sessions are held in Mohan's spacious house in a suburb of Madras near the Bay of Bengal. There are no living accommodations for guests. If you're planning a lengthy stay, you can try to rent a room in a nearby home quite cheaply. For shorter visits, you can rent quiet ocean-view rooms at the nearby Buharis Blue Lagoon Beach Resort Hotel for about Rs 400 a night. There's not much in the way of good restaurants in Pallavakkam.

Schedule

Individually arranged.

Fees

Donation.

Contact Information

A. G. MOHAN
PLOT # 27, VGP LAYOUT, PART-1
PALLAVAKKAM
MADRAS 600 041
TEL AND FAX: 91-44-4925460

How to Get There

Pallavakkam is a suburb just south of the Madras city limits. From Madras, take bus or autorickshaw to Pallavakkam. Call for directions to Mohan's house.

Other Services

There is an STD booth in Pallavakkam, but no fax. The closest hotel is the Buharis Blue Lagoon (about 5 kilometers away, in Neelankarai). All services are available in Madras.

Books and Tapes

Yoga for Body, Breath, and Mind by A. G. Mohan (Rudra Press).

"Whether we want to touch our toes or reach God, there must be movement. This movement is yoga."

—A. G. MOHAN
(from *Yoga for Body, Breath, and Mind*)

Krishnamurti Foundation
Vasanta Vihar Study Centre
Madras, Tamil Nadu

J. Krishnamurti (1895–1986)

Truth is a pathless land, and you cannot approach it by any path what-soever, by any religion, by any sect," proclaimed the philosopher Jid-dhu Krishnamurti. The Vasanta Vihar Study Centre was inspired by Krishnamurti's vision of "a place of learning and austere living with inward discipline and work, without a guru, without a leader, and without a system of meditation or working." In keeping with his rejection of organized religion and spiritual methods, there are no formal programs offered at the Center; however, you can stay in the small guest house on its serene six-acre campus and study Krishnamurti's teachings via books, videos, audio-tapes, unpublished writings, and even CD Roms.

For anyone interested in Krishnamurti, this place—with its flower gardens, groves of coconut and mango, and remarkably solicitous staff—is an ideal retreat from the din of Madras. Krishnamurti was catapulted into the public eye at age thirteen, when a clairvoyant former schoolmaster named Charles Leadbeater—an official of the Theosophical Society (p. 258), which was then making headlines with its occult speculations and investigations of paranormal phenomena—spotted him playing on the beach outside the Society headquarters in Madras. According to Leadbeater, the young boy—whom teachers and relatives dismissed as dimwitted, due to his vacuous manner and inability to concentrate—had the most extraordinary aura he had ever seen and was destined to be an incomparable spiritual teacher. Within months, Krishnamurti had been taken from his parents and taken under the wing of Society president Annie Besant. He was proclaimed to be the vehicle into which the Lord Maitreya, the "World Teacher" whose coming was prophesied by Theosophical scriptures, would incarnate.

Krishnamurti was given a strict British education and indoctrinated into Theosophy's esoteric teachings (including nightly visits to the astral plane, under Leadbeater's guidance, to imbibe the instructions of disembodied Masters). A spiritual group called the Order of the Star was organized around him and attracted thousands of members in Europe and the United States. However, a series of intense mystical experiences—including the classic and often excruciating symptoms of kundalini awakening—led Krishnamurti to question everything the Theosophists had taught him. In 1929 he publically dissolved the Order of the Star, returned all of its assets to the donors, and renounced all formal religious paths. In a speech that summed up the philosophy he would follow the rest of his life, he explained:

"Truth, being limitless, unconditioned, unapproachable by any path whatsoever, cannot be organized; nor should any organization be formed to lead or to coerce people along any particular path. . . . If an organization be created for this purpose, it becomes a crutch, a weakness, a bondage, and must cripple the individual, and prevent him from growing, from establishing his uniqueness, which lies in the discovery for himself of that absolute, unconditioned Truth."

With the death of Annie Besant in 1933, Krishnamurti's last links with the Theosophical Society were broken. Although he adamantly insisted he did not want devotees, he quickly developed a massive following, and for more than fifties years he traveled worldwide giving penetrating, provocative public lectures and interviews. Recognized as one of the century's greatest spiritual philosophers, he aimed to set people free by cutting through the veil of dogma and concepts that kept them from experiencing naked truth with an alert and sensitive mind. He scorned all formal systems of meditation, advocating instead a free-form but rigorous process of observation and inquiry.

"I can't find a strong enough word to deny that whole world of gurus, of their authority, because they think they know. A man who says 'I know,' such a man does not know. Or if a man says, 'I have experienced truth,' distrust him completely," he said. "Systems make the mind mechanical, they don't give you freedom, they may promise freedom at the end, but freedom is at the beginning, not at the end."

Facilities and Food

The Vasanta Vihar Study Centre—the headquarters of the Indian branch of the Krishnamurti Foundation—is a peaceful six-acre campus with flower gardens and coconut and mango groves. A guest house can accommodate about twenty people (in addition to the five permanent residents) in rooms with attached baths. Other facilities include a meditation hall and a laundry service. Vegetarian breakfast, lunch, dinner, and tea are offered.

The guest house is solely for people who want to study Krishnamurti's teachings and shouldn't be treated as a hotel base for sightseeing or business in Madras. As rooms are limited, you're asked to register at least fifteen days in advance of your arrival.

In Krishnamurti's stately former residence is a library containing copies of all of his books (including translations), photocopies of out-of-print books, biographies, and commentaries on his teachings, and bulletins of the Krishnamurti Foundation, as well as other works on religion, psychology, literature, and the arts. There are video and audio consoles for playing tapes of Krishnamurti's talks. Books and tapes can be checked out. An archives building houses photographs and rare unpublished material.

This is a place for individual study; there is no organized program of meditation or lectures. The study center is open to visitors from 10 A.M. to 1 P.M. and from 2 to 7 P.M. every day except Mondays. Occasionally there are spontaneous discussion groups, video viewings, or silent sittings. Every Saturday at 5:30 P.M. there is a video screening that is open to the public.

Fees

Contributions are flexible according to the guest's capacity. The minimum suggested donation is Rs 75 per day; foreign guests are asked to contribute the equivalent of $10 (U.S.) per day.

Contact Information

KRISHNAMURTI FOUNDATION
VASANTA VIHAR STUDY CENTRE
64 GREENWAYS ROAD
MADRAS 600 028 TAMIL NADU
TEL: 91-44-4937803 OR 4937596
FAX: 91-44-4991360

U.S. Contact:
KRISHNAMURTI FOUNDATION OF AMERICA
P.O. BOX 1560
OJAI, CA 93024
TEL: (805) 646-2726
FAX: (805) 646-6674

How to Get There

The Vasanta Vihar Study Centre is located in the Adyar area in the southern part of Madras and can be reached by autorickshaw, bus, or taxi. Tell the driver it's on Greenways Road near Satya Studios.

Other Services

All services are available in Madras.

Books and Tapes

Books and tapes are available for purchase at the Study Centre and through the Krishnamurti Foundation of America. Good introductory works include *The Awakening of Intelligence* by J. Krishnamurti (Harper-SanFrancisco) and *Total Freedom: The Essential Krishnamurti* (Harper-SanFrancisco).

One can see that it is a waste of energy to follow anybody—you understand?—to have a leader, to have a guru, because when you follow you are imitating, you are copying, you are obeying, you are establishing authority and your energy is therefore diffused. Do observe this; please do so. Don't go back to your gurus, to your societies, to your authorities, drop them like hot potatoes. . . . [E]nergy is wasted when you indulge in ideation, in theories: whether there is a soul or no soul, whether there is an Atman, or no Atman—isn't it a waste of time, a waste of energy? When you read or listen to some saint endlessly, or some sannyasi, making commentaries on the Gita, or the Upanishads—just think of it!— the absurdity of it!—the childishness of it! Somebody explains some book which in itself is dead, written by some dead poet, giving to it a tremendous significance.

—J. KRISHNAMURTI
(from *The Awakening of Intelligence*)

Theosophical Society Headquarters
Madras, Tamil Nadu

🐚 *Madame H. P. Blavatsky (1831–1891)*
🐚 *Colonel H. S. Olcott (1832–1907)*

The Theosophical Society Headquarters sits on what's probably the most beautiful piece of property in Madras: a 249-acre tropical park bordered by ocean and river beaches and densely forested with frangipani, mango, bougainvillea, banyan, coconut, rain trees, and other jungle plants. Unfortunately, you have to be an active Society member to stay here; however, visitors are welcome to stroll through the estate (a welcome respite from the pollution of Madras), visit the bookstore and enormous research library, and attend the public lectures offered through the Society's School of Wisdom.

Teachers and Teachings

As stated in its charter, the Theosophical Society has three purposes: "To form a nucleus of the Universal Brotherhood of Humanity, without distinction of race, creed, sex, caste, or color; To encourage the study of Comparative Religion, Philosophy, and Science; To investigate unexplained laws of Nature and the powers latent in man." The tenets of Theosophy— a word that means "divine wisdom"—are strongly influenced by Hinduism, Buddhism, and nineteenth-century Western occultism. However, the Society itself is dedicated to philosophical and spiritual freedom, stressing that "there is no doctrine, no opinion, by whomsoever taught or held, that is in any way binding on any member of the Society, none which any member is not free to accept or reject."

The Theosophical Society was founded in New York in 1875 by Madame H. P. Blavatsky, a dispossessed Russian aristocrat and occultist, and Colonel Henry Olcott, a former attorney and journalist who became Madame Blavatsky's most ardent admirer. At the time of their meeting, Madame Blavatsky was working in a sweatshop making artificial flowers for a living and mesmerizing audiences with tales of her travels in India and Tibet and her apparent abilities to conjure up spirits, materialize showers of flower petals, and produce mysterious rapping noises under séance tables. Under the patronage of the Colonel—who scandalized New York society by setting up house with her, although their relationship apparently remained platonic—she wrote a massive spiritualist opus called *Isis Unveiled,* which she claimed was telepathically dictated to her by an assortment of disembodied "Masters." (These Masters, the astounded Colonel reported, also had a penchant for penning letters that dropped from thin air onto his desk in his study.)

Isis Unveiled laid out the fundamentals of Theosophy, an esoteric stew of American spiritualism, Eastern religion, and evolutionary theory. Theosophy posits, among other things, an all-pervading spiritual force that creates and sustains the world; a divine plan that guides everything from the electron to the stars; and a human soul that incarnates again and again on an evolutionary path toward perfect understanding of its identity with the Absolute. Theosophy stresses the law of karma, the power of thought to shape reality, and the existence of untapped powers—within and without—that can help us along on our spiritual journey. In the Theosophical view, "The soul of man is immortal and its future is the future of a thing whose growth and splendour has no limit."

When its U.S. membership dwindled in the wake of mocking press coverage, Madame Blavatsky and the Colonel moved the Theosophical Society to India, where they hoped its ideas would find more fertile soil. Although public controversy continued until Madame Blavatsky's death—including charges that her purported miracles were cleverly faked stage tricks—the Society attracted leading intellectuals and flourished as a forum for the study of comparative religion and the investigation of paranormal phenomenon. Today, there are over 30,000 members in fifty countries.

In its modern form, the Society focuses on study of the world's wisdom traditions. Each December, the Society holds its week-long international convention at the headquarters in Adyar. The convention is for members only but includes some lectures that are open to the public. For more in-depth study, members can attend the two-and-a-half-month courses offered twice a year through the School of Wisdom, whose syllabus includes studies of the Upanishad, Kabir, mysticism and modern physics, Ramana Maharshi, Krishnamurti, and modern occultism. These courses also include some public lectures.

Facilities and Food

The magnificent gardens include the world's largest banyan tree, with branches and dangling roots covering 40,000 square feet. The Adyar Library, one of the main attractions, has about 250,000 printed books and 17,000 rare palm-leaf and paper manuscripts, as well as some interesting displays of historic texts. There are temples and shrines to many different faiths, including Buddhism, Christianity, Hinduism, Islam, Zoroastrianism, and Freemasonry.

Accommodations are only for members who have some serious spiritual or scholarly work to do at the Society. Members must apply to the Society in India with a recommendation from their branch or lodge in their home country. To become a member, you must apply to your local branch. Enrolling in the School of Wisdom course does not automatically grant you accommodations at Adyar.

Schedule

Visiting hours are 8:30 to 10 A.M. and 2 to 4 P.M. daily, except Sundays and holidays. During these hours you can tour the grounds, get information about the Society, visit the library, etc. The Society's annual convention is held the last week of December and there are public lectures and symposiums at that time. The School of Wisdom courses run from October through mid-December and January through mid-March. During most of the year there are public talks on the first and third Wednesday of every month.

Fees

There is no charge for public lectures or for visiting the grounds. Members should contact their local chapters for information about fees for School of Wisdom courses or accommodations at Adyar.

Contact Information

THEOSOPHICAL SOCIETY HEADQUARTERS
ADYAR, MADRAS 600 020
TEL: 91-44-4912815

U.S. Contact (for books and tapes):
THE THEOSOPHICAL SOCIETY IN AMERICA
PUBLISHING HOUSE
P.O. BOX 270
WHEATON, IL 60189
TEL: (708) 665-0130
FAX: (708) 668-4976

Adyar is a residential area on the southern fringe of Madras, about 10 kilometers from the city center. You can get there by bus, autorickshaw, or taxi—any driver will know where it is.

Other Services

All services are available in Madras.

Books and Tapes

Books and tapes are available from the bookshop or from any Theosophical Society centers worldwide.

THE THREE GREAT TRUTHS

1. The soul of man is immortal and its future is the future of a thing whose growth and splendour has no limit.

2. The principle which gives life dwells in us and without us, is undying and eternally beneficent, is not heard or seen or smelt, but is perceived by the man who desires perception.

3. Each man is his own absolute law giver, the dispenser of glory or gloom to himself; the decreer of his life, his reward, his punishment.

—from *The Idyll of the White Lotus*

Vasavi Yogasram
Madras, Tamil Nadu

Sri Satchidananda Yogi (1908–)

It practically takes yogic siddhis just to *find* the Vasavi Yogasram, a tiny upper-floor apartment sandwiched between silk merchants and electronics shops on a teeming, muddy side street in the heart of Madras's oldest business district. There, in a small room that serves as both practice room and living quarters, the ninety-year-old Swami Satchidananda teaches classical hatha-yoga classes twice a day to local Indians and a few European devotees.

Teachers and Teachings

The walls are plastered with black-and-white photos of the swami some fifty years ago—as a handsome, muscular man in a white loincloth, demonstrating traditional yogic asanas. (Curiously, there are also quite a few pictures of grimacing weightlifters with swollen muscles.) Nowadays Swami Satchidananda uses these old yoga photos as teaching tools, pointing to them without speaking—he took a vow of silence over thirty years ago—and then snapping his fingers imperiously at the student he wants to assume the position. Classes are loosely structured, with each student working on different postures according to the swami's instructions.

Swami Satchidananda has toured in Europe and has an especially devoted following in France, Belgium, and Switzerland—European students often arrange group trips to study with him. He looks the part of an archetypical yogi, with a loose white robe and two meters of yellowed hair bundled around his head. (In the tradition of the ancient rishis, he has never cut his hair.) In addition to leading twice-daily hatha-yoga classes and a weekly puja to the Divine Mother, he gives instruction on mantra, kriyas, and yoga philosophy—communicated by writing on a chalkboard or translated by an Indian woman with whom he communicates in sign language. He stresses the importance of regular fasting to facilitate the flow of prana, which he promises will give "computer-banklike memory, masterly control of one's own senses, and everlasting youth along with bubbling vitality."

Facilities and Food

There are no residential or kitchen facilities; practice is done on woven straw mats in Swamiji's concrete-floored living room. There are many cheap hotels nearby where foreign students can stay. For groups of twenty to sixty people, special classes can be arranged at another location.

Schedule

Hatha-yoga classes for men only: 6 to 8 A.M.
For women only: 4 to 6 P.M.
Sri Devi Puja: Friday 6 P.M.

Fees

Donation only.

Contact Information

VASAVI YOGASRAM
106 GOVINDAPPANAYAK STREET
MADRAS 600 001
TAMIL NADU
TEL: NONE

European Contact:
SYLVIE DEGUIN
SHERIF HOLIDAYS
NO. 1, RUE PAUL COLLOMP
67000 STRASBOURG
FRANCE
TEL: 33-88-256012
FAX: 33-88-371355

How to Get There

The ashram is located on Govindappanayak (sometimes spelled Govindappa Naicken) Street in the Parry's Corner area of Madras. It's not far from the bus station at Parry's Corner, but it's hard to find—expect to ask directions several dozen times on your way there.

Other Services

All services are available in Madras.

Reaching the Unreached
G. Kallupatti, Periyakulam Taluk, Tamil Nadu

🍂 *Brother James Kimpton (1925–)*

The glory of life is to love, not to be loved; to give, not to get; to serve, not to be served," reads the first page of Reaching the Unreached's annual report. If you're interested in doing service work in rural India, you'll find plenty of volunteer opportunities—from digging wells to working in medical clinics—with this multifaceted charitable organization founded by a British Christian monk.

Teacher and Teachings

Although founded by a Christian from Britain, there's no proselytizing at Reaching the Unreached—the organization is run by Indians, and Brother James Kimpton laughs that in his almost forty years in India, he hasn't converted a single person. Instead, RTU focuses on down-to-earth matters—a medical clinic that serves 65,000 people a year; villages for orphans and abandoned children; leprosy clinics; schools and industries for village people. In the past fifteen years they've built over 5,000 low-cost homes and dug over 1,000 wells (with the help of Brother James's natural gifts as a "water witch").

An artist and monk in the De La Salle order, Brother James Kimpton came to India in the early 1960s to start an industrial training school for street children in Madurai. He went on to found a village for destitute village boys, which eventually became the seed of RTU.

The main campus of RTU consists of a foster village (where forty-eight foster mothers care for 250 children) and an administrative complex that includes schools and a medical clinic. From this core, aid flows to more than forty villages in a 1,600-square-mile area.

Almost anyone with a true desire to help can find something useful to do here—you can stay for as short or long a time as you want. Especially needed are people with skills in medicine, carpentry, masonry, or computers.

Facilities and Food

About fifteen volunteers can be accommodated in the guest area of the children's village in single or double rooms with attached baths. Accommodations are limited, so it's best to write in advance. Meals are served in the dining hall.

Schedule

Optional prayer sessions are held every morning and evening. The day is spent doing service work here and in the villages.

Fees

Donation only. Through special programs you can sponsor a child or family or designate funds for a particular type of service work.

Contact Information

REACHING THE UNREACHED
G. KALLUPATTI, PERIYAKULAM TALUK
DIST. MADURAI
TAMIL NADU 95203
TEL: 91-516-6659232
FAX: 91-516-6653349

U.S. Contact:
REACHING THE UNREACHED—USA
MR. JOHN CIOFFI
301 SOUTH SEAS DRIVE, SUITE 302
JUPITER, FL 33477
TEL: (561) 744–6508
FAX: (561) 775–0089

How to Get There

RTU is about 75 kilometers west of Madurai, which is accessible by plane, bus, or train. From Madurai, take a bus or taxi to G. Kallupatti. The first RTU facility you reach will be Anbu Illam (Place of Love Children's Village). Continue about .5 kilometer further to the main center and offices.

Other Services

There are few services available in the nearby villages, but Kodaikanal, a popular tourist hill station, is 50 kilometers away. There you can find restaurants, shops, and accommodations.

Books and Tapes

Two BBC films on Brother James and RTU are available through RTU—USA.

My own philosophy tends to make me concerned about individuals: a lost child, a sick person, a distraught mother, a family in need of everything. For example, a tiny baby girl two days old is brought to us, rescued from certain death (murder) because it was a girl. She is the fifth baby girl to be born to this family. Already the fourth had been killed shortly after birth. We welcomed the tiny child into our ever-growing families of abandoned children. A couple who cannot have children of their own were desperate to have a girl-child. They came a long way, they had waited for many months. And now we have brought them together: a baby girl in danger of swift death and a fine couple who had waited fifteen years for just such a baby.

—BROTHER JAMES KIMPTON

🌀 *Dr. Govindappa Venkataswamy (1918–)*

It's not an ashram or retreat center; the only way to participate is to volunteer your services. But if you're interested in the path of karma yoga—selfless service—there may be no better place to practice in India than the Aravind Eye Hospital, named for the philosopher and yogi Sri Aurobindo. Using a combination of modern medicine, Western management techniques, yogic philosophy, and sheer hard work, the hospital has become the world's largest and most efficient center for curing blindness, each year treating over 700,000 outpatients and conducting more than 90,000 sight-restoring surgeries. It's also a model of self-sustaining service work, providing a revolutionary example of how to help people and empower them at the same time.

Teachers and Teachings

Most of the hospital's patients are poor people—among India's fifteen million blind—who would otherwise be condemned to a life of darkness. "You don't have to be a religious person to serve God. You serve God by serving humanity," says the hospital's director, Dr. Govindappa Venkataswamy (generally known as "Dr. V."). A devotee of Sri Aurobindo and the Mother (p. 271) and a deep admirer of Gandhi, Dr. V. is committed to healing as a spiritual path. As he told *Yoga Journal*, "the goal of life is not to escape from the world to some higher consciousness, but to transform life on earth into a Divine Life."

This is not the place to come for casual tourism; but if you're willing to work, Dr. V. will find something for you to do. The center especially needs volunteers with skills in the area of management, organizational development, and communications. It's best to make arrangements in advance; you can contact Dr. Suzanne Gilbert at the Seva Foundation in the United States for more information (see Contact Information).

Despite hands crippled and swollen by rheumatoid arthritis, Dr. V. trained himself to use a surgeon's scalpel and has regularly performed over a hundred cataract operations a day (by contrast, the usual number for U.S. surgeons is five to ten). His center is a model for what he calls "compassionate capitalism." Over two-thirds of the surgery is provided for free, paid for by the other one-third of the patients (whose fees are also, by Western standards, astoundingly low). Aravind's own laboratory manufactures intraocular lenses—essential for effective cataract treatments—at a fraction of the cost of international suppliers, making sight affordable to millions of people previously doomed to blindness. (In the process, the lab has redefined the world market for such supplies, which was previously dominated by a few corporations whose prices were much higher.) Dr. V. hopes to replicate his hospital all over the world, becoming "the McDonald's hamburgers of worldwide eye care."

With about six hundred beds and hundreds of employees, the hospital is a beehive of activity—squeaky-clean, highly organized, and pulsating with no-nonsense, joyful energy. Associated with the hospital is the Aravind Institute, where people come from Asia, Africa, and other countries to study Aravind's systems and attempt to replicate them in their own countries.

Facilities and Food

There is a small guest house and a hostel near the Eye Hospital and Institute. These are not operated on a commercial basis but are for visiting ophthalmologists, residents, community health workers, and volunters. Depending on the purpose of your visit, it may be possible to stay at one of these facilities by prior arrangement.

Madurai has many hotels and restaurants available.

Schedule

The staff comes in at 6:30 A.M. and works until 6 P.M. or later at least six days a week. Tours are available by prior arrangement.

Fees

Donation.

Contact Information

ARAVIND EYE HOSPITAL
1, ANNA NAGAR

MADURAI 625 020
TAMIL NADU
TEL: 91-452-532653
FAX: 91-452-530986
E-MAIL: 102116.2236@COMPUSERVE.COM

U.S. Contact:
SEVA FOUNDATION
1786 FIFTH STREET
BERKELEY, CA 94710
TEL: (510) 845-7382
FAX: (510) 845-7410
E-MAIL: ADMIN@SEVA.ORG

How to Get There

Madurai is about 500 kilometers south of Madras and accessible by plane, bus, or train. The Aravind Eye Hospital is about 7 kilometers from the famous Meenakshi Temple (at the city center) and can be reached by taxi or autorickshaw.

Other Services

Madurai has a population of approximately 1 million, and all services are available.

Books and Tapes

None.

In our work, though we are confining ourselves to the control of blindness, we are also interested in seeing how we can grow in our consciousness, and whether we can become a new human being, not with a mind groping in darkness, but a human being who is a

*better instrument, an improvement, just as the electron micro-
scope is an improvement upon the ordinary microscope.*

—Dr. Govindappa Venkataswamy

Sri Aurobindo Ashram
Pondicherry, Tamil Nadu

🌿 *Sri Aurobindo (1872–1950)*
🌿 *The Mother (1878–1973)*

I am concerned with the Earth, not with worlds beyond for their own
sake; it is a terrestrial realization that I seek, not a flight to distant sum-
mits," wrote the revolutionary-turned-yogi Sri Aurobindo. The aim of
Aurobindo's "integral yoga" is not to transcend the limited body, mind, and
world in quest of spiritual perfection; but rather, to "draw down" the divine
energy—in a form he calls the Supramental—to create "a divine life in
Matter." His ashram is intended as a laboratory for that work, which he referred to as "the yoga of the cells."

Teachers and Teachings

Founded in the 1920s, Aurobindo's ashram stopped accepting new members in the 1960s, and there is no structured program of spiritual instruction or practice for visitors. Foreign guests who want to immerse
themselves long-term in the practice of Aurobindo's teachings are encouraged to do so at the nearby community of Auroville (p. 276).

However, guests are welcome to stay up to two weeks at one of the
guest houses (by far the best accommodations in Pondicherry); take meals
with ashramites at the collective dining hall; and meditate at the flower-
blanketed, incense-drenched samadhi shrine of Aurobindo and his spiritual
consort, the Mother.

With about two thousand members and four hundred buildings spread
throughout the seaside tourist town of Pondicherry, the ashram today feels

less like a retreat than a conglomerate of spiritually inspired businesses, ranging from handmade paper and steel dinnerware to ayurvedic medicines and the famous Auroshika incense. Don't even bother with the official ashram tour, unless you're dying to buy a hand-loomed sari, some sandal-wood perfume, or a really nice set of teak dining furniture. The tour does an excellent job of busing you around to the various ashram retail outlets, but omits any real insight into the community's spiritual practice.

That's too bad, because behind the scenes are some innovative explorations in alternative education, lifelong physical fitness, creative arts, and cooperative living. According to Aurobindo, human evolution is not yet complete. Just as human beings evolved from animals (a shift that is assumed, by Aurobindians, to be a step forward), so human beings can evolve, through the practice of cellular yoga, into a brand-new species. Man, says Aurobindo, is a "Mental being." The new human, on the other hand, will be fully imbued with the Supramental energy, or Truth-consciousness.

If all this strikes you as hopelessly abstract, this might not be the place for you. There are no gurus or teachers other than Aurobindo and the Mother. The actual methods of integral yoga are somewhat vague—there are no prescribed meditations, mantras, yoga exercises, or rituals, although all of these things can be done to prepare the body and mind for the Supramental descent. If you press a long-term devotee for specifics, you'll be instructed simply to set your sights on the Divine; reject all "undivine" impulses (among which are counted drugs, politics, and sex); and surrender yourself completely to the Divine guidance.

If you come to the ashram as a spiritual seeker, your best bet is to open yourself and trust that the appropriate teaching will be given to you. Advises the ashram receptionist, a forty-year-devotee, "Just sit by the samadhi and let your sense of 'I' evaporate like camphor, and the guidance will be given."

Indians revere Aurobindo not just for his spiritual insights, but for his leadership in the earliest days of India's independence movement. Born in Calcutta in 1872 to a wealthy Bengali family, Aurobindo Ghose was raised, at his father's insistence, with virtually no contact with India or Indians. At age five he was sent to a convent school in Darjeeling run by Irish nuns; at age seven he and his brother were sent to England, where they were raised by a reverend's family.

A brilliant scholar, Aurobindo studied classics at King's College, Cambridge. As a student, despite his father's precautions, he became gripped by the cause of Indian nationalism. At age twenty, he returned to India, where he began working as an educator and administrator in the government of the Maharaja of Baroda. He quickly became a prime instigator in India's budding nationalist movement against the British colonial regime. In 1908, he was imprisoned on charges of sedition, of which he was later acquitted; however, his year-long imprisonment awaiting trial proved transformational. While in jail he began an intensive study of the Bhagavad Gita and the practice of yoga; he saw the jail as an ashram, the guards as gurus, his fellow prisoners as manifestations of Krishna. To the bewilderment of his jailers, he spent the year in ecstasy.

Shortly after his release from prison, Sri Aurobindo withdrew from politics altogether and took asylum at the French colony of Pondicherry, where he devoted himself completely to the study and practice of yoga. His philosophical writings and poetry—lofty and impenetrable to the casual reader—attracted a worldwide following. Primary among them was a Parisian psychic and occultist named Mira Alfassa (whom Aurobindo named "the Mother"), who took over the ashram from its inception in 1926, when Aurobindo retired into complete seclusion. It was the Mother who launched the community of Auroville, which flourishes ten kilometers outside of Pondicherry (p. 276).

Today, the ashram community—almost entirely Indian—consists of thirteen hundred "inmates" handpicked by the Mother herself; five hundred students, aged three to twenty-one, enrolled in a unique "free progress" school designed by the Mother to prepare the next generation for the Supramental descent; and five hundred devotees who work in ashram businesses but make their own living arrangements. Since integral yoga is aimed at transforming the world, not renouncing it, all inmates and devotees work in the ashram businesses, without remuneration, as an essential component of their practice.

Facilities and Food

The whole eastern side of Pondicherry bears the ashram's stamp, with its tidy streets and sidewalks (studded with most un-Indian trashbins cheerfully labeled "use me") and its clean and spacious seaside boulevard. Most of the ashram's buildings house either industries, crafts, or services supplying the essential needs of the inmates (from shoemakers and tailors to plumbers and physicians). Other facilities include medical clinics (both allopathic and ayurvedic); a theater; an art studio and gallery; a dance hall; and a concert hall for both Indian and Western music. (Music and art, in the view of Aurobindo and the Mother, were direct channels to the Divine.)

The spiritual center of the ashram is a complex of four houses, two of which, at different times, were the homes of Sri Aurobindo and the Mother. In a quiet inner courtyard is their samadhi, where their bodies are buried in two chambers, one above the other. The library (with its peaceful reading room overlooking the ocean) and bookstore offer access to the voluminous writings of Aurobindo and the Mother.

As a guest, you can stay up to two weeks in one of the ashram guest houses. The best is the seaside Park Guest House, with immaculate rooms (bearing names like Tranquility, Perfection, and Transformation) and balconies overlooking the ocean. Unfortunately, since this is the best hotel in town, it's often impossible to get a room—in the high season it tends to be packed with guests attracted less by its spiritual affiliation than by its excellent value and daily housekeeping service. Since you can't make reservations in advance (unless you're a longtime donor for the ashram), your best bet is to show up on a weekday and just keep trying, despite the dragonlike demeanor of the reception staff. (The sign outside the office permanently reads "full"—go in and ask for a room anyway.) The International, Cottage, and Garden guest houses are also nice, although they don't have the Park's seaside charm. All guest houses have meditation rooms and dining rooms offering limited breakfast and lunch fare at reasonable rates.

For fifteen rupees a day, you can take your meals at the ashram dining hall along with the two thousand other ashramites. The food is excellent, simple Indian vegetarian, with many vegetables grown on the ashram farm.

Schedule

The samadhi shrine is open to all visitors between 8 A.M. and 6 P.M. daily. Those staying at the guest house are issued a pass that enables them to visit the shrine until 11 P.M. Pass holders may also attend collective meditation in the samadhi courtyard from 7:30 to 7:50 P.M. Mondays, Tuesdays, Wednesdays, and Fridays; and in the playground from 7:45 to 8:15 P.M. Thursdays and Sundays. Provided there are sufficient visitors, an ashram tour leaves the gate of the main building at 8:15 A.M. every day except Sunday.

A tour leaves daily for Auroville at 2:30 P.M., but you might as well skip it—all they do is take you to the Visitors Center and whisk you through the Mantrimandir temple, which you'd be better off visiting on your own (see p. 277).

Fees

This ashram definitely operates as a business—if you can't pay, you can't stay. The Park Guest House is Rs 150 to 250 per night, depending on your room; the International is Rs 50 to 100; Cottage is Rs 50; Garden is Rs 35. Rs 15 per day buys you a meal pass at the ashram dining hall.

Contact Information

Sri Aurobindo Ashram
Rue de la Marine
Pondicherry
Tamil Nadu 605 002
Tel: 91-413-34836

How to Get There

Pondicherry is accessible by bus (from Madras, Tiruvannamalai, Bangalore, Chidambaram, Ooty, and Madurai); and by train, via Villapuram on the Madras-Madurai line.

Other Services

Pondicherry is a major tourist center with a population of 517,000, and all services are available.

Books and Tapes

The writings of Sri Aurobindo include commentaries on yoga, Vedanta, Upanishads, Indian nationalism, politics, poetry, literature, and drama. A good introduction is *Integral Yoga: Sri Aurobindo's Teaching and Method of Practice* (Sri Aurobindo Ashram Press). In the United States, books can be ordered from Auromere Ayurvedic Imports, 2621 West Highway 12, Lodi, CA 95242; Tel: (209) 339-3710; Fax: (209) 339-3715; e-mail SASP@AOL.com.

If we want to find a true solution to the confusion, the chaos, and the misery of the world, we have to find it in the world itself. In fact, it is to be found only there: It exists latent, one has to bring it out. It is neither mystical nor imaginary, but altogether concrete, furnished by Nature herself, if we know how to observe her.

—THE MOTHER

Auroville
Pondicherry, Tamil Nadu

🌀 *Sri Aurobindo (1872–1950)*
🌀 *The Mother (1878–1973)*

There should be somewhere on Earth a place which no nation could claim as its own, where all human beings of goodwill who have a sincere aspiration could live freely as citizens of the world." With those words, the Mother—a French-born psychic and occultist who became the senior disciple of the revolutionary-turned-yogi Sri Aurobindo—launched the utopian community of Auroville in 1968, in the barren countryside just north of Pondicherry. Today, Auroville is an ongoing experiment in communal and ecological living, where about a thousand residents from thirty countries are working together to transform 2,600 acres of eroded and deforested wasteland into a green and self-sufficient community.

Teachers and Teachings

For orthodox Aurovillians, the community is an attempt to fulfill the goal of Aurobindo's "integral yoga"—to manifest "a divine life in Matter" (see p. 271). At its most lofty, it's envisioned as the site of the next evolutionary step for humanity, the place where a new species of humans will come into being.

But you don't have to subscribe to this doctrine to appreciate Auroville, or even to join as a full-fledged member. Many of Auroville's residents have little formal contact with the teachings of Aurobindo and the Mother. Instead, they're drawn here by a more general desire to live the principles of conscious community and deep ecology. Wrote the Mother, "In Auroville, simply the goodwill to make a collective experiment for the progress of humanity is sufficient to gain admittance."

Auroville is a patchwork sprawl of about eighty disparate settlements (each with its own unique flavor and focus) linked by a network of dirt roads and interspersed with Tamil farming villages. Set up as an "international trust" by the Indian government and endorsed by the UNESCO general assembly, Auroville is physically and legally separate from the Aurobindo Ashram.

When the first settlers moved to the land, it was a raw expanse of red earth, seared by the tropical heat and scarred by a web of gullies and ravines carved out by torrential monsoon rains. Once a "tropical semi-evergreen scrub jungle" roamed by tigers and elephants, the land—like most of the surrounding region—had been deforested, clearcut, and overgrazed under centuries of British and French rule.

Today, Auroville has been regenerated into a shady oasis with temperatures averaging several degrees cooler than the surrounding territory. Over two million forest trees, fruit trees, hedges, and shrubs have been planted; native birds and animals have begun to return. An integrated soil and water conservation program includes organic farms and raised earth banks and ditches to catch monsoon rains. The community is committed to renewable energy and appropriate technology and boasts over thirty water pumping windmills, forty biogas plants, several organic wastewater treatment plants, 450 solar photovoltaic panels, and a fleet of solar-powered cookers, water heaters, and food dryers.

For some Aurovillians, though, the community's spiritual core is the Matrimandir ("Temple of the Divine Mother"), a one hundred-foot-high elliptical sphere—partially plated with the polished gold discs—that looks, to a cynical eye, like an enormous golfing trophy. Inside the sphere is an exquisite meditation chamber of pure white marble, with a huge crystal globe at the heart, illuminated by a single ray of sunlight channeled through an opening at the apex of the sphere.

Still under construction after nearly three decades, the Matrimandir—controversial among Aurovillians, some of whom think the community's money would have been better spent on more secular endeavors—draws busloads of gawking tourists each day. To preserve the serenity of the inner sanctum for serious meditators, you need to prove your sincerity by coming back twice to get a special entrance pass for the daily meditation period, a process that can be as complex as getting a resident's visa. It's worth it, though, to experience the profound silence of the pure white chamber, deliberately bare of any external religious imagery, and bathed in the diffused and reflected light of the sun.

For a good introduction to Auroville, stop by the Visitors Center that is open daily from 9:30 A.M. to 5:30 P.M. Facilities include an information center offering books, brochures, and photo displays; a boutique; an art gallery; and a video room. An eleven-minute film about Auroville plays regularly but is somewhat confusing if you're not already familiar with Auroville's history and philosophy. The Visitors Center is also the place to start the process of getting a pass to the Matrimandir.

Getting a more in-depth look at the community is more difficult. Aurovillians in general are busy running their lives and businesses and aren't necessarily willing to accommodate the questions of visitors who are just passing through. Periodically, there are weeklong introductory programs for visitors, in which you'll be given daily tours of different departments and mini-communities. The best way to get an inside look at Auroville, though, is to stay there as a guest in one of the thirty to forty settlements that offer accommodations to outsiders. A couple of these are full-fledged guest houses, where you'll be treated as a lodger; others are working communities with a few spare beds and varying degrees of comfort and facilities, where you'll be expected to join in the daily work.

If you're interested in joining Auroville as a permanent resident, you're advised to make a preliminary visit and get the approval of the Entry Group, who will give you a letter of recommendation. With this letter you can obtain an entry visa (unlike a tourist visa, it can be converted to a permanent visa once you're established in Auroville) that will allow you to come to Auroville as a "newcomer" for a probationary period of one year, during which you participate fully in the work and life of your chosen community. After one year, if there are no objections from your community, you become a full member of Auroville.

Unfortunately, Auroville is not yet self-sufficient—you will need a significant outside income in order to live there and eventually build a house. Plan on working and contributing significantly to the community— Aurovillians don't look kindly on those who view it as a kind of New Age retirement home.

Facilities and Food

Auroville is made up of about eighty different settlements of varying size and sophistication, ranging in focus from appropriate technology and organic agriculture to meditation and creative arts. Close to forty of these communities have facilities for outside guests, although in many cases accommodations are spartan at best. During the peak periods (December–March and July–August), guest rooms fill up months in advance— write well ahead to make reservations. (During the torrid April to June months, though, you can drop in whenever you want.)

Upon request, Auroville provides a list of available housing, which indicates both the level of comfort and facilities and the particular orientation of the community. If you're looking for a full-fledged guest house with all the amenities, shoot for a room in Centre, Kottakarai, Samasti, and Sharnga, which have about sixty beds between them and offer meals and laundry facilities. (Centre and Samasti also rent bicycles; Sharnga has a swimming pool.) These guest houses are great for meeting fellow travelers, but less great for meeting Aurovillians—if that's a priority for you, try one of the smaller places. If you're into tree planting and other eco-activities, check out Fertile East, Fertile Windmill, and Gaia in Auroville's "Green Belt." Verité has a strong vipassana community, a yoga hall, and a meditation room—they have a strong communal life and offer regular workshops in dance, aikido, breath work, psychosynthesis, and other mind-body disciplines. New Creation emphasizes social work and education projects in the local Tamil villages. If you yearn for ocean swimming at pristine white-sand beaches, try the beachfront Quiet Beach, Repos, Sri Ma, and the far-flung Eternity (which you'll probably need a moped to reach).

If you're just visiting for the day, you can purchase meals at several different restaurants and cafes, including the Visitors Center, the Auromodele restaurant, and the gourmet restaurant Upahar.

You'll need a bicycle or moped to get around Auroville. You can rent one in Pondicherry fairly inexpensively; some of the communities also rent them to guests.

Schedule

The Visitors Center is open daily from 9:30 A.M. to 5:30 P.M. The Matrimandir meditation hall is open for viewing from 3:30 to 4:30 P.M.; you'll need to obtain a pass at the Visitors Center. If you want to attend the meditation period from 5 to 6 P.M., you'll have to come back a second day with your pass stamped from the previous day's viewing—this policy is to discourage casual tourists during the meditation time.

Fees

Fees at the various guest houses range from Rs 35 per day (for ultra-basic) to Rs 300 and up (for hotel-style comfort).

Foreigners who join the community are asked to contribute Rs 1,500 per month toward Auroville. In addition, you'll be expected to support yourself and your dependents, which generally costs about Rs 2,000 to 3,000 per month. Since housing is scarce at Auroville, if you become a resident you'll be asked to bear the expense of constructing your own home; if you decide to leave, the house will remain the property of Auroville.

Contact Information

AUROVILLE
VISITORS CENTER
AUROVILLE 605 101
TAMIL NADU
TEL: 91-413-62239
FAX: 91-413-6227
E-MAIL: GUESTS@AUROVILLE.ORG.IN

U.S. Contact:
AUROVILLE INTERNATIONAL (AVI) U.S.A.
P.O. BOX 162489
SACRAMENTO, CA 95816
TEL: (916) 452-4013

How to Get There

Auroville is located 10 kilometers north of Pondicherry, which is accessible by bus (from Madras, Tiruvannamalai, Bangalore, Chidambaram, Ooty, and Madurai); and by train via Villapuram. For a day trip, you can get to Auroville by rickshaw from Pondicherry, but you'll have to get the driver to wait while you do your tour, as it's hard to find a rickshaw going back. Your best bet is to rent a bicycle or moped in Pondicherry and get to Auroville under your own power.

Other Services

Auroville has its own bank, post office, STD, and fax services. All services are also available in Pondicherry.

Books and Tapes

Books, brochures, and videotapes on Auroville, Aurobindo, and the Mother are available at the Visitors Center and through the Auroville International (AVI) centers in Europe, Canada, and the United States.

India has become the symbol representing all the difficulties of modern humanity.

India will be the land of its resurrection, the resurrection to a higher, truer life.

India represents all the terrestrial human difficulties, and it is in India that there will be the . . . cure. And it is for this—it is FOR THIS that I have been made to start Auroville.

—THE MOTHER

International Centre for Yoga Education and Research
Kottakuppam (via Pondicherry), Tamil Nadu

🌀 *Yogamaharishi Dr. Swami Gitananda Giri (1906–1993)*
🌀 *Meenakshi Devi Bhavanani (1943–)*

Swami Gitananda Giri was often called the "lion of Pondicherry"—a blunt, flamboyant, and sometimes controversial guru who was famous, in the words of his wife, for "performing ego-dectomies without anesthesia." Since his death in 1993, the beachside ashram he founded on the outskirts of Pondicherry—now led by his American-born wife Meenakshi Devi Bhavanani—continues to offer six-month, intensive teacher's training courses in "classical rishiculture yoga," with a strong emphasis on purification, concentration, and energy amplification.

Teachers and Teachings

Be prepared for total immersion. Before you even enroll in the program, you're required to complete a fifty-two-week correspondence course in the fundamentals of Patanjali's ashtanga yoga. Once you're at the ashram, you'll live in a close-quartered, family atmosphere with ten to twelve other students—about three-quarters of them foreigners—studying asana, pranayama, kriyas, mudras, meditation, philosophy, Sanskrit, and classical Indian carnatic music and bharat natyam dance from five in the morning till ten at night. With only one day off a week, there's a bit of a pressure-cooker atmosphere.

The program is broken into two three-month sessions (which do not need to be taken back to back, although that's highly recommended). The first month emphasizes cleansing and detoxification, including a five-day fast, coffee enemas, and traditional yogic salt-water intestinal cleanses. The second month emphasizes building physical strength and endurance. In the third month, the physical practices level off and the emphasis shifts to cultivating mental stillness and concentration. In the second three-month session, the whole sequence is repeated on a more intense level.

Because the program is rigorous, you should only enroll if you are in good physical and mental health. Meenakshi Devi stresses that this ashram is not in the business of therapeutic yoga. "We're interested in yoga as a spiritual sadhana," she explains. "It's not our calling to cure people of addictions, cure cancer, that sort of thing—there are other places that do that." The course is geared for younger students (thirties and under), she says, who are "fit and haven't wrecked their nervous systems through drugs and unhealthy living."

Born in India of an Indian father and an Irish mother, Swami Gitananda Giri began studying classical hatha and raja yoga with a Bengali tantric guru at the age of thirteen and received initiation at age sixteen; as an adult, he was also initiated by a south Indian Shaivite master. He was educated in England and lived in the West until he was in his fifties, when he returned to India and put on the orange robes of a swami. He helped rebuild yoga into a national institution, including launching the "yoga sports" movement and asana competitions, and his blend of Western science and classical yoga attracted a large and devoted international following. However, he outraged many local people by his outspoken comments (which included blunt critiques of such local icons as Sri Aurobindo and the Mother) and his marriage to Meenakshi Devi Bhavanani, who was one of his American students.

Since her husband's death, Meenakshi Devi has taken over the running of the ashram and the teacher's training program. Now an Indian citizen, Meenakshi Devi has lived in India since 1968, studying yoga and bharat natyam, the traditional south Indian dance form. She has written four books on yoga and scripted and starred in a ten-part India television serial called *Yoga for Youth*.

Teachings at the ashram are presented in the context of traditional Hindu philosophy and Indian culture, with a strong emphasis on dharma (duty), karma, and the yamas and niyamas (moral and ethical guidelines). Students are asked to wear Indian clothes and are introduced to Indian culture and religious rituals as a backdrop to yogic practices.

The program revolves around practices designed to awaken and increase the flow of energy through the system. You'll practice classic asanas with an emphasis on energy flow rather than physical perfection ("we're not part of the cult of flexibility"); about forty different pranayamas; and about a dozen different flowing series that incorporate asanas, pranayamas, bandhas, and mudras.

Once awakened, the energy is used to fuel meditation and, ultimately, bring about the state of samadhi, which Gitananda taught was dependent upon a purified body and mind. "To reach those subtle states you need a very sensitive nervous system," Meenakshi Devi says. "You can't reach samadhi if you've destroyed your nervous system with drugs and alcohol. Even if you've quit, you have to face the karma of that. But yoga can still help you live a good and useful life and get reborn with a chance to do better next time."

Facilities and Food

Enter here only if you are happy," says a sign over the ashram door. The ashram is in a tropical garden on the Bay of Bengal, with a wide sandy beach and warm, unpolluted water for swimming. Parrots and brilliant blue kingfishers nest in the groves of bananas, mangos, and dates. Asana classes are held on the rooftop patio or on the beach itself.

About twenty students can stay in double rooms with shared bath. Facilities include a stage for dance performances. For pujas and other traditional rituals, students go to Swami Gitananda's samadhi shrine on another piece of property several kilometers away.

Clean drinking water comes from the ashram's own protected well. This is one of the few ashrams in India that serves real "health food" with lots of whole grains, sprouts, salads, and raw (disinfected) vegetables.

There are over 100 "rishiculture yoga" centers worldwide. A complete directory is available from ICYER.

Schedule

The six-month teacher's training course is held annually from October 1 through March 25. The schedule begins with meditation, chanting, and asana at 6 A.M.—a typical day also includes karma yoga, pranayama, yoga therapy, lectures, satsang, and bhajans.

Fees

Required membership in Yoga Jivana Satsangha (includes monthly newsletter subscription): U.S. $40. Refundable bedding deposit: Rs 500. Monthly donation for room, board, teachings: U.S. $500 (or equivalent). Yoga correspondence course: U.S. $400.

INTERNATIONAL CENTRE FOR YOGA EDUCATION AND RESEARCH
16-A, METTU STREET
CHINNAMUDALIARCHAVADY
KOTTAKUPPAM (VIA PONDICHERRY) 605 104
TEL: NONE

U.S. Contact:
YOGACHARYA
BILLY UBER
P.O. BOX 2234
WAUSAU, WI 54402

How to Get There

The ashram is 8 kilometers north of Pondicherry along the road to Auroville. You can take a bus or autorickshaw from Pondicherry, which is accessible by bus (from Madras, Tiruvannamalai, Bangalore, Chidambaram, Ooty, and Madurai) and by train.

Other Services

All services are available in Pondicherry.

Books and Tapes

The monthly magazine *Yoga Life,* books by Swami Gitananda Giri and Meenakshi Devi Bhavanani, and a fifty-two-week correspondence course are available through the ICYER.

You have two choices open to you in your attitude towards life: "iti, iti." Or "neti, neti." "Iti, iti" means "This is God. That is God. Everything is God." "Neti, neti" means "This is not God. That is not God. Nothing is God." It has to be one or the other. Either

*everything is God or nothing is God. Either everything is impor-
tant or nothing is important. Both are correct. But there is no
truth in any in-between.*

—SWAMI GITANANDA GIRI

Sri Ramanashram
Tiruvannamalai, Tamil Nadu

Sri Ramana Maharshi (1879–1950)

"They say that I am going, but where could I go?" the sage Ramana Maharshi said to a devotee grieving his impending death. "I am here."
From the day he first came to the holy mountain Arunachala—as a sixteen-
year-old runaway casting himself into the fire of Self-realization—to the
day of his death in 1950, Ramana Maharshi never ventured more than
two miles away from the base of this rocky red hill. Today, his presence is
still palpable on Arunachala, and his ashram is packed with the hundreds
of devotees who come here to soak up his silent message: that the eternal,
unchanging Self is all that exists.

Teachers and Teachings

According to his biographers, Ramana spontaneously awakened to the
true Self as a schoolboy of sixteen, alone in an upstairs room of his
uncle's south Indian house. Inexplicably seized with the terror that he was
going to die—although he was outwardly in good health—he lay down on
the floor like a corpse, went into a kind of conscious trance, and, over the
course of a few minutes, experienced in every detail the death of his own
body. During this remarkable process, he realized—not as a concept, but as
a lived reality—that his true nature was eternal and not bound up in the
body, mind, or personality.

Unable to continue with his ordinary life, Ramana left a cryptic
farewell note for his family and—with only three rupees in his pocket and
almost no knowledge of the world outside his home—made his way to

Mt. Arunachala, a rugged hill worshipped as a physical expression of Lord Shiva. He took refuge in the ancient Shiva temple at the base of the mountain, stripped off his clothes (only with great reluctance accepting the loincloth that the scandalized priests forced upon him), and lived for months in a vault in the temple basement, absorbed in an ecstasy so profound that he was oblivious of the rats and insects gnawing at his wasting body. Finally returning to physical awareness—but with his knowledge of his true nature unclouded—Ramana took up residence in a cave on Mt. Arunachala, where he lived in solitude for seventeen years, gradually attracting a devoted circle of followers.

In the 1920s, an ashram was built for him at the foot of the mountain. For the last twenty years of his life, thousands of visitors flocked to see him—including the British journalist and mystic Paul Brunton, who first brought his teachings to a Western audience—but despite his increasing fame, Ramana continued to live a simple and largely silent life. His only private possessions were a loincloth (always impeccably white), a water-pot, and a walking stick; he lived and even slept in a communal hall which was open to visitors twenty-four hours a day.

Ramana taught primarily through the sheer impact of his presence. "Instead of giving out verbal instructions he constantly emanated a silent force or power which stilled the minds of those who were attuned to it and occasionally even gave them a direct experience of the state that he himself was perpetually immersed in," David Godman writes in *Be As You Are*. "Throughout his life Sri Ramana insisted that this silent flow of power represented his teachings in their most direct and concentrated form." According to one disciple, Arthur Osborne, "The real teaching was not the explanation but the silent influence, the alchemy worked in the heart."

This alchemy is what pilgrims come to the Ramanashram to experience. Disciples believe that Ramana—though no longer in his body—continues to emit his silent teachings here like an invisible force field. There are no formal meditation sessions, satsangs, or philosophical talks. There are no required work sessions or classes. Instead, you're on your own to meditate in the small chamber where he spent years sitting in silence with devotees; circumambulate his samadhi shrine; do pradakshina (a ritual walk) around Mt. Arunachala; sit in the tiny mountain cave where he lived for seventeen years; and generally steep in his still-powerful vibrations.

If you want something more explicit, you can explore the well-stocked bookstore that contains translations of and commentaries on Ramana's

Mt. Arunachala

"Arunachala! Thou dost root out the ego of those who meditate on thee in the heart, O Arunachala!"

—RAMANA MAHARSHI
(from Hymns to Sri Arunachala)

"Sooner or later, everyone must come to Arunachala," Ramana Maharshi said. "Arunachala is one's own Self." So sacred is Mt. Arunachala in the Hindu tradition that merely to think its name is said to be enough to bring about liberation. And so intense was Ramana's love for this dry, rocky hill that from the day he first came here to the day he died, he never ventured more than two miles away from its base.

Geologically, Arunachala is an upthrust piece of the Earth's igneous crust, far older than the Himalayas. Mythologically, it is Lord Shiva himself—not just his dwelling place, but his actual lingam, the god himself in physical form. According to the Puranas, Brahma (the creator god) and Vishnu (the sustainer) became embroiled in a terrible fight over which of them was the greatest. To resolve the dispute, Shiva appeared as a blinding column of light that reached infinitely into the sky. Believing that the one who found the source of this column would be crowned as the supreme god, Brahma and Vishnu set off looking—Vishnu digging deep in the ground for the base, Brahma soaring high toward the summit. Neither was successful, however, and both had to humble themselves before Shiva. In answer to their prayers, Shiva condensed himself from a column of light into the mountain Arunachala, and decreed that the mere sight or thought of this hill would suffice to neutralize all karma and even bestow the state of ultimate knowledge. Believed to fulfill wishes and bring about miraculous healings, the 2,668-foot mountain has been the home of saints and sages for countless generations.

Homage is paid to Arunachala through "Giri pradakshina"—the devotional exercise of circumabulating the mountain clockwise. On festival days, the thirteen-kilometer Pradakshina Road that rings the mountain is thronged with pilgrims; and every day at dawn at least a few dozen barefoot sadhus and Westerners in Birckenstocks set out on the route, which is punctuated by numerous shrines and temples, each with its own story and significance. (A map available in the ashram bookstore offers information about the various sacred stops.) Take the main, paved road only if you don't mind sharing your pilgrimage with trucks, buses, bicycles, and buffalo carts. Otherwise, try the much more pleasant, unpaved inner path, which is usually almost deserted. To find the inner path, go into the Annamalai Ashram (just up Pradakshina Road from the Ramanashram, on the same side of the street). Behind the ashram you can pick up the trail, which is fairly clearly marked the whole way with white paint on stones. (Women, unfortunately, should not walk alone, as there have been some incidents of attacks.)

"One should go round either in Mouna [silence] or Dhyana [meditation] or Japa [repetition of Lord's name] or Sankeertan [Bhajan] and thereby think of God all the time," Ramana advised. "One should walk slowly like a woman who is in the ninth month of pregnancy." He also suggested walking on the left side of the road, so as not to obstruct the movement of the invisible siddhas and sages who also go regularly around the mountain. (The souls of the dead, it is said, do pradakshina clockwise on the other side of the road.) The walk is traditionally done barefoot—one local rumor holds that the failed monsoon in the last few years is due to foreign pilgrims going around the mountain with their shoes on.

If you want to climb the mountain, you can take the worn stone path that leads from the back gate of the Ramanashram. A half-hour's walk will bring you to the Skandashramam, a peaceful tree-shaded hermitage overlooking Tiruvannamalai, where Ramana lived from 1916 to 1922. A few hundred yards farther, down a hill and across a stream, you can meditate in the Virupaksha cave, believed to be the samadhi site of an ancient yogi, where Ramana lived from 1899 to 1916.

From the Skandashram you can take a branch in the path to Arunachala's summit, a two- to three-hour climb. A silent sadhu lives at the very top, but beware: he often doesn't take kindly to having his meditations disturbed. If you feel compelled to visit, be sure to bring an offering such as fruit or flowers. On the final, full-moon night of the festival of Kartikai Deepam in November or December—which celebrates the union of Shiva and Parvati—an enormous fire is lit on the peak, its flames visible for miles around.

At the foot of the mountain, in the heart of town, is the massive four-towered temple to Shiva, one of the largest temples in south India, the oldest parts of which date to the ninth century C.E. There you can visit the basement chamber where Ramana sat in samadhi when he first arrived in Tiruvannamalai. There are daily pujas at the temple at 7:30, 9:30, and 11:30 A.M. and 5:30, 8:30, and 9:30 P.M.

In recent decades, Arunachala—once the jungly home of cheetahs, elephants, leopards, foxes, and deer—has been almost completely deforested by goat grazing and firewood scavenging. Intensive reforestation work is being done by the Annamalai Reforestation Society, which is planting the mountain with drought-resistant, goat-resistant trees like silk cotton, neem, and jujube. To get involved, contact the Annamalai Reforestation Society, MIG, 95 Thamarainagar, Tiruvannamalai 606 601.

verbal teachings. For those who could not comprehend his silence, Ramana taught the method of "self-inquiry," a practice of rigorous introspection on the nature of what he termed "the 'I'-thought." Ramana instructed his followers to ask themselves, again and again, "Who am I?" When thoughts arise in the mind, he said, we should immediately ask, "To whom do they arise?" In this way we break our false identification of "I" with our body, our mind, our senses, our personality; and direct our attention to the source from which the "I"-thought itself springs. "The thought, 'Who am I?' will destroy all other thoughts, and, like the stick used for stirring the burning pyre, it will itself in the end get destroyed," Ramana said. "Then, there will arise Self-realization."

Today, the Ramanashram is a bustling place—if you're expecting *external* silence, you may be in for a rude awakening. The once-tiny temple town of Tiruvannamalai is growing fast, and you're never far from the honking of horns, the barking of dogs, and the solicitations of the beggars and sadhus who throng the dusty, chai shop–lined road outside the ashram gates. Even inside the ashram, pilgrims and devotees mill in and out; you may well find the sound of an electric sander competing with the Brahmin boys chanting at the samadhi shrine. In recent years, the ashram has been "discovered" by Western devotees of the late Poonjaji—a master who himself achieved Self-realization in Ramana's presence—and the influx of foreign pilgrims has created a thriving social scene. (Asked if he had visited a lot of other ashrams, one long-term seeker said, "I don't need to. Sooner or later everyone comes to the Ramanashram.") But underlying the bustle you can always feel the presence of Arunachala—potent, intense, and profoundly silent.

Facilities and Food

Situated at the base of Mt. Arunachala, Ramanashram is large, well maintained, and busy, with monkeys quarreling in the immense shade trees and peacocks strolling about the grounds. The ashram offers accommodations for over one hundred people in numerous buildings and cottages with one, two, four, or more rooms per building. Most rooms are semiprivate but there are also dormitories and suites for families. Most rooms have attached bathrooms. Bedding is provided. The ashram has a one-day laundry service.

You must write ahead for reservations as the ashram is usually full during the cool winter months. Your letter should state your date of arrival and expected duration of stay. You will receive a confirmation letter, which you will be asked to present upon arrival. If you can't stay at the Ramanashram, there are numerous smaller ashrams and group houses nearby that can accommodate you. You can stay at the Ramanashram for one to two weeks only; if you want to stay longer, you'll have to find outside accommodations.

About a half-hour's walk up the mountain is the Skandashramam, a peaceful tree-shaded hermitage overlooking Tiruvannamalai, where Ramana lived from 1916 to 1922. Slightly further is the Virupaksha cave, believed to contain the ashes of an ancient yogi, where Ramana lived from 1899 to 1916.

The food is superb south Indian fare, served on banana leaves, with excellent curd, buttermilk, and milk from the ashram cows. Meals are only for those actually staying at the ashram. Filtered water is freely available in the dining hall.

Schedule

All scheduled events are optional for guests at the ashram. Those staying elsewhere are welcome to attend any event except meals. The daily routine includes chanting of "forty Verses in Praise of Bhagavan" at 6:45 A.M.; Vedic chanting from 8 to 9:15 A.M. and 5 to 6:15 P.M. at Ramana's samadhi shrine; and chanting of Ramana's Tamil writings from 6:45 to 7:30 P.M.

In addition to major Hindu holidays, special feast days include Ramana Maharshi's birthday in December or January (dependent on the Tamil calendar) and his mahanirvana (the day he "dropped his body") in April or May.

Fees

Donations are not required but are accepted at the ashram office when you are ready to depart.

How to Get There

To get to Tiruvannamalai from Madras, take the bus or train to Tindivanam (122 kilometers) or Villapuram (159 kilometers). Then go by bus or taxi to Tiruvannamalai (about 70 kilometers). You can also get to Tiruvannamalai directly from Bangalore (by bus); Pondicherry (train); or Madurai (train or bus). The ashram is about 2 kilometers from the temple at the center of Tiruvannamalai.

Other Services

Most services are available in this town, which has a population of approximately 100,000. If you need to stay in a hotel, the Trishul Hotel has comfortable accommodations and food for about Rs 300 per night.

Books and Tapes

An excellent introduction to Ramana's life and teachings is *Be As You Are: The Teachings of Sri Ramana Maharshi*, edited by David Godman (Penguin). The ashram has an excellent library as well as a bookstore with books and audio/video tapes in English and several other languages.

There is something in this man which holds my attention as steel filings are held by a magnet. I cannot turn my gaze away from him. My initial bewilderment, my perplexity at being totally ignored, slowly fade away as this strange fascination begins to grip me more firmly. . . . I become aware of a silent, resistless change

which is taking place within my mind. One by one, the questions which I have prepared on the train with such meticulous accuracy drop away. For it does not now seem to matter whether they are asked or not, and it does not seem to matter whether I solve the problems which have hitherto troubled me. I know only that a steady river of quietness seems to be flowing near me, that a great peace is penetrating the inner reaches of my being, and that my thought-tortured brain is beginning to arrive at some rest.

How small seem those questions which I have asked myself with such frequency! How petty grows the panorama of lost years! I perceive with sudden clarity that the intellect creates its own problems and then makes itself miserable trying to solve them. This is indeed a novel concept to enter the mind of one who has hitherto placed such high value upon intellect.

—PAUL BRUNTON,
describing his initial meeting
with Ramana Maharshi
(from *A Search in Secret India*)

Yogi Ramsuratkumar Ashram
Tiruvannamalai, Tamil Nadu

Yogi Ramsuratkumar (1918–)

He refers to himself as a "beggar," and that's what he looks like: a sweet-faced old man bundled in rags, his grey hair wild and bushy. Until a few years ago, the mystic and madman known as Yogi Ramsuratkumar lived on the streets—but so many people were flocking for his blessings that devotees finally began constructing an ashram to accommodate the hordes. But the eighty-year-old yogi barely seems to notice the buildings that are going up around him. Driven to the hall for darshan each day, he sits on his dais in a cloud of cigarette smoke, puffing beatifically away on one beadie after another, while a throng of devotees sings bhajans to him.

Other Local Gurus

Mt. Arunachala has been attracting saints, sages, and spiritual teachers for hundreds of years. Many of them prefer to remain invisible; however, here are a few to look for:

LAKSHMANA SWAMI

Lakshmana Swami is an elderly recluse, said to have been enlightened by Ramana Maharshi, who lives in a large house (with a satellite dish) not far from the Ramsuratkumar ashram and appears for silent darshan four times a year: his birthday (which happens to be on Christmas Day), New Year's Day, Shivaratri (sometime in February or March), and Kartigai Deepam (November or December).

He sticks mainly to silence, and when he does give verbal teachings, they consist of steering devotees to Ramana Maharshi's teachings. A gentle man with a close-cropped white beard, he holds his four annual darshans outside his house under a canopy of flowers. Gates generally open at 9 A.M., but get there earlier if you want to sit up close. He'll sit with you in silence for an hour or so, looking out over the crowd with luminous eyes; then he'll distribute prasad before going back into his house.

V. GANESAN

The grand-nephew of Ramana Maharshi, V. Ganesan was brought up in the presence of the master. As an adolescent, he stood near the entrance to Ramana's room the day Ramana left his body and witnessed the famous "flash of light" that moved toward the top of Mt. Arunachala. Now in his sixties, he leads small, informal satsang six days a week—from 9 to 11 A.M. Mondays through Saturdays—at his home, "Ananda Ramana," a short walk from the Ramanashram.

Ganesan earned a master's degree in philosophy and worked briefly as a journalist, but most of his life has been dedicated to the Ramanashram. He was one of the founders and editors of the *Mountain Path* magazine and worked for the ashram in various administrative positions for over thirty-five years. He punctuates his teachings with stories not only of Ramana, but of all the many saints who have lived in or passed through Tiruvannamalai. To get to his home, turn right out the Ramanashram gate and follow the paved road approximately two kilometers. Turn left just before the large sign for Anudamen Nursery. Follow the orange brick wall about 200 meters to a gate with a white thatched-roof house behind it. Satsang is held on the patio under the thatched roof.

NANNA GARU

Nanna Garu—whose name simply means "respected father"—never met Ramana Maharshi in person, but he says he received the Maharshi's darshan in a dream in 1957, in which Ramana kissed him three times on the cheek. Nanna Garu's main ashram is in Andhra Pradesh, but he spends several months of the year in his newly built Andhra Ashram in Tiruvannamalai on a side street just up the road from the Ramanashram. He has a small group of devotees—including a handful of Westerners—who come to him not for his verbal teachings (he's mainly silent, though he speaks excellent English) but for his warm presence and his piercing glances, which, as an ashram publication puts it, "turn their minds and thoughts from things external towards the Heart Center."

HUGO MAIER

Hugo Maier (known as Appa by his followers) is the German-born founder of Shantimalai Trust, a spiritual community and service organization—funded by donations from the West—whose motto is "Help Toward Self-Help" and whose projects include a medical clinic, an orphanage, a leper colony, a health-care training center for village women, a cooperative farm, and a vocational training program. Hugo Maier came to Tiruvannamalai in 1959 and lived for many years at the Ramana Ashram; he moved out when he began attracting substantial numbers of his own Western devotees. He founded the Shantimalai Trust as a way of showing his gratitude for the teachings he had received from Ramana Maharshi.

About 150 Western disciples spend the winters at Shantimalai, but it's not open to short-term visitors: "We don't want window shoppers," Maier says. He's only interested in seekers who are ready to make a substantial commitment both to Shantimalai's charitable work and to him as a guru. If you're interested in investigating further, you can write him and request an interview with one of his staff: Shantimalai Trust; Shanthimalai, Sivanagar; Tiruvannamalai 606 603.

BENCH SWAMI

No one knows his full name—they just named him for the bench that he sits on in silence, his eyes closed, all day long. The bench is in an enclosed front porch of a little house belonging to a family who cares for the swami, who is in his nineties. Locals say that he's been sitting on that bench for the past twenty-five years (and on various other benches for many years before that). If you sit with him long enough, he may open his eyes and look at you, which is, in itself, supposed to be a kind of blessing.

Originally a postmaster from a nearby town, Bench Swami met Ramana Maharshi in the 1940s. When he asked Ramana for permission to return to his work, Ramana looked at him and said, "Iru." (This is the Tamil imperative for the verb "to be" and "to stay.") The postmaster promptly went into a trance, which he has remained in ever since.

To get to Bench Swami's bench, take the road toward Ramsuratkumar's ashram. At the end of this road (about 300 meters) turn right. On your left will be a pink three-story building, with a green gate just past it on your left. Through the green gate and down the lane, you'll come to a gate to the first house on your right. If the gate is open, it's okay to go inside. The enclosed front porch also has a metal gate that will be open if it's okay to visit. Bench Swami is on the bench inside this porch.

Teachers and Teachings

Yogi Ramsuratkumar gives only one teaching: to surrender to God and chant His name constantly. "All I know is Ram Nam," he says. "Chant the name all twenty-four hours! That's enough for this beggar!" You probably won't get much in the way of verbal teachings from him, although he does speak excellent English. The main reason to attend his twice-daily darshan is just to be near his energy field, which by itself, devotees say, can put you into bliss.

Born near Varanasi in northern India, Ramsuratkumar left home at age sixteen to become a wandering sadhu. In the 1940s he visited the Aurobindo Ashram in Pondicherry and immersed himself in Aurobindo's teachings (see p. 271), then went to Tiruvannamalai for the blessings of Ramana Maharshi (see p. 286). Finally, he became the disciple of Swami Ramdas in Kerala (see. p. 153), who initiated him into the mantra "Sri Ram Jaya Ram Jaya Jaya Ram" and instructed him to chant it twenty-four hours a day. "This beggar had three fathers," Ramsuratkumar likes to say. "Aurobindo started, Ramana Maharshi did a little, and Ramdas finished."

Plunged into ecstasy by the mantra chanting, Ramsuratkumar spent seven years wandering as a beggar and finally arrived in Tiruvannamalai in 1959. He's been there ever since—living in caves and on street corners, eating whatever food was given him, roaming the streets, chanting his mantra, and dancing in ecstasy. He has never claimed any miraculous powers, but people have always flocked to see him, drawn, they say, by the peace and joy they feel in his presence.

Now that the ashram has been built, it's harder to access the yogi than it used to be. It's difficult (though possible) to get a private interview—try leaving a request with the attendent at the front gate. Yogi Ramsuratkumar's routine changes constantly, "as his Father commands." On some days, darshan may consist simply of a drive-by viewing—then you'll walk into an immense, half-completed auditorium (construction was stopped by God's commands), march around a life-size statue of the yogi, and go into a smaller satsang hall for chanting.

Other days, there's a longer darshan, with Ramsuratkumar present. (Be sure to bring an offering of fruit, sweets, or—for this particular guru—cigarettes.) Sometimes Ramsuratkumar will move about the room giving blessings; sometimes he sits doing japa with an invisible mala; periodically he smokes a cigarette cupped in his hand. His smile is sweet and childlike; he occasionally bursts into almost maniacal laughter for no obvious reason. Sometimes he requests particular bhajans: one Christmas, for instance, he asked a group of Americans to sing Christmas carols throughout the darshan. Often, though, he seems almost oblivious to the fact that he is on a dais surrounded by people chanting his name. Remarked one British visitor, "You could set him down in the middle of Trafalgar Square and he'd be doing exactly the same thing."

Facilities and Food

The ashram is still under construction on a quiet, four-acre field with an excellent view of Mt. Arunachala. Six small cottages can house several people apiece, but they are officially reserved for donors and not available for general visitors. The darshan hall seats about five hundred people; an auditorium for 5,000 is being built, though construction is intermittent according to the yogi's directions. No meals are currently available to guests.

Schedule

Darshan is held from 10 A.M. until 12 noon and from 4 to 6 P.M.

Fees

Donation.

Contact Information

YOGI RAMSURATKUMAR ASHRAM
AGRAHARA COLLAI
1833/1, CHENGAM ROAD
TIRUVANNAMALAI 606 603
TEL: NONE

U.S. Contact:
MR. LEE LOZOWICK
c/o HOHM
P.O. BOX 4272
PRESCOTT, AZ 65302
TEL: (520) 778-9189
FAX: (520) 717-1779

How to Get There

The ashram is in Tiruvannamalai on a side street off the main Pradakshina Road about a hundred yards up from the Ramana Ashram (but on the opposite side of the road). The turnoff is marked by a large picture of Yogi Ramsuratkumar.

To get to Tiruvannamalai from Madras, take the bus or train to Tindivanam (122 kilometers) or Villapuram (159 kilometers.) Then go by bus or taxi to Tiruvannamalai (about 70 kilometers). You can also get to Tiruvannamalai directly from Bangalore (by bus); Pondicherry (train); or Madurai (train or bus).

Other Services

Most services are available in Tiruvannamalai.

Books and Tapes

A small booklet about Yogi Ramsuratkumar is available at the ashram office.

Without warning, [Yogi Ramsuratkumar] swatted a fly on the bare counter of the vacant stall with his powerful hand. He picked the creature up by a wing and gave it to me. I tentatively accepted it, trying to appear grateful, and examined the insect in the palm of my hand to see if there was something I had missed. Mangled, oozing, one wing buckled into a squashed abdomen, it looked like any other dead fly I'd ever encountered.

The yogi watched me intently, puffing and counting those invisible beads, a big, generous smile swelling through his high cheekbones.

"Very dirty," he said, nodding at the fly. "Put it there." He indicated the spot where the fly had just met its abrupt end. A tiny stain was still visible on the wood.

I tipped the speck down near the stain.

"What can death be?" the yogi asked.

I shrugged, not about to offer an answer to that.

"It is a question we are interested in—is it not so?"

I nodded.

"Watch." He pointed to the fly.

I watched the raisinlike blob, hearing the yogi's breathing become faster and faster—until it suddenly stopped. He then held up his right hand a yard or so from the fly, becoming incredibly still. This stillness was all the more dramatic after his perpetual motion—and it really was stillness. As I continued to watch, the fly started twitching, shaking its buckled wing out, then getting up, testing its legs with a few unsteady steps. A second later, it flew away.

The yogi remained motionless for another minute, then immediately became his old self again, lighting up and fanning.

My first thought was just how dead the fly had been. Surely I had seen enough dead flies to know the difference. This fly had been crushed, split open.

"How did you do that?" I asked.

He looked over through the gloom, the whites of his eyes sparkling. "Life is a force," he said quietly. "Death is the absence of that force—is it not so?"

"I suppose . . ."

"Fly needs less force than the human—is this true?"

"Probably . . ."

"Can this beggar not give the fly enough force to live?"

I asked how he could transfer his life force and how the fly could repair the damage to its body even if it received new life force.

"Is it not so that God can do anything he wishes?"

"Yes, but . . ." I stopped, because I had the distinct impression that the answers I was looking for weren't available. No words from this yogi were going to explain anything at all.

—PAUL WILLIAM ROBERTS
(from *Empire of the Soul*)

Vellaiyanantha Swami Ashram
Kotthanthavadi, Tamil Nadu

🌀 *Vellaiyanantha Swami (1925–)*

The first thing you notice about Vellaiyanantha Swami is his hair: over twelve feet of matted braids wrapped around his head, draped over his ribs, and spilling to the floor to join in a heap with his equally long beard. His devotees say he has never had it cut. They also say that he has not left the chair he now sits in for twenty-five years and has not eaten or drunk for ten (his protruding belly, they explain, is due to the shakti he has accumulated). Drawn by such stories, increasing numbers of people are coming to darshan in his tiny ashram—really just his house—in a village about thirty kilometers from Tiruvannamalai.

Teachers and Teachings

Vellaiyanantha Swami—also known as Karrumarapatti Swami—has never had a guru. He speaks no English, but through a translator he explains that he had a powerful enlightenment experience when he was about seven years old and currently spends five or six hours a day in meditation.

Married, with three children, the swami still lives with his wife in a small house in a village with no paved roads. Every day devotees come to seek his blessings—mostly local villagers, but in recent years more and more foreign visitors have come by rickshaw or taxi from Tiruvannamalai as a day trip. (One of Swamiji's devotees, an enterprising rickshaw driver, has set up a sort of shuttle service and provides both transportation and translation for foreign spiritual seekers.) You'll be escorted into his room and given a semiprivate audience, in which he'll answer your questions through a translator, give you his blessings, and distribute vibhuti. Don't be surprised if he puts his hands on you quite abruptly (which can be a bit of a shock, since the fingernails on one hand are five inches long).

The swami is playful and energetic, with a ready smile and a quick sense of humor. Asked where his happiness comes from, he replies, "I taste the honey all the time."

Facilities and Food

The ashram is really just Swamiji's house—there are no accommodations or food for visitors either at the ashram or elsewhere in this little village. If you come for the day, be sure to bring all the food or water you will need.

Schedule

You're welcome to join Swamiji in his daily meditations from 3 to 7 A.M. and from 4 to 6 P.M. The rest of the day, he will receive you whenever you happen to show up.

Fees

Donations.

Contact Information

VELLAIYANANTHA SWAMI ASHRAM
P.O. KOTTHANTHAVADI
VIA MANGALAM
KARRUPMARAPATTI
TIRUVANNAMALAI (T.K.) 606 752
DIST. SAMBUVARAYAR
TAMIL NADU
TEL: NONE

How to Get There

The ashram is in a small village about 30 kilometers from Tiruvannamalai. You can take a rickshaw or taxi from Tiruvannamalai (the drivers outside the Ramanashram all know how to find it).

To get to Tiruvannamalai from Madras, take the bus or train to Tindivanam (122 kilometers) or Villapuram (159 kilometers.) Then go by bus or taxi to Tiruvannamalai (about 70 kilometers). You can also get to Tiruvannamalai directly from Bangalore (by bus); Pondicherry (train); or Madurai (train or bus).

The nearest services are in Tiruvannamalai.

None.

PILGRIMAGE SITES IN Tamil Nadu

❧ **Chidambaram.** The city of Chidambaram—a name that means "expanded consciousness"—is the site of a great temple dedicated to Shiva Nataraj, the form of Shiva whose cosmic dance sustains the universe. Along with temples to Vishnu, Parvati, and Ganesh, it forms one of the oldest temple complexes in the south, an exquisite example of Dravadian architecture.

In Tamil sacred geography, the Earth's sushumna nadi—one of the three major energy pathways in the human body—runs through Chidambaram, ending at the power spot of the temple. According to an ancient tantric text: "Straight within the forehead/Between the eyebrows/Is the astral Space vast; Peer, peer within there/the luminous mantra Aum will be . . . That verily is the Holy Temple of Chidambaram." The priests shave one side of their heads to represent the male aspect of god, and grow the hair long on the other to represent the female aspect.

Chidambaram is about 250 kilometers south of Madras, on the main line of the Southern Railway. Food and lodging are readily available.

❧ **Tirupathi.** Probably the most visited city in south India, Tirupathi is actually just over the border in Andhra Pradesh, but the best way to reach it is by bus from Madras. Up to 100,000 devotees each day come to visit the Tirupathi temple of Sri Balaji, an incarnation of Vishnu. The face of the image remains covered because the gaze of Sri Balaji is said to be so powerful it will incinerate onlookers. The faithful believe that wishes made in front of the image will come true. The temple, located on Tirumala Hill, is one of the richest in India, with a dome covered with gold and an annual income of about $15 million.

Pilgrims pay homage to the god by sacrificing their most precious possession, their hair; you'll be met by gangs of barefoot, razor-wielding barbers. The shorn hair is sold by the temple to fund charitable projects.

Non-Hindus can enter the temple for some hassle and a price. During peak season it can take four hours in queue, but off-season only about half an hour (that's if you join the paying queue for about thirty rupees; you can get in for free if you're willing to wait up to twelve hours).

There are many places to stay in Tirupathi, which is a day trip by road from Madras on an express bus.

❧ **Kanchipuram.** This is one of the great southern temple cities and the seat of the Shankaracharya of Kanchi, one of the most important Hindu spiritual leaders in India. (The former Shankaracharya, revered as a saint, died a few years ago at the age of 101.) Boasting over a hundred temples, it dates from the second century and is one of the seven most sacred Hindu cities, along with Dwarka, Mathura, Haridwar, Aydohya, Varanasi, and Ujjain. There are train and bus links from Madras to Kanchipuram.

❧ **Madurai.** Most pilgrims come to the city of Madurai—the second largest city in Tamil Nadu, with a population of 1,100,000—to visit the Meenakshi Temple. This seventeenth-century temple with its thousand-pillared hall is dedicated to the goddess Meenakshi, the wife of Shiva (in his manifestation as Sundareswara, the "Lord of Beauty"). Every night a procession takes an idol of Shiva to Parvati's chamber for the night; it is carried back early the next morning.

There are flights, trains, and buses into Madurai and plenty of places to stay.

❧ **Kanyakumari.** The Bay of Bengal, the Indian Ocean, and the Arabian Sea all meet at Kanyakumari, the southernmost tip of India, where the god Shiva is said to have married the goddess Parvati. It's considered a holy place to bathe, and the moonrise and sunset are spectacular. On a small rock island just offshore is the Vivekananda Rock Memorial, marking the spot where Swami Vivekananda—the man who first brought yogic teachings to America a hundred years ago—sat in meditation and received the inspiration to travel to the West. Trains and buses run regularly to Trivandrum and other major cities.

—LEA TERHUNE

Sadhana Kendra Ashram
Village Domet, District Dehra Dun

🐚 *Chandra Swami (1931–)*

Sadhana Kendra Ashram sits on the banks of the Yamuna River, surrounded by Himalayan foothills and miles of small farms, orchards, and grassy fields—to the dazed traveler straight off the bus, it may seem like you've found the only quiet spot in all of India. Don't confuse the teacher, Chandra Swami, with the more famous jet-setting guru by the same name, whom headlines in Indian newspapers have linked with money-laundering scandals. This Chandra Swami is a warm, unassuming man who has been in mauna (silence) for almost twenty years. But for part of the year, he communicates his teachings via written notes to a small group of Indian and Western devotees (many of whom also observe silence while at the ashram).

Teachers and Teachings

Although its beautiful setting may tempt you to come just for the ambience, this small ashram is only for serious seekers—"This is a place for spiritual effort, not recreation or passing time," state the printed guidelines for visitors. All guests are required to participate in the four scheduled hour-long meditation sessions each day. Chandra Swami gives daily satsang for about half an hour—communicating via written notes that are read by one of the devotees—during which he offers teachings (often in the form of jokes or stories), answers questions, and comments on world events. (He stays current via the TV news, which he follows ardently, often inviting devotees to his room to watch newscasts.) For about six months a year, though (January to February and mid-June to mid-October), he observes a practice of complete silence during which he does not communicate in writing or any other way.

With his long white beard and twinkling eyes, Chandra Swami looks like a picturebook guru—in fact, he was featured as a centerfold (standing dramatically on a rock in the middle of the Ganges) in a 1991 *Life* magazine feature on "Men of God." Chandra Swami was initiated as a young boy in the Udasin order of Baba Bhuman Shah, an Indian mystic saint of the eighteenth century who lived in what is now Pakistan and drew devotees among Hindus and Moslems alike. Midway through a post-graduate degree program in science, he dropped out of school to take vows of sannyas and embarked on eight years of solitary meditation and pranayama in Kashmir. He then spent another eight years in a thatched hut on an island in the Ganges near Haridwar, before devotees persuaded him to take up residence in an ashram so they could seek him out without risk of being swept away by the river.

Since his discovery in the 1970s by a French spiritual seeker—now a well-known teacher in his own right named Swami Anand Chetan—Chandra Swami has attracted increasing numbers of devotees, both Western (primarily French) and Indian (primarily well-educated professionals). But his ashram remains a small, intimate place with a family atmosphere, where your chapattis will be cooked for you right before your eyes and you can easily get a private meeting with the swami. Families with children often stay here (be sure you write ahead to get approval), and Chandra Swami can frequently be seen playing pranks on the children or offering them treats. However, silence is highly valued; there's little unnecessary talking, and many devotees emulate Chandra Swami by observing mauna while they're at the ashram.

Facilities and Food

Built in the early 1990s, this small ashram can accommodate about thirty guests in shared rooms. There are common bathrooms and showers with Western and Indian-style toilets. Bedding and blankets are provided.

Food is non-spicy vegetarian, simple but extremely fresh. Milk and curd come from the ashram cows; some of the vegetables from the ashram garden. A newly planted orchard will soon provide papayas, mangos, bananas, and other fruit.

There are beautiful flower gardens, a badminton court, and a well-organized and diverse library. You can swim in the river, which is clean but swift and very cold. The surrounding countryside is ideal for walks and hikes.

You must write ahead for permission to visit, as accommodations are limited and there's no lodging in the immediate area. Write well in advance, as postal services are slow to this little village.

Schedule

Four required hour-long meditation sessions begin at 4:30 A.M., 9 A.M., 3:30 P.M., and 6:30 P.M. There is a question-and-answer session with Chandra Swami at 11 A.M. and a brief darshan at 4:35 P.M.

Fees

Donation.

Contact Information

SADHANA KENDRA ASHRAM
VILLAGE DOMET (BARWALA)
P.O. ASHOK ASHRAM
VIA VIKAS NAGAR
DISTRICT DEHRA DUN 248 125
UTTAR PRADESH
TEL: 91-1360-2204

How to Get There

Sadhana Kendra Ashram is 48 kilometers northeast of Dehra Dun, near Barwala village, about 10 kilometers from the town of Vikas Nagar. You can take a train, bus, or plane from Delhi to Dehra Dun. From Dehra Dun take a bus or a taxi to the town of Vikas Nagar, then on to Barwala. A taxi directly from Dehra Dun to the ashram costs approximately Rs 300 and takes about one-and-a-half hours. If you use the bus, it's a five- to ten-minute walk from the village to the ashram.

You can also go by bus or taxi straight to Vikas Nagar from Delhi (via Saharanpur).

Once in Vikas Nagar, stop at Amar's Sweet Shop for further guidance (and sweets for Swamiji). Then it's 10 kilometers to Barwala. Just before crossing the river at the Barwala bridge, turn right at the sign for Sadhana Kendra Ashram. The Ashram is about 700 meters up the lane on your right.

Other Services

Barwala is a village of about 250 people. It has tea stalls, limited vegetable and fruit stands, and some basic supplies, but no lodging. Vikas Nagar, about 10 kilometers away, is a town of about 10,000 that has restaurants, limited lodging, and STD booths.

Books and Tapes

Books in Hindi, French, and English are available by writing the ashram. A donation of about U.S. $5 will cover the cost of the book and postage.

When I arrived at Sadhana Kendra Ashram, Chandra Swami was playing badminton. His sixty-five years were pitted against a twenty-year-old. In a fold of his dhoti there were some rupee notes. Chandra Swami was taking bets on the game. A couple of French disciples were cheering his opponent on. Whenever the boy was about to serve, Chandra Swami would make noises or jump about to distract him.

To no avail. When he had lost the match, he went off to the meditation room to lead the evening meditation. Chandra Swami has been in silence for decades, but he speaks volumes with a constant flow of smiles and laughter . . . The same warmth is there all the time, whatever he seems to be doing. It was there in the badminton match, it is there when he eats, or walks down the corridor. He is the same compassionate and immensely joyful presence wherever he is.

Though he will draw on all the different spiritual streams in answer to people's questions, it is evident that his real teaching is the way he leads his life. In the end, Chandra Swami doesn't do anything; he is utterly unselfconscious. Yet his ashram functions with unusual efficiency; he is always giving time to people, overseeing the new building works, signing cheques, answering the mail, living a life—but, it seems, with not a single gesture out of place. He has died into the stream of life.

—ROGER HOUSDEN

(from *Travels Through Sacred India*)

Kainchi Ashram
Naini Tal, Uttar Pradesh

Neem Karoli Baba (189?–1973)

Neem Karoli Baba—known to his disciples simply as Maharajji—became famous in the West as the loving, mischievous, and apparently omniscient guru described by Ram Dass in the counterculture Bible *Be Here Now*. Maharajji died in 1973, a few years after *Be Here Now* came out. But devotees still visit his ashrams all over India, including this one in an isolated river valley near the hill station of Naini Tal. To stay there overnight, you need to be a devotee of Maharajji (it helps to have a letter of recommendation from an affiliated group or a devotee known to the ashram). However, anyone is welcome to visit for the day and participate in the daily round of chanting and devotion.

Teachers and Teachings

There's no guru other than Maharajji, although an Indian woman named Siddhi Ma, who was with Maharajji for many years, has become the de facto manager of most of his Indian ashrams. She's normally in Kainchi from March through September and maintains a strict regimen of chanting and ritual. Every day, ashram residents are required to participate in arati and to chant eleven rounds of the Hanuman Chalisa, a forty-verse hymn to Hanuman that Maharajji taught to all his devotees.

Siddhi Ma offers no formal teachings herself—her only advice is to "remember Maharajji." Devotees mainly come to the ashram to feel, as one person wrote, "the nectar of his presence, the totality of his absence—enveloping us now like his plaid blanket."

Little is known about Maharajji's early life. "Facts are few, stories many," wrote a devotee in *Miracle of Love,* a collection of thousands of anecdotes compiled by Ram Dass after Maharajji's death. "He seems to have been known by different names in many parts of India, appearing and disappearing through the years. . . . He gave no discourses; the briefest, simplest stories were his teachings. Usually he sat or lay on a wooden bench wrapped in a plaid blanket while a few devotees sat around him. Visitors came and went; they were given food, a few words, a nod, a slap on the head or back, and they were sent away. There was gossip and laughter for he loved to joke. . . . Sometimes he sat in silence, absorbed in another world to which we could not follow, but bliss and peace poured down on us."

Ram Dass met Maharajji when he was still Richard Alpert, a Harvard professor, psychoanalyst, and psychedelic adventurer on sabbatical in India. Maharajji astounded him by immediately reading his mind and stating—correctly—that he was thinking about his mother's death of a spleen condition. "I felt like a computer that has been fed an insoluble problem—the bell rings and the red light goes on and the machine stops," Ram Dass wrote. "At the same moment I felt this extremely violent pain in my chest and a tremendous wrenching feeling, and I started to cry. . . . The journey was over. I had come home."

A few days later, Maharajji demanded that Ram Dass bring him "the medicine"—and proceeded to consume 900 micrograms of LSD with no visible effect. (Three years later, he repeated this feat with 1,200 micrograms). "These medicines were used in Kulu Valley long ago. But yogis have lost that knowledge," he explained. "To take them with no effect your mind must be firmly fixed on God."

Maharajji shunned publicity, but several hundred Westerners—and many more Indians—found their way to him before he died. They recount thousands of examples of his ability to read minds, predict the future, protect his devotees, and perform miracles. But most significant were the profound changes of consciousness they experienced in his presence. As Maharajji once said, "The key to the mind is in my hand and I can turn it in any direction."

The ashram is built into the mountainside on a river in a steep, narrow valley—the name Kainchi, meaning "scissors," refers to the jagged road that zigzags down to it. Ochre-and-white buildings with gold trim gleam among the jewel-green hills. Four or five temples sit amidst luxuriant flower gardens.

In the open season (March through September) about 150 guests can be accommodated in shared rooms; however, you must be a devotee and must write in advance for permission. Many people choose to stay in Naini Tal and just visit for the day. Simple food is provided for resident guests only.

Schedule

Devotees may visit during summer and monsoon months (March through September). The rest of the year the ashram is closed to visitors. The mandatory daily schedule consists of morning and evening arati, kirtan, and chanting of the Hanuman Chalisa.

Fees

Donation.

Contact Information

Sankata Mochana
    Hanuman Mandir
P.O. Kainchi, via Bhowali
Dist. Naini Tal
Uttar Pradesh 26313

U.S. Contact:
Neem Karoli Baba Ashram
P.O. Box W
Taos, NM 87571
Tel: (505) 751-4080
Fax: (505) 737-0180

How to Get There

Kainchi is about 30 kilometers from Naini Tal. From Delhi, take the train to Kathgodan; then go by bus to Naini Tal or by taxi straight to

Kainchi. There's also an airport in Pantnagar, 71 kilometers from Naini Tal.

Other Services

Kainchi is an isolated ashram. The nearest services are in Naini Tal (about 30 kilometers).

Books and Tapes

Miracle of Love: Stories About Neem Karoli Baba, by Ram Dass (Dutton).

This is how Maharajji became known as Neem Karoli Baba, which means the sadhu from Neem Karoli (or Neeb Karori). This was many years ago, perhaps when Maharajji was in his late twenties or early thirties.

For several days, no one had given him any food and hunger drove him to board a train for the nearest city. When the conductor discovered Maharajji seated in the first-class coach without a ticket, he pulled the emergency brake and the train ground to a halt. After some verbal debate, Maharajji was unceremoniously put off the train. The train had stopped near the village of Neeb Karori where Maharajji had been living.

Maharajji sat down under the shade of a tree while the conductor blew his whistle and the engineer opened the throttle. But the train didn't move. For some time the train sat there while every attempt was made to get it to move. Another engine was called in to push it, but all to no avail. A local magistrate with one arm who knew of Maharajji suggested to the officials that they coax the young sadhu back onto the train. Initially the officials were appalled by such superstition, but after many frustrating attempts to move the train they decided to give it a try. Many passengers and railway officials approached Maharajji, carrying with them food and sweets as offerings to him. They requested that he board the train. He agreed on two conditions: (1) the railway of-

ficials must promise to have a station built for the village of Neeb Karori (at that time the villagers had to walk many miles to the nearest station), and (2) the railroad must henceforth treat sadhus better. The officials promised to do whatever was in their power, and Maharajji finally reboarded the train . . . And they proceeded.

Maharajji said that the officials kept their word, and soon afterward a train station was built at Neeb Karori and sadhus received more respect.

—Ram Dass

(from *Miracle of Love*)

Satsang Bhavan
Lucknow, Uttar Pradesh

🌀 *Sri H. W. L. Poonja (1910–1997)*

Asked what kind of shrine he would like to commemorate his teachings, the renowned advaita vedanta master H. W. L. Poonja responded, "Not one brick." Poonjaji—or Papaji, as he was called by devotees around the world—died in late 1997. But at his house and satsang hall in Lucknow, about fifty of his long-term Western students still maintain a spiritual center for seekers who come from all over the world to taste the teachings that Poonjaji himself often summed up in two words: "Keep quiet."

Teachers and Teachings

Asked by an interviewer to convey his teachings in a single sentence, Poonjaji answered, "No teaching, no teacher, no student."

"Then what are we doing here today?" the questioner asked.

Poonjaji told him, "To find out who you are."

That answer is typical of Poonjaji's simple but paradoxical message: that we already *are* the freedom we are seeking. Our true nature, he said, is unbounded, limitless consciousness; we simply need to realize this fact. No techniques are needed for this awakening—why should we practice to become what we already are? "Practice is needed when you have some destination, something to attain," he taught. "Abandon this concept of gaining something at a later date. What is eternal is here and now."

Poonjaji himself had his first taste of this truth as an eight-year-old child, but it would take years of spiritual searching before he met the master who would plunge him into it permanently. Disappointed by countless "businessmen disguised as sadhus," he finally came to Ramana Maharshi's ashram in Tiruvannamalai. "Have you seen God?" Poonja asked the sage. "And if you have, can you enable me to see Him?"

"I cannot show you God or enable you to see God because God is not an object that can be seen. God is the subject. He is the seer," Ramana told him. "Don't concern yourself with objects that can be seen. Find out who the seer is. You alone are God."

"Under that spellbinding gaze I felt every atom of my body being purified," Poonja would recount years later. "A process of transformation was going on—the old body was dying, atom by atom, and a new body was being created in its place. Then, suddenly, I understood. I knew that this man who had spoken to me was, in reality, what I already was, what I always had been."

In recent years, thousands of people sought out Poonjaji in Lucknow—braving the smog and grit of this once grand city—because it was possible, they said, to experience this nondual consciousness directly while sitting in his presence. Accounts of dramatic awakenings—many of them by teachers who have gone on to collect their own worldwide followings—attracted throngs of seekers, drawn by the enticing message that you don't have to *do* anything to get enlightened.

Some seekers report that Poonjaji's powerful presence still pervades his home and satsang hall, which are open for meditation daily. You can also watch daily videos of Poonjaji's dynamic satsangs and interviews, in which he answers questions ranging from the philosophical ("Is freedom from thought really freedom from ego?") to the logistical ("I like to sleep with many different women. Is that okay?"). In every case, Poonjaji—blunt, clear, funny, occasionally caustic—eventually guides the seeker back to the ultimate query: Who is it who is asking the question, anyway? "Going within means just listening to your own Guru. And this Guru is your own Self," he taught. "You don't know him, you don't recognize him, you don't understand his language of silence. The real Guru will introduce you to the Guru within and ask 'you' to keep quiet."

Facilities and Food

Satsang Bhavan is a large suburban home that Poonjaji's students have rented and converted into a satsang hall. Poonjaji's former residence, about a mile from Satsang Bhavan, is open daily to visitors. There's no official ashram housing, but there are several Western-managed guest houses nearby, as well as larger hotels in the central part of the city. Your best bet is to go to Satsang Bhavan as soon as you arrive and ask for assistance.

Excellent Western-style vegetarian food prepared by students is served for lunch and dinner at the "Papaji Restaurant" on the roof of Satsang Bhavan. There are also several good local vegetarian restaurants within walking distance from Satsang Bhavan.

Schedule

Videotapes of Poonjaji's satsangs are shown daily at Satsang Bhavan from about 10 A.M. to 12 and 8 to 10 P.M. Poonjaji's former home is open to visitors from about 9 A.M. to 9 P.M. daily. Because Poonjaji only recently died, activities and schedule may change—it's advised that you call or fax in advance.

Fees

Meals at Satsang Bhavan generally run about Rs 50, depending on what you order. There are no charges or donations requested to visit or attend the daily video screenings.

Contact Information

SATSANG BHAVAN
A 306
INDIRA NAGAR
LUCKNOW 226 016
UTTAR PRADESH
TEL: 91-522-381189
FAX: 91-522-388578

How to Get There

Lucknow is approximately 490 kilometers southeast of Delhi. Take a taxi, autorickshaw, or tempo (group autorickshaw) to Indira Nagar, Sector A. If you take a tempo, get off at tempo stop Shalimar Crossing and ask directions to Satsang Bhavan, a few minutes' walk. If you take a taxi or autorickshaw, ask them to take you directly to Satsang Bhavan, which is near Shalimar Crossing—by now all the drivers know where it is, and you're likely to be accosted as soon as you get off the train.

Other Services

Lucknow has a population of approximately 1.8 million. All services are available. In the area of Satsang Bhavan are numerous restaurants and markets. Bicycles and motor scooters are available for rent.

Books and Tapes

Books, audio and videotapes of Poonjaji's life and the satsang sessions are available at Satsang Bhavan or by contacting:

POONJA JI VIDEOS
2888 BLUFF STREET, SUITE 390
BOULDER, CO 80301-9002
TEL: (303) 440-9607
FAX: (303) 494-8060

A good introduction to Poonjaji's teachings is *Papaji: Interviews* (Avadhuta Foundation) or the video *Call off the Search. Nothing Ever Happened* by David Godman (Avadhuta Foundation) is a three-volume biography of Poonjaji.

You are already here and you are already free. You think or have a notion that you have to search for something, to meditate. You have been told this many times. Now just for a short while, sit quietly and do not activate a single thought. You will discover

*that what you were searching for through methods or sadhanas
was already there. It was what was prompting you to meditate.
The desire for freedom arises from freedom itself.*

*Most meditation is only mind working on mind. You are
somewhere where the mind cannot trespass.*

—Poonjaji

(from "Plunge Into Eternity," *Yoga Journal*)

Dargah Hazrat Inayat Khan
New Delhi

Hazrat Inayat Khan (1882–1927)
Murshid Hidayat Inayat Khan (1917–)

Tucked amid the winding, congested alleys of one of Delhi's Moslem districts is the Dargah, or tomb, of Hazrat Inayat Khan, the musician and Sufi teacher who first brought Sufism to the West. In this small, grassy compound—walled off from the din of the surrounding streets—you can meditate, listen to *qawwali* (sacred music sung in Hindi, Persian, or Urdu, designed to transport the listener into communion with God), and study the teachings of Sufism, which Inayat Khan defined as "the message of love, harmony, and beauty."

Teachers and Teachings

Sufism, insisted Inayat Khan, is not just the mystical branch of Islam, as is commonly thought. It is a universal philosophy, a path of the heart, that can be practiced by followers of any religion. As formulated by Inayat Khan, Sufism emphasizes the quest for God within the heart; the primacy of "the sacred manuscript of Nature, the only Scripture that can enlighten the reader"; the universality of all religions; and the sacredness of beauty, art, and music as expressions of the soul. (However, some Moslems do not consider his teachings to be genuine Sufism, as they do not insist upon orthodox Islamic laws and practices.)

Born in 1882 into a family of mystics and musicians, Hazrat Inayat Khan traveled throughout the United States and Europe giving concerts and founding branches of a group he called the International Sufi Movement. Today, the main teacher at the Dargah—and the head of the ISM—is Hazrat's younger son, Pir Hidayat Inayat Khan. He lives in Europe but visits the Dargah three or four times a year to offer teachings.

The highlight of the Dargah is the weekly qawwali, a concert of sacred music that often features some of India's finest musicians. Since music is so central to Inayat Khan's message, other meditative music programs are also offered regularly, including Indian classical music and music from other religious traditions.

Each month the Dargah offers a "service of universal worship," which includes readings from the scriptures of the world's religious traditions.

Facilities and Food

The Dargah is in the heart of Basti Hazrat Nizamuddin, a poor Moslem district that takes its name from a great Sufi saint—Hazrat Nizammudin Aulia—who is also buried there, and whose tomb draws pilgrims from all of India. Across the street, ragpickers sort through the rubble of a garbage dump; the tiny alleys are a gridlock of vegetable vendors, bullock carts, and donkeys. But the Dargah courtyard itself is tranquil and green, showered, in the spring, with tiny yellow flowers from a massive acacia tree.

The main focus is Inayat Khan's rose-decked tomb. Around the tomb is an airy domed meditation hall with marble latticework quarried from the same source as the marble of the Taj Mahal. There are no accommodations or meals offered at the Dargah, but there are many hotels in the area.

A small library and information center is open to the public. The Dargah's charitable trusts operate a school and a dispensary for the local community.

Schedule

The Dargah is open from sunrise until about 9:30 P.M. If the gate is closed, just ring the bell. During most of the year there are daily prayers and meditations and weekly qawwali (every Friday evening just after sunset). The Service of Universal Worship is held roughly once a month; there are regular concerts of Indian classical music and regular lectures and courses on modern Sufism. Contact the Dargah for specific information.

Donation.

Contact Information

DARGAH HAZRAT INAYAT KHAN
129 BASTI HAZRAT NIZAMUDDIN
NEW DELHI 110 013
TEL: 91-11-462-5833
E-MAIL: BPBWALISUFI@COMPUSERVE.COM

THE INTERNATIONAL HEADQUARTERS OF THE SUFI MOVEMENT
24 BANSTRAAT
2517 GJ THE HAGUE
NETHERLANDS
TEL: 31-70-365-76-64
FAX: 31-70-361-4864

U.S. Contact:
MAHARAJ JAMES MCCAIG
1613 STOWE ROAD
RESTON, VA 22094-1600
TEL AND FAX: (703) 709-6983
E-MAIL: JMMCAIG@WORLDWEB.NET

How to Get There

The Dargah is about 5 kilometers from the center of Delhi and can be reached by taxi, bus, or autorickshaw. Ask for the Basti Hazrat Nizamuddin district, then ask directions to the Dargah once you are in the right area. Women traveling alone should be vigilant as this can be a rough neighborhood.

All services are available in Delhi.

Books and Tapes

Books on Sufism are available in most bookstores in the psychology/religion section, often including books by Hazrat Inayat Khan (such as the fourteen-volume series *The Sufi Message*). Books are also available through the International Headquarters of the Sufi Movement (see Contact Information) or through the electronic bookshop (jmmcaig@world-web.net).

> *Sufis and Yogis can respect each other, as the only difference between the Yogi and the Sufi is that the Yogi cares more for spirituality and the Sufi more for humanity. The Yogi thinks that it is better to be God; the Sufi thinks that it is better to be man, because if one is only spiritual, there is always the danger of a fall . . . the Sufi says that as all the needs and desires of this body and its senses exist, one should satisfy them; he says that we should have whatever we can have, but if we cannot have it, we should not care.*

> —HAZRAT INAYAT KHAN
> (from *Sufi Teachings*)

Gobind Sadan Institute for Advanced Studies in Comparative Religion
Gadaipur, New Delhi

Baba Virsa Singh Ji (1943–)

Don't be intimidated by the imposingly academic name: Gobind Sadan is primarily an interfaith spiritual community, intended as "a practical demonstration of God's love," where people of all religions come for meditation and teachings. The leader, Baba Virsa Singh, is a Sikh peasant preacher who has gained a worldwide following—despite the fact that he can neither read nor write—with his simple example of hard work and trust in God.

Teachers and Teachings

Life is work; work is worship; those who do not work neither live nor worship," reads one of Gobind Sadan's slogans. As a visitor, you're encouraged to join in the daily work of this community—whose forty acres of green, self-sufficient farm and dairy land were coaxed forth from the barren terrain south of Delhi—and you're more likely to find Baba Singh digging in the gardens than courting the adulation of devotees in the meditation hall. "I am just trying to be a better human being," he says, shrugging off the title of guru. "What I say is not new. I just repeat the commands of God so that people will remember them." Nonetheless, religious and political leaders from all over India seek him out at Gobind Sadan, drawn by what one American devotee describes as "spiritual powers of biblical proportion."

Baba Singh models himself on the lives and teachings of the Sikh Gurus (p. 237). As a spiritual discipline, Sikhism has two basic components: a daily discipline of meditation and prayer combined with social service and action. Sikhs are commanded to rise early in the morning and sit quietly invoking the name of God. At Gobind Sadan, early really means *early*—prayers and kirtan start at 2 A.M., followed by meditation at 4 A.M. Meditation, prayer, and scriptural readings continue on a twenty-four-hour basis to create a devotionally charged atmosphere.

Babaji stresses the universality of all religions, insisting that "religion is one, love is one, humanity is one, existence is one." People of all faiths come to Gobind Sadan, as Babaji's teachings support all spiritual paths. He works to bring people closer to God by using examples from their own traditions, quoting equally from the Koran, the Bible, and the Hindu scriptures.

At Gobind Sadan's farms, previously barren land (marked as "wasteland" in government surveys) has been reclaimed to produce record-breaking crops of sugarcane, wheat, rice, and mustard seed. Crop surpluses are donated to the poor, and the community uses the crop income to run services for the villagers, including a free medical clinic, school, and kitchen.

An adjunct to the community is the Gobin Sadan Institute—designed to bring religious research back to its spiritual roots—which sponsors semiannual conferences on comparative religion that attract scholars from all over the world. Although there's no formal curriculum of study, there are generally a few scholars in residence, and anyone is welcome to use the library.

Facilities and Food

The interfaith community has about fifty permanent residents who take care of the farms, dairy, communal kitchen, and devotional program. About ten to fifteen people can be accommodated in five rooms with bath in a special complex for foreign guests; a few more guest rooms with Indian-style bathhouse are sometimes available in the central community. You must write ahead for permission to visit. If you want to stay longer than three days, you need special permission from Babaji.

Although several thousand people may come to special functions—Gobind Sadan celebrates the holidays of all religions with great fervor—there are normally fewer than a hundred people in residence.

Most of the community food is grown on their own farms.

Schedule

The day begins with kirtan at 2 A.M. followed by prayers and more kirtan. There are morning and afternoon sessions of volunteer service, followed by kirtan, prayers, and a lecture in the evening. Babaji is often in seclusion, but sometimes audiences can be arranged by appointment.

Fees

Donation.

Contact Information

GOBIND SADAN
GADAIPUR
VIA MEHRAULI-MANDI ROAD

New Delhi 110 030
Tel: 91-11-680-2937, 2251
Fax: 91-11-680-1653

U.S. Contact:
Gobind Sadan, U.S.A.
Sikh Information Center
Box 383, RD 2 Graves Road
Central Square, NY 13036
Tel: (315) 676-2308
Fax: c/o Ralph Singh, (315) 449-3030

How to Get There

The Institute is located in Gadaipur, a suburban area of small farms south of the Delhi airport. The best strategy is to take an autorickshaw or taxi to Gadaipur and have the driver telephone for instructions once you are near the Institute.

Other Services

All services are available in New Delhi.

Books and Tapes

Books and tapes are available at the ashram or by contacting the Syracuse, New York, center (see Contact Information).

There are many yogic postures and methods of meditation, but even by practicing them you cannot attain God unless you feel the longing of love. God is Love, and God is too great for any method. It is God who pulls us to meditate, and it is God who teaches us how to love him.

The only method of meditation that works is to offer God constant love . . . Begin like this, and then God will show you the way. Make no demands, except for One: "Oh God, make me as You want me to be."

—BABA VIRSA SINGH
(from *Loving God*)

Sawan Kirpal Ruhani Mission (Kirpal Ashram)
Science of Spirituality
New Delhi

Sant Rajinder Singh (1946–)

The "Science of Spirituality" group is an offshoot of the Radha Soami movement, a mystical path whose primary teaching is "surat shabd yoga," the meditation on the inner Light and Sound. Unlike the Radha Soami group in Beas (p. 233), the Kirpal Ashram in Delhi—the headquarters of the Science of Spirituality organization—is open to non-initiates; the only requirement is that approximately six months before coming to the ashram you adopt a strict vegetarian diet, begin to spend 10 percent of your time in meditation, and give up alcohol and other intoxicants. (If you find these requirements daunting, this probably isn't the right place for you; it doesn't get any more lenient once you're inside.)

Teachers and Teachings

Like other Radha Soami branches, the Science of Spirituality group refers to their path as Sant Mat, "the teachings of the saints." The essence of the Sant Mat teachings is the meditation on inner Light and Sound. According to surat shabd yoga, God's creative power manifests in the world as Light and Sound, which flow in a divine stream through all the planes of existence. At the time of initiation, the Sant Mat master opens the disciple's inner ear to hear the celestial melody, giving a firsthand taste of the bliss it provides.

When you sit in meditation, you're instructed to repeat five "charged words" (given to you at your initiation) and concentrate your attention at the third eye, the seat of the soul, located between and behind the eyebrows. By concentration on this point, it is said, the initiate comes in contact with the inner Light and Sound. "By daily practice, students can transcend physical consciousness and explore inner realms of radiant Light," says a Science of Spirituality brochure. "This meditation method enables them to transcend the physical limitations of this world and experience the beauty of dimensions undreamed of."

The current guru, Sant Rajinder Singh, represents his family's third generation of Sant Mat teachers. He received initiation from his grandfather at age sixteen, then went on to earn a degree in electrical engineering and pursue a twenty-year career in the field of communications, electronics, and computers. While working for a communications company in the Chicago area, he began delivering spiritual discourses at the centers his grandfather had established throughout the Midwest. Since his father's death in 1989, Sant Rajinder Singh has assumed leadership of the entire Science of Spirituality organization, which now boasts 850 centers around the world (including sixty-two centers in Delhi alone).

The Kirpal Ashram is a large-scale operation, attracting close to 20,000 people—mainly well-educated professionals—to its Sunday satsang and meditation. Satsangs are in Hindi but translated into five or six other languages. When the guru is in residence, there are usually fifty to one hundred Westerners staying at the ashram. The atmosphere is disciplined and strict, with a high emphasis on morality and clean living; service work is encouraged though not required. Guests are asked to fill out a daily "introspection diary" checking off their observances (or lapses) of virtues such as non-violence, truthfulness, humility, and chastity (in thought, word, and deed) and recording the time spent in selfless service and meditation. (The back of the form features a helpful checklist of inner sounds you might have heard during meditation, ranging from "whistle or siren" to "vina or bagpipe.")

Facilities and Food

Up to four hundred people can be accommodated in dormitories and semiprivate rooms. There's a wide-ranging spiritual library (which even stretches to include books by Shirley MacLaine) and several large meditation halls. The grounds are quite limited; however, within two kilometers there are two more Sant Mat ashrams that have more open space and grounds for walking.

Schedule

Be prepared to get up early: the first four-hour meditation period begins at 3 A.M. Most of the day is spent in meditation, with satsang in the late afternoon and darshan in the early evening.

Each year Sant Rajinder Singh spends several months at the ashram and several at the U.S. headquarters near Chicago. He is normally at the ashram the last week of January until March; from May into early June; and September through October. He regularly tours in the United States, Europe, and India giving talks and meditation seminars.

Fees

Donation only.

Contact Information

KIRPAL ASHRAM
ATTN: SECRETARY
2 CANAL ROAD
VIJAY NAGAR
DELHI 110 009
UTTAR PRADESH
TEL: 91-11-722-2244 OR 3333
FAX: 91-11-721-4040

U.S. Contact:
SCIENCE OF SPIRITUALITY CENTER
4 S. 175 NAPERVILLE ROAD
NAPERVILLE, IL 60563
TEL: 630-955-1200
FAX: 630-955-1205

How to Get There

The ashram is located about 8 kilometers from the center of New Delhi and can be reached by taxi, bus, or autorickshaw.

Other Services

All services are available in Delhi.

Books and Tapes

A recommended introductory book is *Inner and Outer Peace Through Meditation* by Sant Rajinder Singh. In the United States you may order books, audiotapes, videotapes, and photographs directly from the Science of Spirituality Center (see Contact Information).

The Master, at the time of initiation, opens our inner ear to hear the Celestial Melody. This Sound is the God-into-expression Power, the Word or Naam, which brought all creation into being. On hearing the divine Melody, the soul, which is of the same essence as God, is magnetized to the Sound Current. Then we can travel on this Sound Current through the higher regions.

—Sant Rajinder Singh
(from *Ecology of the Soul*)

Sri Ram Ashram and Orphanage
Shyampur Village, near Haridwar, Uttar Pradesh

 Baba Hari Dass (1923–)

Baba Hari Dass first caught the eye of Western spiritual seekers as a character in Ram Dass's 1960s spiritual classic *Be Here Now*, in which

Ram Dass describes him as an "incredible fellow," a silent sadhu who had been living with a renunciate sect in the jungles since he was eight years old. In 1971, Baba Hari Dass left India for California, where he still presides over the Mount Madonna Center, a flourishing yoga community in the redwoods outside Santa Cruz. But from mid-January to the end of March each year, you can find him at the ashram and orphanage he founded in the countryside near Haridwar.

Teachers and Teachings

It's essential to make arrangements to visit this ashram in advance through Mt. Madonna Center (see Contact Information), as the staff is not prepared to handle drop-in visitors. Although Baba Hari Dass gives satsang and teaches classes when he is in residence, ashram officials stress that his main focus is the children at the orphanage.

Baba Hari Dass has been in silence for about forty years—he dispenses his teachings via a chalkboard hung around his neck, hundreds of letters to devotees, and an assortment of books that range from philosophical treatises to adventure stories for children. His teachings center on the classic eight-limbed (ashtanga) yoga of Patanjali, with a strong emphasis on karma yoga, the path of service.

"The spirit of karma yoga is performing duty with love, compassion, and enthusiasm," says Baba Hari Dass, who himself is legendary for the avidness with which he tackles physical work. (Among other things, he's an excellent rock mason who "lifts the rocks just with one-pointedness of mind," according to Ram Dass.) "There is no end to selfless service—the more you give the more you want to give."

When Baba Hari Dass is in residence, the Sri Ram Ashram is a busy place, with about seventy-five Western guests and a steady stream of Indian visitors. The ashram's orphanage houses up to fifty children from all over India—these children are not put up for adoption but are cared for and educated until age eighteen, when they are old enough for jobs or marriages to be arranged. Guests at the ashram may visit with the children as much or as little as they like. Guest quarters are separate from the orphanage, but many visitors enjoy playing with the children and helping to teach them English.

The program includes daily hatha-yoga asanas, pranayama, and purification techniques; devotional singing; meditation; and classes on yoga philosophy. You'll be expected to adhere to Indian mores about dress, behavior, and—when interacting with the children—child rearing. The ashram revolves around the orphanage, and formal spiritual practices are just a backdrop to this work. As one ashram spokesperson put it, "We're practical people doing a practical job. The spiritual part comes from the inside."

Facilities and Food

The ashram can accommodate up to seventy-five people in a combination of private, semiprivate, and dormitory rooms. The setting is rural—the four-acre property includes gardens where wheat, rice, and vegetables are grown. There's a meditation temple and a library with books for both children and adults. In addition to the orphanage, the ashram operates a school that serves both the orphans and children from a local village.

Meals are vegetarian, with milk from the ashram cows.

Schedule

The daily schedule begins at 6 A.M. and includes prayers, yoga classes, karma yoga, and devotional singing.

Fees

Rs 100 per day is the suggested minimum donation for lodging and meals.

Contact Information

SRI RAM ASHRAM
ANATH SHISHU PALAN TRUST
VILLAGE SHYAMPUR, KANGRI
DIST HARIDWAR 249 402
UTTAR PRADESH
TEL: 91-1364-451134

U.S. Contact:
SRI RAMA FOUNDATION
P.O. BOX 2550

SANTA CRUZ, CA 95063
TEL: (408) 847-0406
FAX: (408) 847-2683

How to Get There

The ashram is near Shyampur Village on Najibabad Road, approximately 9 kilometers from Haridwar. It can be reached by taxi or autorickshaw. (It's in an isolated area, so if you're just going for a day trip, keep the taxi or rickshaw waiting at the ashram.)

Other Services

All services are available in Haridwar.

Books and Tapes

For a good introduction to Baba Hari Dass's teachings, try *Silence Speaks* or *Ashtanga Yoga Primer*.

If you think the burden of the world is on your shoulders then you begin to feel the burden, and in a few years you become hunchbacked. Then one day you realize that the world is existing by itself, and your mind has made it a burden. But the hunchback has already formed. Ninety percent of pain is self-created. You can either accept your duties and responsibilities with a smile or reject them with tears. It doesn't make any difference to the world, but it makes a difference in your contentment.

—BABA HARI DASS
(from *Silence Speaks*)

Swami Dayananda Ashram
(Sri Gangadhareswar Trust)
Rishikesh, Uttar Pradesh

🌀 *Sri Swami Dayananda (1931–)*

This traditional Vedantic ashram is in a prime location right on the banks of the Ganges, surrounded by Himalayan foothills. Founded by a former disciple of Swami Chinmayananda of the Chinmaya Mission (p. 106), the ashram offers classes in Vedantic studies in English, Hindi, and Sanskrit. It's primarily meant for devotees of the founder, Swami Dayananda, especially the renunciates enrolled in his three-year Vedantic training course in south India. However, other people sincerely interested in Vedanta are welcome to stay if space is available.

Teachers and Teachings

All that you require to be free is to know yourself," Swami Dayananda explains. "Vedanta says that you are already free. It does not condemn you and call you a sinner."

In the "nondual" teachings of Vedanta, the individual soul (atman) is identical with the cosmic consciousnes (brahman). The world is an illusion; the only true reality is the unchanging, eternal Self.

Swami Dayananda's spiritual journey began in his twenties, when he began covering spiritual topics as a reporter for an Indian news agency. He studied Vedanta and Sanskrit with a variety of masters and eventually took monastic vows with the Chinmaya Mission, where he quickly rose through the ranks—in fact, he was widely expected to become the successor of the renowned Swami Chinmayananda. However, instead he left the Chinmaya Mission to found his own organization. For over three decades he has taught Vedanta all over India and the West. He has established Vedanta training centers in India, the U.S., Brazil, and Australia; spoken at universities such as Princeton and M.I.T.; lectured the United Nations on the immorality of the arms race; and expounded Vedanta on American cable TV. His 2,000-page commentary on the Bhagavad Gita is available to the public as a home study program.

The teachings of Vedanta have been laid out in centuries-worth of philosophical speculations, and these texts form the program of study at the

Rishikesh and Haridwar

The holy cities of Rishikesh and Haridwar mark the place where the sacred Ganges River descends from the mountains into the plains of Uttar Pradesh. Both are major Hindu pilgrimage centers—however, many Western travelers prefer to stay in the smaller and less congested town of Rishikesh, surrounded by Himalayan foothills, where the bottle-green Ganges foams (as yet relatively unpolluted) over white boulders.

According to legend, the ancient king Bhagirath invoked the goddess Ganga to descend from heaven by performing austere penances for thousands of years. Moved by his supplication, Ganga descended with such torrential force that Lord Shiva had to curb the deluge by entangling her mighty stream among the matted locks of his hair. He released her gradually, starting high in the Himalayas—at Rishikesh and Haridwar, her descent from heaven becomes complete.

RISHIKESH

Known as "the gateway to the land of the gods," Rishikesh is a place of great natural beauty, with its rushing water, giant trees, and fortress-like boulders. Views of majestic, snowclad Himalayan peaks can be reached in a few hours drive.

The launching point for pilgrimages to the sacred sites of the Himalayas—such as Badrinath, Kedernath, and Gangotri—Rishikesh is renowned in its own right as "the yoga capital of the world," as government tourist brochures like to call it. Yogis have inhabited its banks for centuries. In the main ashram district of Muni-ki-Reti, wall-to-wall ashrams crowd the riverbanks, ranging from gaily painted, multistory temple complexes that feed and shelter hundreds of Hindu pilgrims to dilapidated huts with weathered signs advertising "homely rooms, modern facilities." Bhajans blare from boom boxes and megaphones. Sandalwood smoke wafts from spiritual bookstores. Along the paths and bridges, ochre-robed sannyasins rattle begging bowls or lean silently on tridents. Throngs of devotees bathe and offer puja on the cement steps of the ghats. On boulders and sandy beaches, sadhus sit cross-legged in silent meditation—which they will sometimes abandon to offer their insights and advice to passing tourists.

Numerous ashrams provide instruction in yoga, meditation, Indian classical music and dance, Hindi, and Sanskrit. You can also stay in simple hostels where you can pursue a personal practice, free from ashram obligations and schedule. In addition to the ashrams described in detail in these pages, some places of interest are listed below:

Gangha Ghat, in the center of Rishikesh, is the main ghat where devotees perform religious rites and ceremonies. In the evening, arati is performed to the river.

Bharat Mandir, the oldest temple in the Rishikesh area, is in the center of town. Lord Vishnu is worshipped as an image carved from a single black saligram stone, beneath a Sri Yantra representing Lakshmi, his divine consort.

Kailash Ashram, a traditional Hindu ashram and home of many sannyasins, is a ten-minute walk beyond the Sivananda Ashram. It's renowned as a place for Sanskrit and Vendantic studies. Each evening, an arati to Shiva in the main temple fills the hall with voices singing Sanskrit prayers.

Mast Ram Baba Ashram is on the opposite bank, a short walk beyond the Lakshman Jhula bridge. You can visit the cave among the rocks and the sand where this contemporary saint lived for many years. The ashram blends so well with the natural environment that the sound of cymbals and chanting is the only landmark to help you find it.

Neelkantha Mahadev Mandir, about ten kilometers above Rishikesh, is a temple marking the spot where Shiva meditated after he swallowed poison to save the world.

Shakti Peethas (Goddess Shrines) include three famous temples near Rishikesh—Kunjapuri, Surkanda, and Chandrabadini—where Sati, the consort of Lord Shiva, is worshipped. According to tradition, Sati immolated herself after her father insulted Shiva by not inviting him to a great sacrifice. In mourning, Shiva flew all over India carrying Sati and parts of her body dropped at these three places, among others.

Neem Karoli Baba Ashram, one of several in India honoring the guru made famous to Westerners in Ram Dass's *Be Here Now* (p. 327), is just outside Rishikesh along the road to Haridwar. A forty-foot statue of the monkey god Hanuman towers above the ashram. Devotees are welcome to visit but there are no accommodations.

One of the four sites that host the Kumbh Mela festival (p. 58) every twelve years, Haridwar is brimming with temples and ashrams. Particularly noteworthy:

Akhara means "seat" and refers to the place where sadhus reside. Every major Hindu sect has established an akhara in Haridwar where sadhus gather in a kind of ongoing convention. Anyone is welcome to come and sit at their fires.

Sri Ananda Mayee Ma Ashram, located in the Kankhal area of Haridwar, was the main ashram of this Bengali saint who gained Western fame after her story was told in Yogananda's *Autobiography of a Yogi.* The ashram is maintained by devotees.

Har ki Pairi is the most sacred site in Haridwar, where the footprints of Lord Vishnu are imprinted on the wall underneath the water of the Ganges. Don't miss the arati to the Ganges held here every evening at sundown. Priests wave many-tiered lamps with flaming wicks to the accompaniment of bells, gongs, and conches. Pilgrims light candles and float them on the river in tiny boats fashioned from stitched leaves, creating a procession of fire that flickers into the night.

—SITA SHARAN

Dayananda ashrams. A lively and down-to-earth teacher, Swami Dayananda divides his time between this ashram, his school in Coimbature, and his ashram in the United States. Ongoing daily classes in English are conducted by a senior disciple. You can also arrange private tutorials with resident renunciates.

In addition to the classes, the schedule includes daily pujas and the ongoing chanting of Rama Nama Sankirtanam (singing the name of God) from morning till evening. The atmosphere is serious, but the residents are genuinely friendly to sincere seekers. The ashram seems to attract primarily well-educated, upper middle-class Indians. There's a high attention to detail; the staff is alert and focused; and standards seem high on every level, from the maintenance of the buildings to the quality of the instruction.

Facilities and Food

The ashram has fifty shared guest rooms with attached baths, a lecture hall, and a library. Simple vegetarian meals are provided.

Schedule

The day begins with prayers, meditation, and arati at about 5 A.M. Classes on Vedanta are conducted daily.

Fees

Donation.

Contact Information

Dayananda Ashram
Purani Jhadi
Rishikesh 249 201
Uttar Pradesh
Tel: 91-0135-430769

U.S. Contact:
Arsha Vidya Pitham
P.O. Box 1059
Saylorsburg, PA 18353
Tel: (717) 992-2339
Fax: (717) 992-7150

How to Get There

The ashram is a few kilometers north of Rishikesh, just behind the Andhra Ashram, across the Chandrabhaga bridge. A small tar road leads to the the ashram (also locally known as the Purani Jhadi or the Seesum Jhadi) on the banks of the Ganga.

To get to Rishikesh from Delhi, take an express train to Haridwar, then a taxi or autorickshaw to Rishikesh; or take a bus directly to Rishikesh.

Other Services

In the general area of the ashram are restaurants, tea stalls, fruit vendors, shops, and some lodging. Most services are available in Rishikesh and Haridwar.

Books, Tapes, and Affiliated Centers

Books and tapes are available through the ashrams in the United States and India. Swami Dayananda also has an ashram in Coimbatore, 200 kilometers south of Madras.

Vedanta does not promise anything. It does not promise liberation or salvation. It says only that "You are the solution." This means that you do not need to do anything to become free because you are already free.

The very fact that you are struggling, choosing, and searching in order to become free indicates that you have committed an error about yourself. No other tradition tells you this. They say only that you will be saved if you follow this or that. Vedanta does not say this. It says you are already saved and you do not know it.

—Swami Dayananda Saraswati

Jeevan Dhara Sadhana Kutir
Rishikesh, Uttar Pradesh

Vandana Mataji (1924–)

At the entrance to Jeevan Dhara Sadhana Kutir sits a statue made by a village sculptor: Jesus Christ in lotus position. If you're interested in "Christian yoga," a good place to find it is this tiny Christian ashram founded by Vandana Mataji, the author of *Gurus, Christians, and Ashrams* and one of the first Indian Catholic nuns to pioneer a truly Indian form of Christianity.

Teachers and Teachings

"What is it to practice yoga? Is it different from living according to the Gospel?" asks Vandana Mataji. "A yogic way of life helps harmonize or 'unite' not only me to myself (my body, psyche, and spirit 'oned') but also harmonizes my practice of Christian spirituality with that of my own country's culture and religious practices."

Born into a Parsi family, Vandana Mataji (formerly known as Sister Vandana—the title Mataji simply means Respected Mother) converted to Catholicism as a young woman and became a nun in the Society of the Sacred Heart. She went on to recognize Swami Chidananda of the Sivananda Ashram (p. 343) as her guru, and in recent years her teachers have included Buddhist monk Thich Nhat Hanh.

From the beginning, Vandana's mission has been to fuse Christian spirituality and theology with Indian culture so that the Church of India could find a genuine Indian identity and absorb the riches of other faiths, particularly Hinduism. Now a trim, energetic woman in her mid-seventies, she holds a master's degree in history and politics and a post-graduate degree in Hindustani classical music; she has founded several ashrams, written over a dozen books, and has traveled regularly to teach in Europe.

The practice at Jeevan Dhara ashram combines six classical yoga paths: jnana (wisdom), karma (service), bhakti (worship), raja (meditation), hatha (physical exercises and breathing), and japa (recitation of God's name)—all done with a Christian focus, but integrating other traditions as well. For example, the liturgy includes Christian scriptures and readings from works like the Upanishads and the Bhagavad Gita. Says Vandana Mataji, "Reading other scriptures often throws light on our own; they illumine texts with which one has long been familiar, yet which one has not yet really begun to fathom." Ashram rituals incorporate Hindu practices such as arati (the offering of fire) and feast days such as Deepavali, the festival of lights.

This is a place for dedicated seekers only, particularly those with a strong attraction to Christian as well as Hindu practices. You need to write well ahead of time asking for permission to stay.

Facilities and Food

The ashram is in a quiet residential area with peeks at the Ganges from some of the rooms and a full view from the rooftop terrace. Only three guests can be accommodated, each in a private room. Facilities include a small chapel and a good library. All meals are served at the ashram.

Schedule

There are four one-hour meditation periods daily, and group satsang is held once or twice a week. In addition, Mataji is available for private meetings. In the afternoons, you can do seva (work practice) in the garden or library.

The ashram is in silence each morning until lunch and all day on Friday. (In addition, Mataji is silent one full month every year.) On silent days, breakfast is the only meal served (although liquids such as tea or juice are available throughout the day).

Fees

Suggested donation for Westerners is Rs 90 per day.

Contact Information

Jeevan Dhara Sadhana Kutir
P.O. Box Tavovan Sakai
Via Shivanandanagar PO
Rishikesh 249192
Tel: None

How to Get There

The ashram is not far from Rishikesh in the Lakshman Jhula area. From Rishikesh go past the Sivananda Ashram about 1 kilometer. Just before reaching the Lakshman Jhula bridge, you'll see a sign on your left for the "Lupin-Herbal Research Center." Just before the sign, turn left down a small lane. When you can't drive any further, walk another 300 meters to the ashram.

To get to Rishikesh from Delhi, take an express train to Haridwar, then a taxi or autorickshaw to Rishikesh; or take a bus directly to Rishikesh.

Other Services

There are a variety of small shops and other services in the Lakshman Jhula area. All services are available in Haridwar and Rishikesh.

Books and Tapes

Books by Vandana Mataji are available through the ashram, including *Nama Japa: Prayer of the Name in the Hindu and Christian Traditions* and *Find Your Roots and Take Wing*.

Living in a religiously pluralistic country like India, one's theologising cannot be but constantly challenged. If one is rooted in Christ, it can be an exciting exploration, an opening into wider horizons, a climbing into deeper depths in "the cave of the heart."

—VANDANA MATAJI

Saccha Dham Ashram
Rishikesh (Lakshman Jhula), Uttar Pradesh

🌀 *Maharajji Hans Raj Swami (1924–)*
🌀 *Shantimayi (1950–)*

Sri Hans Raj Swami, known to his devotees as Maharaj, was unknown in the West until a few years ago, when his teachings were taken on tour by his disciple and spiritual heir, an American woman named Shantimayi. Now Maharaj and Shantimayi are accumulating a growing flock of

Western disciples who come to daily satsangs and bhajans at Maharaj's small, nonresidential ashram overlooking a crook in the Ganges.

Teachers and Teachings

As a married American woman—blunt and unabashedly Western—Shantimayi tends to attract Western seekers who want a guru who can relate to their cultural programming. Her daily satsangs are often preceded by spirited chanting sessions, with devotees accompanying the singing on guitars—these sessions tend to turn into bliss-fests, with devotees rocking, swaying, weeping, and glowing as they sing along to bhajans with a distinctly folksy beat.

Shantimayi first came to Rishikesh in the mid-1980s, as a dharma-hungry seeker who was, in her words, "desperate for a guru. I was desperate from the moment I first heard the word God." After investigating various teachers, she was steered to Maharaj by an Indian friend who owned a clothing store across the street from Saccha Dham (a name that means "abode of truth"). She spent the next seven years living at the ashram, soaking up Maharaj's energy—he gives very little verbal teaching—and spending most of her days sitting in silence on a meditation platform overlooking the Ganges. At the end of that time, Maharaj—now in his late seventies—sent her to Europe as his spiritual ambassador.

In Maharaj's advaita vedanta lineage, no formal practices are taught or even recommended—because there is no spiritual goal toward which one must progress. "I see everything as intrinsically pure," Shantimayi says. "If you like to do sadhana [spiritual practices]—which I love!—do sadhana. But not for a result. We Westerners have forgotten a lot about doing things just for the sheer love of doing them."

Instead of formal practices, Shantimayi stresses the importance of surrendering to the unconditional love of a guru, through which one can contact the limitless love of Being itself. Teachings consist of simply being in the presence of Maharaj or Shantimayi. When Shantimayi is in town, she gives formal satsangs; when she is not there, Maharaj is sometimes available for silent darshan (although he is not as generally accessible as Shantimayi). When Shantimayi is on tour, the ashram empties out and there is generally no formal schedule, although it's sometimes still possible to see Maharaj.

The ashram is perched on a bluff overlooking the Ganges. Satsang, darshan, and chanting take place outdoors on a concrete platform—also an especially nice place to enjoy the sunset. There are no residential facilities or meals—students must stay in neighboring ashrams or hotels (a nearby branch of the Om Karananda ashram is a popular choice). Because Sacchadham is a traditional Vedic ashram, Westerners are advised to be particularly careful to observe traditional rules of dress and behavior.

Schedule

When Shantimayi is in town, there is generally darshan with Maharaj from 10:30 A.M. to noon and satsang with Shantimayi at 4 P.M. When Shantimayi is not there, there is no formal schedule.

Fees

Donation.

Contact Information

SACCHADHAM ASHRAM
ATTN: SWAMI MIDDHA JI
TAPOVAN SARI
TEHRI-GARHWAL 249 192
TEL: 91-1364-30989 OR 32881 (OFFICE)
91-1364-31132 OR 31898 (RESIDENCE)
FAX: 91-1364-32621 (ALWAYS INCLUDE "C/O SACHA DHAM ASHRAM")

U.S. Contact:
PREM
1750 30TH STREET, #223
BOULDER, CO 80301
TEL: (303) 530-0732
FAX: (303) 786-7073

European Contact:
TERRE DE SACHA
CAN PINOUS
CORSAVY
66150 ARLES SUR TECH
FRANCE
TEL: 33-468392009

How to Get There

The ashram is near the Lakshman Jhula bridge a few kilometers north of Rishikesh. Take a rickshaw to the market near the Lakshman Jhula bridge, then ask directions to the ashram.

To get to Rishikesh from Delhi, take an express train to Haridwar, then a taxi or autorickshaw to Rishikesh; or take a bus directly to Rishikesh.

Other Services

Restaurants, lodging, tea stalls, and STD/ISD booths are available within walking distance of the ashram.

Books and Tapes

Audiotapes of interviews with Shantimayi, chanting tapes, and a video of satsang on the Ganges are available at Sacha Dham or through the foreign contacts.

I actually don't have a teaching. I tell people that they are That, and no matter what they do, That cannot change, and if they realize it, okay, but if not, still it's so. You can purify if you want to purify, but it doesn't make you any more That than you already are. And there is nothing that is not That; there has never been anything that is not That; it is not possible to be anything other than That; and this is the point to realize. And when this is real-

ized all the extraneous garbage—whatever that means—falls
away.

—SHANTIMAYI

Sivananda Ashram
Divine Life Society
Rishikesh, Uttar Pradesh

Swami Sivananda (1887–1963)
Swami Chidananda (1916–)
Swami Krishnananda (1912–)

The teachings of Swami Sivananda and the Divine Life Society are concisely summed up in the slogan over the altar in the samadhi shrine room: "Be Good, Do Good." Swami Sivananda was one of the yogic giants of this century, and his teachings have shaped the way yoga is taught not just in India, but around the world. Since his death in 1963, the ashram he founded—one of the largest and best known in India—has continued under the guidance of two elderly disciples, Swami Chidananda and Swami Krishnananda, both now in their eighties.

Teachers and Teachings

This not a place you can casually drop in and get a room. Anyone is welcome to attend the daily meditations, gentle hatha-yoga classes (not always available), and lectures on yoga philosophy (usually given by the crusty Swami Krishnananda, famous for his bluntness, humor, and keen intelligence). But if you want to actually stay at the ashram, you have to write to Swami Krishnananda to get permission in advance. Your letter should indicate a sincere interest in the teachings of Swami Sivananda and the Divine Life Society, which emphasize morality, self-discipline, generosity, and, above all, devotion to God. "Your only duty is to realize God. This includes all other duties," Swami Sivananda wrote. "The purpose of man's life is to unfold and manifest the Godhead which is eternally existent within him."

Born to an educated Brahmin family in Tamil Nadu, Swami Sivananda trained as a medical doctor and spent ten years working as a physician in Malaysia. Looking for spiritual answers to the suffering and death he saw daily, he abandoned his medical career, gave away his possessions, and returned to India as an itinerant, rag-clad seeker. He was initiated into sannyas in Rishikesh and devoted the next decade to intense yogic practice, living in caves and tumbled-down shacks and subsisting on a diet of only rotis (Indian bread) and Ganges water.

Not content with a solitary practice, Swami Sivananda soon began caring for sadhus suffering from fever, dysentery, cholera, smallpox, and malnutrition. He drew on his savings from his earlier life to establish a charitable dispensary that administered medicines to pilgrims, sannyasins, and local villagers. Disciples began gathering around him, and in 1932 he established the Sivananda Ashram in an abandoned cowshed on the banks of the Ganges.

Sivananda's teachings were distinguished by their practicality, universality, and emphasis on service. He wrote over three hundred books in English, making available on a mass scale ideas and practices that had previously been accessible only to Sanskrit pundits. He strove to make yoga accessible to householders, emphasizing ways to incorporate yogic practices into everyday life.

A revolutionary for his era, Swami Sivananda invited untouchables into his home and ashram, advocated yoga for women as well as men, gave sannyas through the mail, and railed against "superstitious" practices that detracted from the essence of spiritual life. ("Matted hair and emaciated bodies," he wrote, "have nothing to do with the divine life.") He stressed the essential unity of all religions and emphasized cultivating the body as the home of the spirit, rather than destroying it with ascetic practices.

Many of Sivananda's disciples went on to teach in the West, including Swami Chidananda, the president of the Divine Life Society since Sivananda's death in 1963; Swami Satchidananda (of Woodstock fame), whose Integral Yoga Society has branches throughout Europe and the Americas; the late Swami Vishnudevananda (p. 163), an early emissary of yoga in the West and the founder of the Sivananda Yoga Vedanta Centers; and the German-born Swami Sivananda Radha, the first Western woman to take vows of sannyas.

Today, his Divine Life Society boasts about ten thousand members, with over two hundred branches in India and abroad. The Sivananda Ashram itself has grown to a community of several hundred monks, lay residents, and short-term guests, with a large library, a free medical clinic, and a free thirty-bed hospital.

Since residency at the ashram is restricted, the easiest way to participate in ashram activities is to rent a room nearby and attend part—or all—of the daily program, which generally includes meditation, bhajans, a morning lecture or question-and-answer session, evening satsang, and a variety of special services and ceremonies. (Stop by the main office on Lakshman Jhula road to pick up a current schedule.) The daily question-and-answer sessions with Swami Krishnananda—now in failing health—are a delight, though be prepared to be challenged: the swami is known for ruthlessly cutting through jargon and spiritual pretentiousness.

You'll also be welcome at the special celebrations, which include all the major festivals of all the major faiths. On Christmas Eve, there's caroling and Bible reading; for Sivaratri, there's an eight-hour puja; there are celebrations for Buddha's birthday and Guru Nanak Day. As one resident put it, "Any excuse to draw your mind to God, we'll use it."

With the approval of Swami Krishnananda, serious students may be given permission to stay at the ashram for up to several months free of charge. Longer-term residency must be negotiated on an individual basis, and is reportedly much more difficult to arrange for women than for men. Of the close to three hundred residents, only about twenty-five are Westerners, and of those, only a handful are women. This is the place for a self-motivated seeker—while there are plenty of opportunities for study, meditation, chanting, worship, and service work, there are no required activities or formal training programs.

Facilities and Food

The ashram's rambling yellow-painted buildings sprawl on both sides of the road to Lakshman Jhula, just north of the Muni-Ki-Reti rickshaw stand. Facilities include a free medical clinic, an extensive library and bookstore, and an ayurvedic dispensary. Meals and shared rooms with private baths are available for pre-approved guests only.

Schedule

Morning meditation begins at 5 A.M. A lecture or question-and-answer session with Swami Krishnananda is generally held around 10 or 10:30 A.M. Stop by the ashram for a current schedule of pujas and meditation.

Fees

Donation.

Contact Information

SIVANANDA ASHRAM
DIVINE LIFE SOCIETY
P.O. SIVANANDANAGAR
DIST. TEHRI-GARHWAL 249 192
TEL: 91-1364-31190
FAX: 91-1364-31190

U.S. Contact:
DIVINE LIFE SOCIETY
6606 HARDWOOD LANE
KEEDYSVILLE, MD 21756
TEL: (301) 432-4918

How to Get There

The ashram is near Ram Jhula bridge just north of the autorickshaw stand in the Muni-ki-Reti district of Rishikesh. To get to Rishikesh from Delhi, take an express train to Haridwar, then a taxi or autorickshaw to Rishikesh; or take a bus directly to Rishikesh.

Other Services

There are restaurants, tea stalls, fruit vendors, shops, and lodging in the area near the ashram. Most services are available in the towns of Rishikesh and Haridwar.

Books by Swamis Sivananda, Krishnananda, and Chidananda are available at the ashram, at Sivananda centers abroad, and in many spiritual bookstores.

TWENTY INSTRUCTIONS FROM SWAMI SIVANANDA

[These aphorisms on the yogic life are inscribed on a pillar in the courtyard of the Sivananda Ashram.]

1. *Get up at 4 A.M. daily. Do japa and meditation.*
2. *Sit in Padma or Siddha Asana for Japa and Dyana.*
3. *Take sattvic food. Do not overload the stomach.*
4. *Do charity 1/10 of your income or one anna per rupee.*
5. *Study daily one chapter of the Bhagavad Gita.*
6. *Preserve virya [vital force]. Sleep separately.*
7. *Give up smoking, narcotics, intoxicants, drink, and rajasic food.*
8. *Fast on holy days or take milk and fruit only.*
9. *Observe mouna [silence] two hours daily and during meals also.*
10. *Speak the truth at any cost. Speak a little, sweetly.*
11. *Reduce your wants. Lead a happy, contented life.*
12. *Never hurt the feelings of others. Be kind to all.*
13. *Think of the mistakes that you have done [self-analysis].*
14. *Do not depend upon servants. Have self-reliance.*
15. *Think of God as soon as you wake up and when you go to bed.*
16. *Have always a japa-mala on your neck or in your pocket.*
17. *Adhere to the motto: Simple living and high thinking.*
18. *Serve the sadhus, sannyasins, and the poor, the sick, and the suffering.*
19. *Have a separate meditation room under lock and key.*
20. *Keep a spiritual diary and stick to your routine.*

These twenty spiritual instructions contain the essence of yoga and Vedanta. Follow them strictly. Do not be lenient to your mind and you will attain supreme happiness.

🌀 *Swami Shankardas (1947–)*

The Tut Walla Baba Ashram is really just a series of caves in the side of a forested hill, some of which have been roughly refurbished with wood and sheets of metal. The resident yogi, a bright-eyed, bearded man named Swami Shankardas, is as humble as his housing. He makes no attempt to publicize himself or his teachings, but there are generally two or three young Westerners staying with him for personal, largely informal instruction in the basics of yoga and meditation.

Teachers and Teachings

The daily schedule is quite flexible—"We have a variable program and it depends on what people want to learn," Shankardas says. You can stop by and visit with him any time; if you want to stay at the ashram, you can pursue your own meditation practice, help prepare the common meals, and ask Shankardas questions when he's not in meditation.

Shankardas himself came to the ashram as a boy of nineteen, after spending six years as a itinerant seeker driven by a quest for "God in a human form" that had obsessed him since childhood. Wandering in the forest above Rishikesh, he came across the cave he now lives in, where a man was sitting with long, dredlocked hair. Thinking he had stumbled upon Shiva himself, the boy retreated in a panic; however, the next day he summoned the courage to return, and was invited to stay by the long-haired man, who turned out to be a yogi named Tut Walla Baba.

Shankardas stayed with Tut Walla Baba for over a decade, serving him and the occasional visitors who came to the cave. After his guru's death in 1974, Swami Shankardas stayed on in the cave, pursuing his own practice and offering his insights to the pilgrims who come to him—most of them youthful Westerners looking for a taste of authentic yoga. His teachings, while rooted in traditional Hinduism and yoga philosophy, are informal and largely based on his own experience. Because there are so few people there, the teachings can be tailored to your own needs and you'll get plenty of personal interaction with the teacher; that, coupled with the roughness of the facilities, gives you at least the illusion of participating in an old-style guru-disciple relationship.

A maximum of ten people can stay in two or three spartan huts with dormitory-style cots. Bedding is not provided. The meditation cave can accommodate only one person at a time. Other nearby caves and wooded areas provide a place for quiet contemplation.

Food is prepared communally, or you can cook your own if you prefer.

Schedule

Because the ashram is so small, the schedule is determined by the residents. Typically, there's a morning meditation between 4 and 6 A.M., which is done on your own. Breakfast is between 8 and 9 A.M., lunch between 12 and 1 P.M. and dinner before sunset.

Sometimes Shankardas is busy writing or doing a personal meditation retreat and is not available. Occasionally, he will lead hatha-yoga instruction, upon request.

Fees

Donations are accepted but not solicited.

Contact Information

TUT WALLA BABA ASHRAM
P.O. SWARGASHRAM
RISHIKESH 249 304
TEL: NONE

How to Get There

Cross the Ram Jhula bridge in Muni-ki-Reti to the Swargashram area. Wind through the Swargashram area by the Choti Walla Restaurant and past the post office. This road goes uphill past some colorfully painted ashrams until you come to an arch entrance which says "Bhutna Kaliashananda Mission." Continue on this ten-foot-wide stone path going uphill. You will pass a large, very prominent ashram on your left. Eventually you will come to a small bridge that goes over a stream. Cross that bridge and continue up the road about 350 yards. There you will see a small gravel and stone pathway on your left. Climb some stone steps to a brick and tin-covered building that covers the front entrance of the cave. A small sign identifies the ashram. Ask people along the way to make sure that you're going in the correct direction.

To get to Rishikesh from Delhi, take an express train to Haridwar, then a taxi or autorickshaw to Rishikesh; or take a bus directly to Rishikesh.

Other Services

In the Swargashram area are restaurants, tea stalls, fruit vendors, shops, and some limited lodging. Most services are available in the towns of Haridwar and Rishikesh.

Books and Tapes

None.

International Vishwaguru Yoga-Vedanta Academy
(Sri Ved Niketan Dham)
Rishikesh, Uttar Pradesh

Sri Vishwaguruji Maharaj, Mahamandaleshwar (1904–)

The enormous Ved Niketan is the Best Western of Rishikesh ashrams, a two-story orange-and-yellow structure with hundreds of cell-like rooms arranged around a central courtyard. This ashram has been popular among Western tourists ever since it made the Lonely Planet guidebook; because attendance at yoga and meditation classes is not required and there is no minimum stay, it tends to attract some travelers who are more interested in low-budget tourism than in spiritual practice. However, it's also a popular yoga-training ashram with a solid introductory program for foreigners.

Teachers and Teachings

Nothing is mandatory at this ashram: If you want to stay in your room and practice bamboo flute all day, no one here will bother to stop you. On the other hand, you can drop in any day for ongoing classes in hatha yoga, meditation, and Hindu philosophy. The ashram also regularly offers comprehensive one-month introductory yoga courses.

The resident guru is Sri Vishwaguruji Maharaj Mahamandaleshwar, now in his nineties, described in the ashram literature as "an ascetic yogi of great repute." However, on a practical level, you won't have much contact with him: he only appears for special ceremonies and to initiate students into mantra practice at the completion of the hatha-yoga courses. The actual courses are primarily taught by Swami Dharmananda, a yogi from Calcutta who has been living at Ved Niketan for over a decade. In point of fact, he is not literally a swami—he is a retired army officer who has never taken vows of sannyas. However, he has spent the last fifteen years studying yoga and meditation with the SRF (p. 390) (he considers Yogananda his primary guru), Sai Baba (p. 69), the Vivekananda Kendra (p. 134), and the Sivananda Ashram (p. 163).

Swami Dharmananda is a popular teacher among Westerners; his English is fluent, and his lectures on Hindu philosophy are well organized, accessible, and even funny (which is rare among ashram yoga teachers). The hatha-yoga classes are gentle, Sivananda-style; Dharmananda cautions that they are "not meant for advanced hatha-yoga students." In addition to asana and pranayama, the one-month course includes study of the Bhagavad Gita and an introduction to the principles of raja, bhakti, karma, and gnana yogas.

The ashram is a peaceful place to stay from September to April. From May to August, it fills up with Indian families on pilgrimage, and the environment can become quite raucous.

Facilities and Food

The ashram is in a prime location right on the Ganges. There are about a hundred double and single rooms with private or communal bathrooms and a large hall for yoga and meditation. Three Indian vegetarian meals per day are offered.

Schedule

One-month yoga courses are conducted during February, March, April, September, October, November, and December.

Outside visitors are welcome to participate in any part of the daily schedule, which includes pranayama and meditation from 6:30 to 8 A.M., a lecture from 9 to 10:30 A.M., hatha yoga from 5 to 6:30 P.M., and bhajans and/or satsang from 8 to 9:30 P.M.

Fees

A single room is Rs 50 per night; double is Rs 75 per night. Meals are Rs 15 each. The one-month course is Rs 1,200.

Contact Information

SRI VED NIKETAN DHAM
P.O. SWARGASHRAM 249 304
RISHIKESH
TEL: 91-135-430279

How to Get There

The ashram is on the eastern side of the Ganges across the Ram Jhula bridge. From the autorickshaw stand, cross the Ram Jhula bridge (foot traffic only) and turn right; follow the road along the river. The ashram is the last one on your left.

To get to Rishikesh from Delhi, take an express train to Haridwar, then a taxi or autorickshaw to Rishikesh; or take a bus directly to Rishikesh.

Most services are available in Rishikesh and Haridwar.

None.

Yoga Niketan
Rishikesh, Uttar Pradesh

Swami Yogeshwaranand Saraswati (dates unknown)

Ever since Yoga Niketan was featured on Japanese public television a few years ago, it has been especially popular among Japanese tourists looking for an introduction to the yogic life. A collection of simple, white-washed cottages perched on a hillside overlooking the Ganges, the ashram offers yoga courses geared for beginning students. It also attracts travelers who are weary of being tourists and want some meaningful structure to their stay in Rishikesh.

Teachers and Teachings

The center was founded by the late Swami Yogeshwaranand Saraswati, but he and his teachings are rarely mentioned; the asana and meditation classes are taught by a variety of visiting swamis, usually imported from the Bihar School of Yoga (p. 89). Outside visitors can drop in for classes and to use the library, but if you want to stay at the ashram, you have to stay at least fifteen days and attend mandatory yoga and meditation classes every morning and evening. The rest of the day you are free to sightsee in town, although some visitors prefer to stay on retreat in the ashram itself.

This ashram is definitely run as a business; it feels more like a Western retreat center than a traditional spiritual community. But it's a good place for the beginning student to get a gentle introduction to yoga. The meditation sessions focus on simple breath-awareness techniques. The asana classes consist of vigorous practice of basic postures, with pranayama and chanting scattered throughout. Guests comment that the twice-daily group practice helps create a contemplative atmosphere and a sense of community.

Facilities and Food

Yoga Niketan is perched on a hillside just south of the Sivananda arch in Muni-ki-Reti. Roses bloom in quiet courtyards; cement benches tucked under the neem trees invite you to sit and look out over the Ganges. Double or single rooms are available. The meditation hall is spacious and marble-floored with cotton rugs for asana practice.

Meals are your basic rice, dahl, and vegetables—extremely bland, in keeping with yogic teachings.

The ashram also has branches where pilgrims can stay in Gangotri and Uttarkashi.

Schedule

Meditation sessions are from 5:30 to 6:30 A.M. and 6 to 7 P.M. Asana classes are from 7 to 8 A.M. and 4:30 to 5:30 P.M.

Fees

Rs 130 per day covers lodging, food, and classes.

Contact Information

YOGA NIKETAN
P.O. MUNI KI RETI
RISHIKESH 249192
TEL: 91-135-430227 OR 433537

How to Get There

Yoga Niketan is just south of the Sivananda arch in Muni-ki-Reti, Rishikesh, at the top of a steep stone path. To get to Rishikesh from

Delhi, take an express train to Haridwar, then a taxi or autorickshaw to Rishikesh; or take a bus directly to Rishikesh.

Other Services

Most services are available in Haridwar and Rishikesh.

Books and Tapes

None.

The Yoga Study Center
Rishikesh, Uttar Pradesh

❧ *Brahmacharya Rudra Dev (1956–)*

If hatha yoga is your main interest, the Yoga Study Center is probably your best bet in Rishikesh. This nonresidential teaching center at the south end of town was founded by Brahmacharya Rudra Dev, a senior student of B. K. S. Iyengar (p. 221) who spent ten years as monk at the Sivananda Ashram. The daily asana classes are conducted in old-school Iyengar style—tough, precise, military, and vigorous. But Rudra solidly grounds the physical practice in the context of classical yoga philosophy, speaking with equal authority of the psoas muscle and the kundalini, the prana and the organ systems.

Teachers and Teachings

As a young boy in southern India, Rudra turned to hatha yoga to help him correct chronic health problems, including obesity and a crooked spine. At age nineteen, he joined the Ramakrishna Mission, and began studying Sanskrit and yoga philosophy. Shortly after coming to the Sivananda ashram in 1980, he met B. K. S. Iyengar, and began traveling regularly to Pune to study with him. His hatha-yoga classes at the Sivananda ashram soon developed a glowing reputation among Westerners, and in 1990 he opened the Yoga Study Center to accommodate the influx of enthusiastic students.

Hand built by Rudra and student volunteers, the center is an unheated brick building with high ceilings, a cement floor, and a donated collection of well-worn mats, straps, and blankets. Rudra—who adheres to renunciate vows of simplicity and celibacy—lives in one tiny room just off the main studio. In addition to the twice-daily classes (one in English for Westerners and one in Hindi for local students), Rudra leads three-week intensive courses three times a year, which are generally well attended by European Iyengar students who don't want to wait three or more years for a space to open up in Pune. (Thus far, Rudra has resisted his students' entreaties to go on a teaching tour in the West, on the grounds that it would interfere with his own sadhana.)

If you're a woman, don't show up for class in a leotard—"ladies are especially requested to dress decently," says the schedule. Male or female, be prepared to work hard. When Rudra barks out orders (in fluent but heavily accented English that's hard to understand at first), you're expected to jump, and even advanced students may be challenged by some of the postures. "Yoga is a purificatory process," he says as he strides through the room adjusting postures with a slap here, a kick there. "If you want to control the river of prana, you have to build a strong dam." But don't be fooled by the gruff presentation—tune in, instead, to the quick smile and the warm eyes. "This is not *my* center, I am the servant of this center," Rudra likes to say. "I am not a teacher, I am a seeker."

Facilities and Food

The Yoga Study Center is nonresidential but there is plenty of lodging nearby. (Many students stay nearby at the "University of Peace," an oddly named hostel on the banks of the Ganges that offers rooms for about Rs 50 a night.)

Schedule

Three-week intensives are offered February 8 to 28, April 4 to 25, and September 2 to 24. Asana classes of varying levels are offered several times a day from July to November—check the current schedule for details. The center is closed four months a year: from mid-December to mid-January, and all of March, May, and June.

Fees

All classes are offered free of charge. Voluntary donations are accepted.

Contact Information

The Yoga Study Center
Br. Rudra Dev
Ganga Vihar, Haridwar Road
Rishikesh 249201 (Dist. Dehradun)
Tel: 91-1364-31196

How to Get There

The Yoga Study Center is at the southern end of Rishikesh just off the main road. Most rickshaw drivers know where it is.

To get to Rishikesh from Delhi, take an express train to Haridwar, then a taxi or autorickshaw to Rishikesh. You can also take a bus directly to Rishikesh.

Other Services

Most services are available in Haridwar and Rishikesh.

Books and Tapes

None.

Varanasi: City of Light

City of Thieves, City of Light, City of Final Liberation, Varanasi—also known by its more ancient names of Benares and Kashi—is a magical city and the heart of Hindu India. Whatever sins you may have committed in any of your 84,000 births, tradition holds that all can be instantly wiped away by breathing the air of Benares, feeling the dust of its earth on your feet, and stepping into the Ganges from the bathing ghats (steps) that line its banks. A dip in the Ganges here, it's said, can wash away seven generations of bad karma.

Varanasi is famous for death—after all, it's the territory of Shiva, whose favorite haunt is the cemetery and whose favorite outfit is a thick layer of ashes from the funeral pyre. Hindus believe that dying in Varanasi ensures liberation for the soul (on your deathbed here, Shiva himself will whisper a mantra in your ear that ensures your safe passage to the other side). The city is located at the only place in the Ganges' course where it takes a sharp bend and turns to flow north, before resuming its southern eastward course. In metaphysical parlance, this signifies that the human being—always headed toward the south, which is the realm of Yama, the god of Death—at Varanasi alone is afforded the opportunity to turn back.

Every day, the population of Varanasi nearly doubles (from approximately 1 million to nearly 2 million) through the influx of pilgrims and tourists—along with the thousands who come to Banaras simply to die. There are, in fact, many older people who refuse to leave the city precincts—even for medical help at the nearby modernized health facilities at Banaras Hindu University—for fear that the god of Death may try to trick them and take their lives outside the sacred city.

As the oldest continuously inhabited city in the world, Varanasi has been host to a steady stream of famous holy men and women. In fact, for at least the last ten centuries, no aspiring saint or sage could be said to have completed his spiritual course without a pilgrimage to Varanasi. The Buddha himself wandered through the streets of Varanasi in the sixth century B.C.E. and gave his first sermon at nearby Sarnath (p. 94).

Exploring the riches of Varanasi could take several lifetimes. The following are just a few tips:

Boat ride on the Ganges. To watch the sun rise over the river means you have to get up by 5:30, but you get a spectacular view of ancient temples turned gold by the dawn and pilgrims bathing in the river. (You can float within viewing range of the burning ghats where the dead are cremated, but *do not* take photos.) Boatsmen line the riverbanks—you can generally bargain the price down, but you will generally have better luck if you don't start your journey from the central ghat, Dasashvamedh. Be sure to arrange for early morning boat rides the day before.

A couple of hints for those bold enough to take the holy bath: Water tests have shown that the middle portion of the river has minimal amounts of bacteria, whereas the shore areas tend to have high readings. You can take a boat ride out to the middle for a swim; however, you must be an expert swimmer, and during the monsoon months the current is so strong that not even the best swimmers should try it. In the hot season, swimming across the width of the river is not too strenuous. However, the majority of the devout content themselves with three dunks in the more shallow water near the shore.

Kala Bhairava Nath. The pilgrim's traditional first stop in the city of liberation, this temple is located in a maze of winding narrow alleys to the northeast of Chauk Ghat. The deity Kala Bhairava is the city's divine chief of police—it's said that you can't attain any of the merit of visiting the holy city if you do not first announce your presence and ask his permission to be there.

Annapurna Mandir. Located in an alley off the main Dashashvamedh Road, this temple—dedicated to the goddess who bestows an abundance of food—is another traditional stop for pilgrims. Depending on the mood of those watching the door and the attire of entering Westerners, it is sometimes closed to foreigners and—on a lucky day—sometimes not.

Dhundi Raj. This is a very famous image of Ganesh (the elephant-headed god of new beginnings) that lies on a pathway off Vishvanath Gali (alley). Along this alley and in the nearby environs you can find every imaginable piece of puja paraphernalia, including silver, copper, brass, and stone images of different deities; sandalwood paste; rudraksha beads; brass, copper, and silver vessels; and colored powders.

Durga Mandir. For those who are devotees of the Goddess, the Durga Mandir—located near Assi Ghat near Ravindrapuri crossing on Kurudshetra Road—is a wonderful visit. It's sometimes called the "monkey temple" because of the profusion of monkeys running inside and on the roof, waiting for a chance to snatch and eat the flower garland offering of an unwary pilgrim. During Navaratri (a nine-day celebration to the Goddess in October) the temple is packed with local residents who will spend hours sitting and reciting the Devi Mahatmya, Hymn to the Greatness of the Goddess.

Vishalakshi Mandir. This scripturally very famous temple is a tantric peetha ("seat") of the Goddess. It marks the site where the eyes of the Shiva's wife fell as Shiva, mad with grief, carried her corpse around India, while the god Vishnu cut the body apart piece by piece to prevent Shiva's sorrow from destroying the universe. It is located on the main road alongside the Ganges River between Dashashvamedh and Chauk Ghats.

Sankata Mochana. One of the city's most popular temples is this one to the monkey god Hanuman, located in the southern part of the city about two miles west of Assi Ghat. The temple's priest heads the "Swatcha Ganga" campaign to clean the Ganges of pollution and has established elaborate water testing in attempts to get the government to implement more stringent pollution guidelines for drainage into the river.

Ramananda Ashram. Located on Pancaganga Ghat and looking right out over the river, this ashram marks the place where the Muslim-born poet Kabir lay waiting on the steps before sunrise for the saint Ramananda to come for his morning bath. Ramananda accidentally stepped on him and in surprise shouted "Ram!" Kabir took it as his initiation into the mantra. The current residents speak very little English.

Tailang Swami Ashram. Near the Ramananda Ashram, through the winding alley toward the center of the city, is the ashram that once belonged to Tailang Swami, a famous teacher who reputedly lived three hundred years (from the sixteenth to the nineteenth century) and performed numerous miracles. The ashram houses his samadhi shrine, which is a very nice place for meditation, as well as an extremely large Shiva lingam, which apparently—by some miracle or other—was able to come through a door several times smaller than it is.

Kriya Yoga Center. The great grandson of Lahiri Mahasay (the guru of Yuk-teshwar, who was the guru of Yogananda, the author of *The Autobi-ography of a Yogi*) lives in one of the alleys off Chauthasi Ghat (near Chauthasi temple), where he teaches kriya yoga and periodically gives initiations.

Aghora Ashram. This peaceful ashram—located about a few kilometers di-rectly north of the Durga Mandir—draws a fair number of Western vis-itors. Previously a site of tantric practice, its rituals were somewhat tamed by the late guru Bhagavan Ram.

Krishnamurti Center. A branch of the headquarters in Madras (p. 254) lo-cated at the farthermost northern ghat, the facilities here are extensive and the entire environment is green and spacious, with amenities to accommodate Westerners.

Mumuksha Bhavan. This traditional ashram located to the south of Assi crossing can accommodate Westerners even for an extended stay.

Ramakrishna Mission Ashram. Located on Ramakrishna Road in Luxa, this beautiful ashram—a branch of the main headquarters in Calcutta (p. 382)—has a very spirited evening arati.

Anandamayi Ma Ashram. Housed in a beautiful building overlooking the Ganges near Tulasi Ghat, this ashram has a devotional and moving evening puja.

Hindi and Sanskrit Programs. If you would like to learn some Hindi while in Banaras, contact the International Institute of Languages: B-31/27-K Ratnadeep, Lanka, Varanasi 221005. Tel: 91-542-311723. Fax: 91-542-313965.

For a crash course in Sanskrit with a Banaras pandit, contact Vagyoga Chetana Peetham; B 3/131 A, Shivala; Varanasi 221001. Tel: 91-542-311706.

—LORILIAI BIERNACKI

Yoga Sadhana Kendra (Centre for Yoga)
Banaras Hindu University
Varanasi, Uttar Pradesh

🌀 *Program Coordinator: Dr. R. H. Singh*
🌀 *Instructor: Dr. Krishna Murari Tripathi*

Located in a small classroom building on the sprawling campus of Banaras Hindu University, the Yoga Sadhana Kendra is officially described as an "interdisciplinary academic institution for study, instruction, and research in all aspects of yoga, both theoretical and applied." The Kendra arranges lectures on yoga and related topics; sponsors research on philosophical, psychological, and medical aspects of yoga; and runs a four-week part-time certificate course (largely practical) and a four-month part-time diploma course (largely theoretical), both of which are open to foreigners.

Teachers and Teachings

The best thing about these programs is that they're based in Varanasi, one of the oldest and most sacred cities in India and a center of Hindu culture for thousands of years. (See p. 358.) The courses only meet for an hour or two each day, so you can get an academic, scientific introduction to the history and practice of yoga while still having plenty of time to soak in the magic and mysticism of the "city of light."

Aside from that, there's not much mystical about this program, which is staffed by professors, not sannyasins, and prides itself on being strictly rational and objective. "We avoid discussion of religion and God," explains Dr. K. M. Tripathi, an instructor at the Yoga Sadhana Kendra. "We approach yoga as a universal science, free of any religious impressions." According to the program literature, "All books and traditions of Yoga as well as the lives and works of all celebrated Yogis at all times and all over the world are studied reverentially, but critically and dispassionately at this Centre."

The four-week certificate courses—known as "Yogic Practices for Better Living"—are modeled on the programs developed by the Yoga Institute of Santa Cruz (p. 187) and Kaivalyadhama (p. 202), which stress the practical, therapeutic value of the yoga practices. Courses meet one hour a day, six days a week, for four weeks. Most of the classes consist of instruction in the fundamental psycho-physical yoga techniques, including about two dozen basic asanas; simple breathing exercises that prepare you for pranayama; mudras, bandhas, and relaxation exercises. In addition, there are about a dozen lectures on philosophical and scientific aspects of yoga, such as the eight-limbed yoga of Patanjali, yoga therapy, and medical research on yoga techniques.

The four-month diploma program—which is mainly attended by Indians enrolled at BHU but reserves five seats for foreigners—consists of in-depth courses in the foundations of yoga (covering the Upanishads, the Bhagavad Gita, the Yoga Sutras, the tantric and hatha-yoga traditions, and the development of yoga techniques in the Hindu, Jain, Buddhist, Sufi, and Sikh traditions); yoga for health (forcusing on physiological and psychological studies of yoga practices); and contemporary yoga (especially the work of Vivekananda, Gandhi, and Aurobindo).

Once you're enrolled in the program, you can sometimes tailor it to suit your own needs by drawing on the resources available through related BHU departments, such as Sanskrit, philosophy, and Indian history.

Facilities and Food

This program is nonresidential, except for students already enrolled in BHU. Food and lodging are easily available in Varanasi.

Schedule

Certificate courses are generally conducted twice a year, the first in September/October and the second in March/April. Classes meet an hour a day, six days a week.

The four-month diploma course runs once a year and generally starts shortly after the fall festival of Deepavali.

Fees

Certificate course: Rs 100
Diploma course: Rs 500

Reunion in Banaras

I first met Charan Das ten years ago, in Santa Fe, New Mexico, when he knocked on the door of my adobe cabin one frosty November night. The wind was sharp and the churned mud of my driveway was frozen into icy ruts, but he was dressed only in sandals and a brown cotton shawl and lungi; his hair hung in matted dreadlocks past his shoulders.

"We just met your roommate at the Lama Foundation," he said. "She said we could stay at your house for a few days."

"Of course." I peered past him into the dark. "How many of you are there?"

He gave me a radiant, gap-toothed smile. "Just this one," he said.

Over almond tea in front of the wood stove, Charan Das explained that he was a sadhu, one of India's millions of wandering ascetics who live on alms as they travel from village to village in pursuit of God-realization. In a previous incarnation, though, he had been a Texas college student who had gone to India on a research grant. Ten years later, he had come back to the States for the first time, to visit his somewhat alarmed family and the sacred sites of the Southwest. He referred to himself in the plural, he explained, as an ego-deflating spiritual practice. "Our we," he said, "includes you too."

Over the next few days, Charan Das told me stories about sadhus: how they live without possessions, entirely dependent on the generosity of strangers; how they never stay anywhere longer than a few days to avoid becoming attached to places and people (and to spread spiritual teachings as widely as possible); how they often adopt extreme ascetic practices for cycles of twelve years at a time, such as holding one arm continually up in the air, or hanging upright in a sling from a tree branch instead of lying down to sleep. He covered my kitchen table with snapshots of throngs of naked babas plunging into the Ganges at the Kumbh Mela, the world's largest religious celebration. I teased him from time to time—referring to him as "they" and offering him a rafter to hang a sleeping sling from (which he declined in favor of a couch)— but I became quite fond of him, and when he left I expressed regret that his itinerant lifestyle meant I'd have no way of finding him if I ever made it to India.

"Oh," he said, cheerfully. "We only wander half the year. The other half, we have a lady friend in Banaras."

And it was in Banaras that I next ran into him, just a few days ago, sipping chai on the rooftop of the Hotel Ganges View. I recognized him right away, though his dreadlocks have turned gray and a new pair of wire-framed spectacles perched unsteadily on his nose. The lady friend seemed to have dropped out of the picture—he had come to Banaras for just a few days, he told me, to celebrate the Shivaratri festival with his guru and fellow-saddhu, Kathia Baba.

I told him that I was in India researching a spiritual guidebook, and would appreciate his expert insights.

"We were working on a spiritual guidebook, too!" he said in delight. "That's why we originally came to India twenty years ago."

Somewhat alarmed, I asked him what had happened to his project.

"Our notes were all locked up in a friend's house in Banaras," he said. "A whole trunkful of them, on hundreds of ashrams all over India. But the friend died many years ago. The trunk was moved, and we're not sure where."

He began to laugh—a zany, low-pitched chortle that went on long after my own laughter had stopped—and I knew that for him, a spiritual guidebook had long since lost all relevance. My publisher would be alarmed, I'm sure, at how uplifted that perspective made me feel.

—ANNE CUSHMAN
(dispatch from India)

Contact Information

YOGA SADHANA KENDRA (CENTRE FOR YOGA)
MALAVIYA BHAVAN
BANARAS HINDU UNIVERSITY
VARANASI 221 005
TEL: (91-542) 310291
TELEX 0545 304 BHU IN

How to Get There

Banaras Hindu University is at the southern end of Varanasi and can be reached by bus, taxi, or rickshaw. Once there, ask directions to the Malaviya Bhavan building, where the Yoga Sadhana Kendra is located. (Autorickshaws are not permitted on campus, and it's a long walk from the campus gate; you might want to hire a bicycle rickshaw to take you there.)

Varanasi can be reached by air or by train from Delhi.

Other Services

All services are available in Varanasi.

Books and Tapes

None.

International Society for Krishna Consciousness (ISKCON)
Vrindaban, Uttar Pradesh

❋ *A. C. Bhaktivedanta Swami Prabhupada (1896–1977)*

In 1965, an elderly swami arrived by steamship in Boston Harbor, his only possessions a few sets of robes, seven dollars worth of rupees, a typewriter, some translations of Hindu scriptures, and a stack of leaflets proclaiming Krishna as the Supreme Lord of the Universe. Within a few years, A. C. Bhaktivedanta Swami Prabhupada's Hare Krishna mantra had become one of the soundtracks to America's flower-child revolution, and his International Society for Krishna Consciousness (ISKCON) soon swelled to an immense and wealthy spiritual superpower. Splintered by scandals and in-fighting after Prabhupada's death, ISKCON nonetheless continues to attract hundreds of thousands of followers worldwide. Its ashram in Vrindaban, Krishna's sacred city, is a bustling place—replete with magnificent marble and gold-leaf temples—that's open to short-term visitors as well as serious devotees.

Teachers and Teachings

The Hare Krishnas have gotten a lot of negative press over the years; if you're like most people, you mainly know them through newspaper headlines and their enthusiastic proselytizing in airports. If you've been turned off by this group in the past, the Vrindaban ashram may come as a surprise; although missionary zeal is in evidence, you won't get too much of a hard sell, and you're free to participate or not in daily activities. (In fact, the guest house is run more like a hotel than an ashram, and you can come and go as you like.) There are daily lectures in English by senior swamis; however, the main spiritual activity is the round-the-clock chanting of the Hare Krishna mantra: "Hare Krishna, Hare Krishna, Krishna Krishna, Hare Hare, Hare Rama, Hare Rama, Rama Rama, Hare Hare."

By chanting this mantra, Swami Prabhupada taught, the devotee comes into direct communion with Lord Krishna—in traditional Hinduism, one of nine incarnations of the god Vishnu—who is seen, by Hare Krishnas, as the "Supreme Personality of Godhead." "Krishna consciousness is already there at the core of everyone's heart. But because of our materially conditioned life, we have forgotten it," he explained. "The process of chanting the Hare Krishna maha-mantra . . . revives the Krishna consciousness we already have." The more you chant this mantra, Hare Krishnas believe—whether silently or aloud—the more blissful you become. In addition to chanting, ISKCON devotees are asked to follow four basic rules: a strict vegetarian diet; no gambling; no intoxicants; and no illicit sex life (with illicit sex defined as sex outside of marriage).

The "Krishna Consciousness" path is an offshoot of the ecstatic Vaishnavism (Vishnu worship) proclaimed by the fifteenth-century saint Chai-

Lord Krishna's City

Even the dust of Vrindaban is sacred: the entire "Krishna lila," the divine dance of the god Krishna's life, was enacted throughout the city and the surrounding areas of Vraja. Krishna was born in Mathura and raised in Gokul; he held the nearby Govardan mountain on his finger to protect the cows and people from Indra's furious rains. Although he eventually left Vrindaban to rule his kingdom from Dwarka on the coast of Gujarat, his presence is still felt here.

Vrindaban was named after the delicate tulsi plant that is the symbol of Radha, Krishna's beloved mistress. Devotees still invoke her name in greeting. Pilgrims come here to take the barefoot walk along the "parikrama" (holy walk) path around the city. The path no longer meanders along the Yamuna River, which once flowed beneath Vrindaban's majestic ghat; it has changed its course. But the river's waters still sparkle in the moonlight beside sandy silver banks, evoking those nights when Krishna enraptured the milkmaids with his flute music.

Song and dance are integral to the bhakti tradition of Vrindaban. During celebrations, temples sponsor concerts and devotees parade through the narrow alleys, echoing Radha's passion for her Lord. The town is full of countless temples—Behari-ji Mandir is the most famous, along with the nearby Radha Raman and Radha Vallabha. Everywhere narrow cobblestone alleys lead to medieval courtyards through great portals fashioned for elephants. Gardens hidden behind towering walls fill the evening air with the scent of jasmine. Peacocks call from giant trees and flocks of parrots fill the sky. In one garden, it's said, the Krishna lila continues: each night he comes after dusk, and anyone who remains there will go mad. Even the monkeys depart this garden at sunset.

The Radha Krishna devotees embrace blissful surrender to the divine lover—asceticism is not their path. However, today Vrindaban has become a center for sadhus. Several famous saints of this century also have ashrams in Vrindaban. The following are some places of special interest:

Neem Karoli Baba Ashram is located on the parikrama path before it intersects the main road. The ashram's principal temple is to Hanuman, but the ashram complex also includes temples to Sita Ram and

Durga and the samadhi shrine of Neem Karoli Baba, or Maharaji, the guru made famous by Ram Dass in *Be Here Now* (see p. 327). Maharaji's room is also open for devotees to sit, chant, or contemplate. Everyone is welcome to visit and encouraged to take meals at the ashram and attend the evening arati. Westerners often live there during winter months. Accommodations are available either at the ashram or at the Goenka guest house next door, upon request.

Ramakrishna Mission, with its landscaped lawns and flower gardens, is on the main road. Morning and evening worship is directed to the images of Ramakrishna and his wife, Sarada Devi (see p. 386). This ashram runs a hospital and has developed an extensive horticulture outreach program in conjunction with the World Wildlife Federation.

Ananda Mayee Ma Ashram, also on the main road, has undergone little or no change since the beloved woman saint from Bengal lived in this peaceful compound. Bengali devotees worship the image of Krishna in the temple.

Jai Singh Ghera is an ashram beyond the bazaar toward the river. Due to the dedicated efforts of its director, Srivatsa Goswami, Jai Singh Ghera has become the center for an environmental project called "Friends of Vrindaban." Committed to protecting and preserving Vrindaban's fragile natural resources, this grassroots effort has introduced extensive tree planting, a project to clean the Yamuna River, and environmental education in local schools.

Deoria Baba Ashram stands apart on the opposite bank of the Yamuna River and may be reached by boat or (during the dry season) bridge. The samadhi shrine of the famous sadhu is built beside his traditional grass hut. His two senior disciples speak some English and give informal teachings that have attracted Western visitors. Accommodations are not available.

Katyayani Peeth Mandir, just beyond the main post office, is a temple where the goddess Sati, Shiva's consort, is worshipped in the ancient form of Katyayani. According to the famous story of Krishna's tryst with the gopis, the young women invoked her blessing in order to secure their union with the god.

—SITA SHARAN

tanya. The consumnate bhakti yogi, Chaitanya taught that the path to God was through the heart and encouraged his followers to worship Krishna through ecstatic trance, poetry, and song. According to Swami Prabhupada, his own guru was a direct descendant in the line of Vaishnavite gurus initiated by Chaitanya.

Dismayed by what he saw as India's drift away from traditional devotional values toward the lure of the materialistic West, Swami Prabhupada became convinced that the way to set India back on the path to God was to persuade Westerners to walk that path. Offered free passage by a devotee who ran a shipping firm, he took his message to the United States, where "Krishna Consciousness" captured the imagination of the blossoming counterculture. When he was featured alongside the Grateful Dead at a rock concert in Golden Gate Park, the swami was on his way to spiritual superstardom. Tens of thousands of young people—including George Harrison—became his devotees, captivated by the idea of chanting and dancing their way to a permanent high.

He went on to write more than sixty volumes of translation and commentaries on the religious and philosophical classics of India and build ISKCON into a worldwide confederation of over a hundred ashrams, farms, schools, and temples before his death in 1977. Attracting new members is still a major goal of devotees, and the Vrindaban ashram is no exception. On the other hand, if you don't mind a little proseltyzing, the ongoing chanting and devotional atmosphere can definitely bliss you out. There's really no reigning guru at ISKCON—instead, there's a governing board that makes administrative decisions and fifty to sixty senior swamis who are authorized to give initiation to new disciples. Many of the senior swamis joined as former hippies in the 1960s and 1970s, making them a fairly youthful group. Devotees are about half Western and half Indian. The ashram offers regular courses in Vedic literature, ayurveda, and related topics—courses range from four weeks to six months.

Facilities and Food

The ISKCON guest house has about forty-five private rooms with attached bath and one twenty-bed dormitory. Bedding is provided. If the guest house is full, they will arrange lodging with other local guest houses. The vegetarian restaurant is run on a cash basis.

The temples and shrines are exquisitely worked marble, with statues covered in gold leaf—it's said that the intent was to surpass the Taj Mahal. The meditation hall—which is used for chanting, not silent meditation—can hold up to five hundred people. Other facilities include classrooms, a museum, and housing for renunciates. ISKCON also runs a boarding school for children of devotees from all over the world. The ashram has farmland about half a kilometer away, with vegetable gardens and a dairy that supplies milk for the ashram.

The other main center of the Hare Krishnas in India is the world headquarters, just outside of Calcutta. Up to 5,000 people can stay there, and there's a bus day tour of the ashram from Calcutta. The address is Shree Mayapur Chandrodaya Mandir, P.O. Shree Mayapur Dham, District Nadia, Mayapur, West Bengal.

Fees

The guest house costs Rs 200 to 600 for a private room with bath. A full lunch or dinner runs about Rs 40 to 50.

Lifetime membership in ISKCON costs Rs 9,999 in India (in the United States it's $1,111).

Schedule

The temple schedule basically consists of round-the-clock chanting, dancing, and worship. Contact ISKCON for more information about course schedules.

Contact Information

ISKCON
RAMAN RETI
VRINDABAN
MATHURA DIST. 281 124
UTTAR PRADESH
TEL: 91-5664-82478

U.S. Contact:
ISKCON
3764 WATSEKA AVENUE

Los Angeles, CA 90034
Tel: (310) 836-2676
Fax: (310) 839-2715

How to Get There

From Delhi take the train or bus to Mathura (141 kilometers). From Mathura it's 10 kilometers to Vrindaban by autorickshaw, taxi, bus, or steam train. Once in Vrindaban, ask directions to the ashram.

Other Services

Vrindaban has most services available. Mathura, which is 10 kilometers away, has additional choices for food and lodging.

Books and Tapes

Books and tapes in fifty languages are available through the ashram, the 300 centers worldwide, or the Krishna Culture Vedic Resources Catalog: P.O. Box 926337, Houston, TX 77292; Tel: (800) 829-2579. A good introduction is *The Science of Self-Realization*.

My dear Lord Krishna, You are so kind upon this useless soul, but I do not know why You have brought me here. Now You can do whatever You like with me.

But I guess You have some business here, otherwise why would You bring me to this terrible place?

Most of the population here is covered by the material modes of ignorance and passion. Absorbed in material life, they think themselves very happy and satisfied, and therefore they have no taste for the transcendental message of Vasudeva. I do not know how they will be able to understand it.

But I know Your causeless mercy can make everything possible, because You are the most expert mystic...

Oh Lord, I am just like a puppet in Your hands. So if you have

brought me here to dance, then make me dance, make me dance.
Oh Lord, make me dance as you like.

—SWAMI PRABHUPADA,

upon first arriving in the United States

(from *Science of Self-Realization*)

PILGRIMAGE SITES IN *Uttar Pradesh*

 Allahabad. The city of Allahabad is one of the best places to take a sacred dip, where the holy Ganges, Yamuna, and (invisible) Saraswati rivers converge. One of the most important pilgrimage places in India, it is the site, every twelve years, of the Kumbh Mela, when over twelve million Hindus come to bathe (p. 58).

Allahabad has many interesting temples, including the Patalpuri Temple, home of a tree said to never die, even when the entire world is destroyed. Allahabad can be reached by train or bus. There is plenty of lodging in all price ranges.

 Chitrakut. Located about 130 kilometers from Allahabad near the border with Madhya Pradesh, Chitrakut (literally, "bright peak") is a site made sacred by the god and goddess Rama and Sita, who lived here for eleven years of their fourteen years in exile. It's a town that attracts few foreign visitors, although busloads of Indian pilgrims arrive every day to visit its more than thirteen temples and circumambulate the forested hill where Rama is said to have lived. The Madhya Pradesh Tourist Bungalow offers a brochure in English about the various sites in the area. Chitrakut can be reached by bus or train. The closest train station is Chitrakut Dhama Karvi on the Jhansi-Manikpur main line.

 Badrinath. This important pilgrimage site is one of the "Char Dhama"—four sacred shrines—located deep in the beauty of the Garhwal Himalayas. According to one ancient muni, "even if a person who is full of sins happens to get a holy sight of Shri Badrinathji, he becomes free of worldly bondage and secures a seat in Heaven." The ancient shrine sits on the banks of the Alaknanda River, one of the tributaries to the

Ganges. Some say the shrine is as old as the Vedas; it was a Buddhist sacred site for centuries, and was then reclaimed for Hinduism by the sage Shankaracharya, who made a pilgrimage there in the ninth century A.D.

The site is snowbound much of the year; the temple generally opens between the last week of April and the first week of May and closes sometime in October. Plenty of cheap, basic lodging is available. Buses run directly from Haridwar and Rishikesh to Badrinath. If you're interested in a foot pilgrimage, it's possible to trek (from May through September) from Badrinath to the other three sacred shrines of Gangotri, Yamunotri, and Kedarnath. Trekking information and guides are available through tourist agencies in Rishikesh.

🌀 **Kedarnath.** Forty-two kilometers from Badrinath, Kedarnath is the second of the Char Dhama and one of the twelve most sacred places to worship Shiva. According to the Mahabharata, the five Pandava brothers pursued Shiva to the Himalayas after their great clan war to be absolved of the sin of killing their cousins. Unwilling to give them his darshan, Shiva disguised himself as a bull; however, one brother identified him and caught hold of his hump. Pleased with the brothers' determination, Shiva granted them absolution and decreed that his hump be worshipped here in the temple of Shri Kedarnath.

The simple stone shrine sits at 11,500 feet, facing the Mandakini valley against a backdrop of Himalayan peaks. It's generally open from late April or early May to October.

To get to Kedarnath, you have to walk 14 kilometers from Gaurikund, the nearest town. (You can stay overnight, if you wish, at the halfway point at Rambara.) Once there, there are a number of basic lodges where you can stay. Gaurikund can be reached by bus from Badrinath, Haridwar, or Rishikesh.

🌀 **Gangotri and Gomukh.** The third of the Char Dhama, a temple to the goddess Ganga sits beside the Bhagirathi River (which later joins the Alaknanda to become the Ganges) to mark the place where King Bhagirathi did penances for eons to convince the gods to send the goddess Ganga from heaven to earth. Pleased with Bhagirathi's penances, Shiva released the river Ganga from his matted hair, and she descended in a torrent to the earth.

Centuries ago, the Gangotri temple at about 10,500 feet marked the glacial source of the Ganges; now, the glacier has retreated, and the actual origin is a 19 kilometer hike—and 3,000-foot climb—further into the mountains at Gomukh, "the cow's mouth." In ideal weather, it can be done as a day hike, but it's more fun to bring gear and camp at the Chirbasa campground halfway there. The trails to Gomukh will be packed with day-hikers in season; however, serious trekkers can find solitude—and stunning scenery—in the mountains beyond.

A dip in the Ganges at Gangotri or Gomukh is said to be especially potent. The temple generally opens sometime in early May; however, depending on the snows, the path to Gomukh may not be clear until later. There's plenty of cheap, basic lodging at Gangotri; in the high season, be prepared for mobs. Buses run to Gangotri from Haridwar and Rishikesh; the trip takes about twelve hours but can be broken, if you choose, in Uttar Kashi.

Yamunotri. The fourth of the Char Dhama, the Yamunotri temple honors the origin of the Yamuna River. It sits on the riverbanks at 10,000 feet, near a hot spring spurting boiling water hot enough for pilgrims to cook their food in. It's traditional to tie some rice or potatoes loosely in a cloth, dip it in the water, and take it home as prasad (blessed food) when it is cooked. You can also take a holy dip in the nearby Jamuna Bai Kund, which is pleasantly warm.

The temple opens between the last week of April and the first week of May, and closes in the fall on the sacred holiday of Diwali. Cheap, basic lodging and food are available in season.

To get to Yamunotri, you have to walk 14 kilometers uphill from the end of the road at the town of Hanuman Chatti. The climb is steep with spectacular views, but don't carry too much on your back. It's also possible to be carried up in a palanquin or on the back of a pony.

Buses run to Hanuman Chatti from Rishikesh and Haridwar.

—Lea Terhune

Lokenath Divine Life Mission
Calcutta, West Bengal

❧ *Swami Shuddhananda (1949–)*

The *Miami Herald* once described Swami Shuddhananda as "a male counterpart of Mother Teresa—with a twist." If you're interested in doing service work in Calcutta, there are plenty of opportunities through his Calcutta-based Lokenath Divine Life Mission, whose activities range from street schools for homeless children to free hearse services for slum residents.

Teachers and Teachings

Unlike Mother Teresa, says Swami Shuddhananda, "We don't want to bring religion into service. We want to inspire the god within each person to take care of themselves and do service which helps people realize their infinite potential." The LDLM emphasizes education rather than charity: "If you fill someone's begging bowl, fifty years later they will be standing there with fifty children behind them." The group sponsors schools, medical services, handloom industries, fisheries, and many other social and economic programs in 140 poor villages in West Bengal. They also work with local banks and government agencies to develop credit and technical assistance for village groups and entrepreneurs.

Virtually no money goes into facilities and equipment. Rather, in their "street schools," they fund one teacher for every thirty-five children—the teacher then finds space for a school, whether under a tree, in a shed, or in a vacant lot. For sheer inspiration, it's well worth a visit to one of these schools, which teach hygiene, manners, reading, writing, and nonsectarian prayer.

A former business professor at a Hyderabad University, Swami Shuddhananda met his guru at the age of sixteen, and eventually resigned from the college to be with him full time in his ashram in South Calcutta. "I knew I couldn't continue teaching at the university and at the same time continue my deep longing for the truth," Shuddhananda says.

After a series of spiritual visions—in which, he says, he was visited by the great nineteenth-century saint Baba Lokenath, who gave him instructions to spread his teachings worldwide—he moved out of the ashram to wander the Himalayas for several years. In 1987 he launched the LDLM ashram, followed by his first social project, a clinic in the Calcutta slums. A personable man who speaks excellent English, he regularly tours the United States and Europe giving spiritual teachings and presentations on his service work.

Westerner volunteers can serve in a variety of projects, including the mobile clinic and the hearses that take bodies to the burning ghats. You can also participate in the ashram's daily schedule of meditation, pujas, and discourses.

Facilities and Food

The LDLM does charitable work on a very small budget, partly by not investing in buildings or other facilities. There are no residential or dining facilities at the ashram, which consists of a one-room temple on the second floor of a residential building in Calcutta. Several hotels and many restaurants are available within a few minutes' walk.

Schedule

Volunteers are welcome (but not obligated) to participate in the daily schedule at the ashram. You can also visit the ashram without volunteering. There's meditation and puja from 8 to 11 A.M. and 4:40 to 6:30 P.M., followed by bhajans or a discourse from 6:30 to 7 P.M. Swami Shuddhananda gives satsang on Thursday evening from 6:30 to 7:30 and Sunday evening from 7 to 7:30. Satsang is generally in Bengali, but if Westerners are visiting he will repeat significant portions in English.

Fees

Donation. (A donation to this group gets a lot of work done.)

Contact Information

Lokenath Divine Life Mission
P-591 Purna Das Road
Calcutta 700 029
West Bengal
Tel: 91-33-464-3570
Fax: 91-33-464-1587

U.S. Contact:
Lokenath Divine Life Fellowship
Mr. Paul Juneja
211 Gunther Lane
Belle Chasse, LA 70037
Tel: (504) 393-9455
Fax: (504) 433-1406

How to Get There

The ashram headquarters is in the Gol Park area at the southern end of Calcutta.

Other Services

All services are available in Calcutta.

Books and Tapes

A biography of Baba Lokenath by Swami Shuddhananda is available at the ashram.

I never practice anything very difficult. I always thought God is simple and I should reach Him in a path that is simple, humble, and innocent surrender.

—Swami Shuddhananda Brahmachari

Missionaries of Charity
Calcutta, West Bengal

Mother Teresa (1910–1997)

"One cannot say, 'Love God, not your neighbor,' " the Catholic nun Mother Teresa said in her Nobel Peace Prize acceptance speech. "How can we love the God whom we do not see if we do not love our fellow human being whom we do see? Whom we can touch? With whom we live?" For almost half a century, Mother Teresa's Missionaries of Charity order has been serving the "poorest of the poor" in the Calcutta slums. Volunteers are welcome to join in their efforts, which the nuns perform not as social work, but as "an expression of our love for Christ."

Teachers and Teachings

We can't do great things, Mother Teresa liked to say; only small things with great love. Mother Teresa died in 1997, but the Missionaries of Charity continue her work in Calcutta.

As a volunteer with the Missionaries of Charity, you'll be put to work immediately—serving meals, scrubbing floors, changing bedpans, picking maggots out of festering flesh. You'll be assigned to one of several different facilities, such as the home for the dying at Kalighat, the leprosy center, the children's home, or the home for TB sufferers and the mentally handicapped. Although a long-term commitment is appreciated, the nuns will work with whatever they get—if you only drop in for a couple of days, they'll find a way to make you useful.

"Volunteers who come and work with us must have an open mind and be available for any work, because that is how God wants everyone to be," said one nun who works with volunteers. You'll get your training on the job, in the moment. What's most important is not what you do, but that you do it with love. As Mother Teresa said when asked what her sisters offered the dying, "First of all we want to make them feel that they are wanted, we want them to know that there are people who really love them, who really want them, at least for the few hours that they have to live, to know human and divine love."

Born in Albania as Agnes Bojaxhiu, Mother Teresa went to India as a missionary nun at the age of nineteen and spent nearly twenty years teaching in a convent school. In 1946, she says, while on a train to Darjeeling, she heard the voice of God. "The message was clear: I must leave the convent to help the poor by going to live among them."

With the permission of the Pope, she left the convent, exchanged her robes for a white sari with a blue border, and went to live in the Calcutta slums, where she began her work by caring for one dying person she found on the streets. Today, her Missionaries of Charity—a religious order that she formed in 1950 with the blessing of the Vatican—has more than four thousand brothers and sisters worldwide. In addition to the usual vows of poverty, chastity, and obedience, Missionaries of Charity make a fourth vow: "service to the poorest of the poor." Writes Mother Teresa, "The more repugnant the work, or the more disfigured or deformed the image of God in the person, the greater will be our faith and loving devotion in seeking the face of Jesus, and lovingly ministering to him in the distressing disguise."

There are usually a couple of dozen Western volunteers at the Calcutta centers, ranging from dedicated Catholics—not surprisingly, you'll find a lot of Irish volunteers—to the merely curious. If you want to volunteer, go first to the Mother House, where you'll be assigned a place to work based on your preferences and skills and the needs of the moment. The whole operation is extremely well organized and efficient. If you're not comfortable working directly with patients, you can request to help out in the kitchen or the laundry instead.

The work can be intense—with no previous experience, you'll find yourself helping to clean a wound or carry a paralyzed woman to the bath. But volunteers report that it's transformational. "All you have to have is a willingness to help," reflects one volunteer. "That is one of the things about Mother's work—to let people come in contact with the poor. It's as much for our sake as for theirs. We've crossed this enormous divide, you know—it's not just these 'millions' of people, but somebody you've actually touched."

Facilities and Food

The administrative offices are in the Mother House, where the nuns live. Projects of the Missionaries of Charity include schools, clinics, shelters, and homes for lepers, the dying, the handicapped, and sick or abandoned children. It's possible to visit the Children's Home (a few minutes from the Mother House on Lower Circular Road) or the Home for Dying Destitutes (about half an hour away by taxi).

Many volunteers stay at the Salvation Army on Sudder Street or in other cheap hotels in the Sudder Street area. The Mother House distributes a list of inexpensive accommodations, including the Paragon Hotel (2 Stuart Lane), the Modern Lodge (1 Stuart Lane), the YWCA (1 Middle Row), and the Astoria Board (6/2 and 6/3 Sudder Street).

Breakfast for volunteers is available at the Mother House.

Schedule

Volunteers are welcome but not required to join in the daily prayer and Mass at the Mother House. Prayers are at 6 A.M. and 6 P.M. The volunteer work is divided into morning and afternoon shifts; you can work either or both, for as many or few days as you would like.

Fees

None.

Contact Information

MISSIONARIES OF CHARITY
54 A.J.C. BOSE ROAD
CALCUTTA 700 016
WEST BENGAL
TEL: 91-33-2447115

U.S. Contact:
MISSIONARIES OF CHARITY
335 EAST 145TH STREET
BRONX, NY 10451
TEL: (718) 292-0019

How to Get There

The Mother House can be reached by taxi, bus, or autorickshaw.

All services are available in Calcutta.

Books, Tapes, and Affiliated Centers

Books and tapes about the work of Mother Teresa and the Missionaries of Charity are available in most spiritual bookstores. The Missionaries of Charity have facilities all over India that may need volunteers.

In twenty-five years we have picked up more than 36,000 people from the streets and more than 18,000 have died a most beautiful death. . . . A few nights ago we picked up four people. One was in a most terrible condition, covered with wounds, her body full of maggots. I told the sisters that I would take care of her while they attended to the other three. I really did all that my love could do for her. I put her in bed and then she took hold of my hand. She had such a beautiful smile on her face and she said only: "Thank you." Then she died. There was a greatness of love. She was hungry for love, and she received that love before she died. She spoke only two words, but her understanding love was expressed in those two words. I have never seen a smile like that.

—MOTHER TERESA
(from *Total Surrender*)

Ramakrishna Math and Mission
Calcutta, West Bengal

🌀 *Sri Ramakrishna (1836–1886)*
🌀 *Swami Vivekananda (1863–1902)*

As a young priest at a Kali temple just north of Calcutta, Sri Ramakrishna so alarmed temple authorities with his frenzies of devotion to the Divine Mother that they relieved him of his duties and sent him home to be married, hoping that matrimony would cure him of his delusions. By the end of his life, however, this goddess-intoxicated mystic was widely acclaimed as an avatar, a human incarnation of God; and after his death, his teachings were spread worldwide by his leading disciple, Swami Vivekananda, the first emissary of Vedanta philosophy to the United States. Vivekananda was the founder of the Ramakrishna Mission, a worldwide institution whose centers in Calcutta offer the chance to study the life and teachings of the master in the city where he spent most of his life.

Teachers and Teachings

The Ramakrishna Mission actually has two Calcutta facilities that are open to visitors. The monastery known as Belur Math, the headquarters of the Ramakrishna Order of monks, sits on the banks of the Ganges across the river from the Ramakrishna's beloved Kali temple at Dakshineswar. The Institute of Culture is an enormous cultural and educational complex in the southern part of the city. (There's also a nunnery called Sarada Math, but it's virtually closed to foreign guests.) The monastery is quieter and more oriented toward spiritual practice; its guest house is primarily intended for devotees already affiliated with the Ramakrishna Order and its Vedanta Society, although other sincere seekers can sometimes be accommodated if you write to get permission in advance. (Anyone can visit for the day, however, and a steady stream of devotees pays homage to the shrines of Ramakrishna, his wife Sarada Devi, and Vivekananda.) The Institute of Culture, which is open to the general public, has a more academic and artistic flavor; it's the place to go if you want to do serious research (they have an excellent library) or attend lectures and seminars on Ramakrishna's life and Vedantic teachings, as well as other religious and cultural topics.

For many pilgrims, though, these centers are just a base camp from which to visit the Kali temple at Dakshineswar, where Ramakrishna spent thirty years in spiritual ecstasy (see sidebar on Kali temple, p. 384). Ramakrishna's mystical tendencies became apparent in childhood—it's said that while playing the role of Shiva in a school play, he fell into a spontaneous trance so unshakeable that the performance had to be stopped. At age sixteen, he went to Calcutta and trained as a Brahmin priest, eventually taking charge of the newly built Dakshineswar temple. Consumed with

Daksineshwar Kali Temple and
Other Ramakrishna Pilgrimage Sites

The Dakshineshwar Kali Temple, where Ramakrishna spent thirty years worshipping and teaching, sits on the eastern bank of the Ganges about four miles north of Calcutta. The image of Ma Kali in the temple is a young, beautiful girl full of charm and joy—even though she holds a sword and a bloody demon's head in her hands. Her name is "Ma Bhavatirini," Savior of the World.

Not much has changed since the days of Sri Ramakrishna—although the temple (built in 1855) is beginning to show its age, worship continues in a similar fashion. In the Hindu ritual, Kali is treated as an honored and beloved relative. She gets awakened at 4:30 A.M., bathed, clothed, and decorated with flowers. The morning puja starts around 9:30 A.M. The priest performs purification mantras and mudras, chants hymns to glorify the goddess, and offers light, incense, water, clothes, food, and fans. Cooked food is offered around 12:30 P.M. Arati (evening fire ceremony) is around 6 or 6:30 P.M., depending on the season. Once a month, priests perform a special amavasya (dark night of the moon) puja. During this puja, a he-goat gets worshipped and beheaded; then its meat is cooked, offered to Kali, and distributed among devotees as prasad.

Pilgrims sometimes stand in line for hours to catch a moment's glimpse of Kali. In their passionate devotion they'll cry, laugh, sing, shout, and—most of all—push you in an attempt to see Ma faster. Tuesdays and Saturdays are dedicated to Mother worship and are especially crowded and boisterous—the temple does have ushers trained in crowd control, but if mobs make you nervous, you'd be better off visiting on some other day.

The Dakshineswar Kali Temple is accessed via road or river. For a special treat, you can rent a country boat and arrive at the temple's bathing ghat where Sri Sarada Devi, Sri Ramakrishna's wife, used to bathe. But most people arrive by bus or car for convenience. A parking lot within the temple compound charges a nominal fee. Shoes are not allowed in the temple, so it's a good idea to leave them in the car or deposit them with a shopkeeper in one of the little stalls that line the road leading to the temple.

No official guided tours are sponsored by the temple, so you'll have to fend for yourself. It's customary to first bow to the Divine Mother Kali before visiting the other shrines. Most pilgrims purchase a "puja basket" from one of the many stalls, which usually contains sweets, flowers (hibiscus garland a must), and incense. Taking this basket to the inner shrine of Kali, the pilgrim hands it to a priest who then, muttering some mantras, offers it to the Great Mother Goddess and returns a portion to the pilgrim as prasad. This is considered a great blessing. Adjacent to the Kali temple is the Vishnu temple, where you can make a similar offering. If you have time, you can visit all twelve Shiva temples and even pour Ganges water over each of the Shiva lingams.

In the northwestern corner of the temple compound is the room where Sri Ramakrishna lived for fifteen years. Though the room is often very crowded, you can usually find a corner to meditate. North of Sri Ramakrishna's room is the Nahabat where Sri Sarada Devi lived, and further north are the Panchavati and Panchamundi areas where Sri Ramakrishna practiced tantra and had many visions.

All the shrines in Dakshineswar have large offering boxes, but if you want to do something more elaborate, you can talk to temple employees in the office and pay for a puja in the Kali temple. If time permits, you can also visit another Kali temple in the village of Dakshineswar named Adyapith. Though smaller and less famous, this temple has its own following. Almost adjacent to the Adyapith Kali temple is Sarada Math, the convent of the Ramakrishna Order. Also nearby is the beautiful ashram of Paramahansa Yogananda (p. 390).

Devotees of Sri Ramakrishna may want to spend some time in north Calcutta and visit the places Sri Ramakrishna frequented, such as the house of Balaram Bose, a beloved householder disciple whom Ramakrishna used to visit regularly. The room that is today the shrine room was the room used for kirtan and entertainment. The swamis of the Ramakrishna Order, which owns the house today, will permit you to sit and meditate on the same floor where Sri Ramakrishna and his disciples danced in ecstasy.

The house where Sri Sarada Devi lived is also in the same area. A short drive away are Swami Vivekananda's birth home and the house belonging to M, the schoolmaster who wrote the famous *Gospel of Sri* passion for Kali, he began desperately praying to receive a vision of her—he took to meditating naked in the nearby burial grounds, beating his head on the ground, weeping in longing for the Mother of the Universe.

His intimate love for the Kali image in his temple resulted in most unorthodox behavior. Recounted his nephew, "I saw how Uncle's chest and eyes were always red, like those of a drunkard. He'd get up reeling from the worshipper's seat, climb onto the altar, and caress the Divine Mother, chucking her affectionately under the chin. He'd begin singing, laughing, joking, and talking with her, or sometimes he'd catch hold of her hands and dance." Soon he ceased to attend to the external image at all, feeling the Divine Mother present with him always; sometimes he would decorate his own body with flowers and sandalwood, as if confusing it with the idol.

Appalled, the temple authorities sent him home to be married. However, the marriage—to a six-year-old girl named Sarada—was never consummated; Ramakrishna believed Sarada to be an incarnation of the Divine Mother, and worshipped her as such. (Later in life, Sarada Devi herself attracted hundreds of devotees, who addressed her as "Holy Mother.") He soon returned to Dakshineswar, where he walked a variety of paths to ecstasy. He learned tantric disciplines with a woman ascetic, who was both his devotee and his mentor. He dressed as a woman so he could become swept away by desire for Krishna. Finally, he was initiated into sannyas by a Naga sadhu, who taught him to meditate on the formless Absolute. Ramakrishna spent six months oblivious to the world, in the state called "nirvikalpa samadhi," in which all traces of individual identity are erased and the meditator experiences himself as one with the Absolute. Returning to consciousness at the calling of Kali, he lived the rest of his life immersed in the knowledge that the world and its phenomena were simply waves emanating from the Cosmic Mind.

"The nameless, formless Reality, the transcendent awareness in which you are now permanently awake, is precisely the same Reality that you perceive blossoming around you," he told a sadhu who came to him for instruction. "The perfectly peaceful Absolute is not different from the playful relative universe."

This was the vision brought to the West by Swami Vivekananda, Ramakrishna's spiritual heir, who electrified audiences at the World Parliament of Religions in Chicago in 1893. Vivekananda traveled throughout the United States and Europe preaching Ramakrishna's Vedantic vision, which held that all religions led to the same goal and that Jesus, Allah, Buddha, and Kali were merely different aspects of one Reality.

Today, the Ramakrishna Order has two branches: the Ramakrishna Math, or monastery, and the Ramakrishna Mission, which is mainly devoted to philanthropic activities. Vedanta Societies in the West are also part of the Ramakrishna Order. Like most large spiritual groups, it has become somewhat institutionalized; don't expect a lot of personal attention, especially at the Institute of Culture. At the more contemplative Belur Math, you can seek out swamis to give you instruction. But the best way to get a direct experience of Ramakrishna's energy is to visit the Kali temple in Dakshineswar; Ramakrishna's birthplace in the village of Kamapukar; or one of the other sites associated with his life around Calcutta (see sidebar p. 384).

Facilities and Food

Belur Math is a leafy, beautifully maintained monastery and temple complex on the banks of the Ganges. The ashes of Ramakrishna, Sarada Devi, and Swami Vivekananda are enshrined here; you can also visit the building where Vivekananda lived and died, which contains relics such as his bed, sandals, and turban.

There's a comfortable guest house with about twenty rooms with attached Western-style bathrooms. The guest house is for members of the various Vedanta societies and for devotees of Sri Ramakrishna. Others may stay up to two days if they write ahead of time.

The Institute of Culture is a four-story U-shaped building around a central courtyard with manicured lawns and flower gardens. Guests are housed in about sixty semiprivate guest rooms with attached bath. Cultural and educational facilities include a school of world religions, a school of foreign and Indian languages, concert and lecture halls, a theater, an excellent library, an art gallery, a small museum, and a children's art school. Food is available in a Western-style dining room.

Schedule

Belur Math maintains a regular schedule of meditation and puja, which guests can participate in as they please. Guests can make day trips outside the monastery but are requested not to leave the premises in the evenings.

The Institute of Culture is open from 10 A.M. to 8 P.M. all working days. Lectures—in English and Bengali, on topics such as the Gospel of Ramakrishna, the Upanishads, and other aspects of Indian philosophy—are generally held in the afternoon from 5:30 to 7:30 P.M. In addition, there's an ongoing schedule of performances in music, dance, and theater.

Fees

Staying at Belur Math is by donation only.

At the Institute, accommodations and meals in the Scholar's House (for long-term residents) cost Rs 290 per day for single occupancy and Rs 400 for double. In the Guest House, which has more space and air-conditioning, the charges are from Rs 460 for one person to Rs 660 for two people, including meals.

Contact Information

BELUR MATH:
SWAMI ATMASTHANANDA, GENERAL SECRETARY
RAMAKRISHNA MISSION
P.O. BELUR MATH, 211202
DIST. HOWRAH, WEST BENGAL
TEL: 91-33-654-1146, 1180, 1144, 5391, 9581, 9681
FAX: 91-33-654-4346

INSTITUTE OF CULTURE:
All correspondence
Attn: SWAMI LOKESWARANANDA, SECRETARY
RAMAKRISHNA MISSION INSTITUTE OF CULTURE
GOL PARK
CALCUTTA 700 029
TEL: 91-33-74-1303, 1304, 1305
FAX: 91-33-74-1307

RAMAKRISHNA MISSION INSTITUTE OF CULTURE
ADVAITA ASHRAMA
5 DEHI ENTALLY ROAD
CALCUTTA 700 014
WEST BENGAL
TEL: 91-33-440898
FAX: 91-33-2450050

U.S. Contact:
SWAMI PRABUDDHANANDA
VEDANTA SOCIETY OF NORTHERN CALIF.
2323 VALLEJO STREET
SAN FRANCISCO, CA 94123
TEL: (415) 922-2323

How to Get There

The Ramakrishna Mission Institute of Culture is located in the southern part of Calcutta and can be reached by bus, autorickshaw, or taxi. If in doubt, telephone for directions.

Belur Math is across the river from Calcutta on the western bank of the Ganges. It's about 8 kilometers from the Howrah train station, but gridlock can make getting there a nightmare; it's best to take an autorickshaw to maneuver through the traffic. From Belur Math you can take a boat across the river to Dakshineswar, or go by bus, which takes 10 or 15 minutes.

Other Services

Calcutta has a population of approximately 10 million. All services are available.

Books and Tapes

A good introduction to Ramakrishna's life and teachings is *Ramakrishna and His Disciples* by Christopher Isherwood (Vedanta Press). A wide assortment of books and tapes is available from Vedanta Society centers around the world.

What do I care for sophisticated philosophical arguments about the irreality of the world? You alone are manifest through all phenomena, O Mother. Even Shiva, sheer transcendent Knowledge, when awakening from the peaceful trance of Great Yoga, arises and dances powerfully, crying KALI KALI KALI.

—SRI RAMAKRISHNA

(from *Great Swan*, by Lex Hixon)

Yogoda Satsanga Society of India (Self-Realization Fellowship) Dakshineswar, Calcutta, West Bengal

Paramahamsa Yogananda (1893–1952)

First published in the 1940s, Paramahansa Yogananda's now classic *Autobiography of a Yogi* introduced a whole generation of Westerners to the esoteric science of kriya yoga, a system of breathing exercises and visualizations that's claimed to accelerate a million-fold the process of spiritual evolution. The Yogoda Satsanga Society is the Indian wing of the Self-Realization Fellowship, the worldwide organization founded by Yogananda. Yogoda Satsanga's original—and largest—ashram is actually in

Ranchi, Bihar, but it's not really set up to accommodate foreigners—it's primarily a training facility for Indian male renunciates (although you can attend the morning and evening meditations). However, foreign guests—with the exception of women traveling alone—are welcome at the smaller, somewhat sleepy ashram in Dakshineswar.

Teachers and Teachings

Aside from the Sunday satsang led by a resident swami, there's not a whole lot happening at the Dakshineswar ashram. But it's a lovely place to pursue your own sadhana, with quiet grounds on the banks of the Ganges and stately old buildings dating from the 1870s. For those sincerely interested in Yogananda's teachings, resources are available—you just have to be prepared to take charge of your own education.

One of the first Indian teachers to bring yoga to the West, Paramahansa Yogananda taught a system he called kriya yoga, which had been passed down to him through three generations of gurus from the elusive master Babaji, who rediscovered this long-hidden technique. (Babaji, whose mastery of kriya yoga has purportedly granted him physical immortality, is said to still be alive in a remote Himalayan cave.) As Yogananda himself described it in *Autobiography of a Yogi*, kriya yoga is "a simple, psychophysiological method by which human blood is decarbonated and recharged with oxygen. The atoms of this extra oxygen are transmuted into life current to rejuvenate the brain and spinal centers. By stopping the accumulation of venous blood, the yogi is able to lessen or prevent the decay of tissues. The advanced yogi transmutes his cells into energy."

According to Yogananda, the energy thus generated is capable of accelerating the process of spiritual evolution so that "in three years, a kriya yogi can thus accomplish by intelligent self-effort the same result that Nature brings to pass in a million years." Through gradual practice of kriya techniques, the body becomes fit to handle higher and higher voltages of this energy, and is "finally fitted to express the infinite potentials of cosmic energy, which constitutes the first materially active expression of Spirit."

The specific kriya techniques are not available in written form—they must be taught in person by an authorized kriya yogi. Although there are no formal courses available at the ashram, information may be available through one of the resident swamis.

Facilities and Food

The ashram is primarily a men's facility—women are admitted only if accompanied by another woman or a husband, brother, or father (or a plausible facsimile). The ashram has a guest house with eleven shared rooms, nine with attached bath and two with outside bathrooms. There are about twelve to fifteen permanent residents.

The guest house is primarily intended for members of the SRF and the Yogoda Satsanga. Write ahead well in advance for permission to stay. Your initial visit can be up to three days; to stay longer, you'll need special approval. Outside guests are welcome to attend the daily morning and evening meditations and the Sunday morning satsangs.

Schedule

Daily meditations are held at 6:30 A.M. and 5:30 P.M., except on Sunday, when there is satsang from 10:30 to noon with one of the resident monks. The administrative office is open 9 A.M. to 4 P.M.

Fees

Donation only.

Contact Information

YOGODA SATSANG SOCIETY OF INDIA
YOGODA SATSANGA MATH
21, U.N. MUKHERJEE ROAD
DAKSHINESWAR
CALCUTTA 700 076
WEST BENGAL
TEL: 91-33-553-1931
FAX: 91-33-553-2208 (6:30 A.M. TO 9:30 A.M. ONLY)

U.S. Contact:
SELF-REALIZATION FELLOWSHIP
3880 SAN RAFAEL AVENUE

Los Angeles, CA 90065
Tel: (213) 225-2471

How to Get There

The ashram is 15 kilometers from the center of Calcutta. Take a local train from Sealdah Station to Dakshineswar Station, or a bus to Dakshineswar; then go by autorickshaw to the ashram.

Other Services

All services are available in Calcutta.

Books and Tapes

Books, tapes, and instruction are available through the Self-Realization Fellowship, which has many branches worldwide (see Contact Information). *Autobiography of a Yogi* is available in most spiritual bookstores in India and abroad.

The Northern Himalayan crags near Badrinarayan are still blessed by the living presence of Babaji, guru of Lahiri Mahasaya [the guru of Yogananda's guru]. The secluded master has retained his physical form for centuries, perhaps for millenniums . . .

The deathless guru bears no mark of age on his body; he appears to be a youth of not more than twenty-five. Fair-skinned, of medium build and height, Babaji's beautiful, strong body radiates a perceptible glow. His eyes are dark, calm, and tender; his long, lustrous hair is copper-colored . . .

Swami Kebalananda, my saintly Sanskrit tutor, spent some time with Babaji in the Himalayas.

"The peerless master moves with his group from place to place in the mountains," Kebalananda told me." His small band contains two highly advanced American disciples. After Babaji has been in one locality for some time, he says, 'Dera danda

uthao.' ('Let us lift our camp and staff.') He carries a danda (bamboo staff). His words are the signal for moving with his group instantaneously to another place. He does not always employ this method of astral travel; sometimes he goes on foot from peak to peak . . .

"On [one] occasion Babaji's sacred circle was disturbed by the arrival of a stranger. He had climbed with astonishing skill to the nearly inaccessible ledge near the guru's camp.

" 'Sir, you must be the great Babaji.' The man's face was lit with inexpressible reverence. 'For months I have pursued a ceaseless search for you among these forbidding crags. I implore you to accept me as a disciple.'

"When the great guru made no response, the man pointed to the rock-lined chasm below the ledge. 'If you refuse me, I will jump from this mountain. Life has no further value if I cannot win your guidance to the Divine.'

" 'Jump then,' Babaji said unemotionally. 'I cannot accept you in your present state of development.'

"The man immediately hurled himself over the cliff. Babaji instructed the shocked disciples to fetch the stranger's body. After they had returned with the mangled form, the master placed his hand on the dead man. Lo! he opened his eyes and prostrated himself humbly before the omnipotent guru.

" 'You are now ready for discipleship.' Babaji beamed lovingly on his resurrected chela."

—Paramahansa Yogananda
(from *Autobiography of a Yogi*)

PILGRIMAGE SITES IN *West Bengal and Assam*

Ganga Sagara. Sacred as the place where the Ganges flows into the Bay of Bengal, Ganga Sagara—also called Sagar Island—is south of Calcutta, at the mouth of the Hoogly River. At the time of the winter solstice, hundreds of thousands of Hindus come for a purificatory bath during a three-day festival, hoping to be liberated from rebirth. A road links Calcutta and Diamond Harbor, a resort about 50 kilometers from Calcutta, and ferries run from here to Sagar Island. Lodging is available both at Diamond Harbor and on Sagar Island.

✺ Navadipa.

North of Calcutta on the Hoogly River is Navadipa, an important pilgrimage site for the Vaishnava sect. Chaitanya, a great mystic, considered by some to be an incarnation of Vishnu, was born in the Navadipa area. After receiving a powerful vision of Lord Krishna, he became a devotee, and wandered around the countryside singing and chanting the name of Krishna and striving for ecstatic union with the god. He left no written teachings, but his teachings were transmitted orally by close disciples.

Vaishnavite minstrels called Bauls carry on Chaitanya's tradition. They renounce ordinary lives, even their names, and wander the country singing and dancing to devotional verses. They usually dress in orange robes and turbans, sometimes wearing colored patchwork cloaks. They go in groups on foot, carrying the small hand drums with which they accompany their performances. They may often be seen about the temples at Navadipa, particularly in February, when there is an annual gathering of Bauls.

Navadipa is 114 kilometers north of Calcutta, accessible by road and rail. Across the river from Navadipa is Mayapur, the site of a massive ISKCON (p. 366) center.

✺ Kamakhya.

From West Bengal you can travel by train or air to the state of Assam to visit a major tantric pilgrimage site. About 10 kilometers from Gauhati in the state of Assam, Kamakhya is the site of the Kamakhshi Mandir, the shrine marking the place where the yoni (genitals) of Sati fell as Shiva carried her dead body around India (p. 333). Tantric practitioners are attracted to Kamakhya because it is known throughout India as a power place conducive to magic, mantra, and yogic powers.

Kamakhshi Mandir is situated on Nilachal hill near the Brahmaputra River. You can walk up from the base of the hill to the temple. Inside the shrine is a cave through which the river flows. During the monsoon season the river turns reddish and the Goddess herself is believed to be menstruating—this is the height of the pilgrimage season. There is no image of the Goddess in the temple—instead, she is represented by a stone in the form of a yoni that is kept moist by a natural spring. Male animals are sacrificed and offerings of flowers and leaves are put on the yoni.

Gauhati can be reached by rail, road, or air and has hotels in a variety of price ranges.

—LEA TERHUNE AND JANET CHAWLA

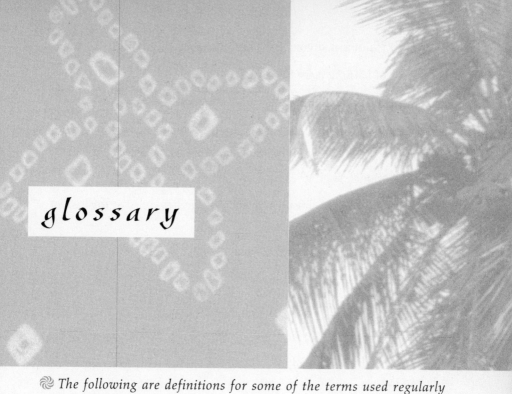

glossary

🌀 *The following are definitions for some of the terms used regularly throughout this guidebook:*

arati (arti, arathi): a Hindu ceremony offering light and fire to a deity

asana: the physical postures associated with the practice of hatha yoga

ashtanga yoga: the eight-limbed path prescribed by Patanjali; also known as raja yoga

Atman: the true Self, the individual soul

avatar: human incarnation of the divine

bhajan: devotional song

bhakti: worship or devotion

brahmacharya: celibacy

Brahman: the Absolute, the cosmic Consciousness

chakra: literally, wheel; an energy center in the body

darshan: the sight or viewing of a guru or deity

dharma: in Hinduism, divine law; the spiritual teachings of the Buddha

ghat: steps or bathing place by a river

japa: repetition of a mantra

hatha yoga: the path of yoga that emphasizes the physical body as a vehicle for awakening

kirtan: devotional singing

kundalini: powerful psychospiritual energy that lies coiled at the base of the spine

lama: a Tibetan Buddhist monk

lingam: the phallic symbol of Shiva

mahasamadhi: the death of a saint

mandir: temple

mantra: a sacred sound used for meditation, traditionally given by a guru to an initiate

math: monastery

mudra: ritual hand gesture used in yoga and meditation to direct energy

nadis: energy circuits throughout the body

prana: the life-force energy

pranayama: the breathing techniques associated with the practice of hatha yoga

prasad: food that has been offered to and blessed by a guru or deity

puja: literally, "respect"; a ritual of worship to a deity

raja yoga: *see* ashtanga yoga

rishi: a seer or sage

sadhana: spiritual practice

sadhu: a wandering ascetic or holy person

samadhi: the blissful union of the individual consciousness with the Absolute; also, a shrine containing the ashes or body of a saint

sannyas: vows of renunciation

sannyasin: a renunciate or ascetic

satsang: gathering where teachings are given by a guru

seva: literally, service; in an ashram, work as a spiritual practice

siddhi: magical powers acquired through the practice of yoga

sutras: spiritual teachings presented in verse form

swami: a Hindu holy man who has taken monastic vows

Vedas: Hindu holy scriptures

Vedanta: literally, the end of the Vedas; the vast body of metaphysical speculation based on the mystical Upanishads, the closing books of the Vedas

vibhuti: sacred ashes

vipassana: a form of insight meditation taught by the Buddha

yatra: pilgrimage

yoga: systematic practices designed to bring about union with the Absolute

index to people, places, and practices

❧ NOTES ❧

❧ NOTES ❧

❧ NOTES ❧

❧ NOTES ❧

❧ NOTES ❧

❧ NOTES ❧

❧ NOTES ❧

❧ NOTES ❧

Anne Cushman is editor-at-large at *Yoga Journal* magazine and a certified yoga teacher. She has a degree in comparative religion from Princeton University, and has written for the *New York Times*, the *San Francisco Chronicle*, and the *Utne Reader*. She is writer-in-residence at the Kripalu Center for yoga and health in Lennox, Massachusetts.

Jerry Jones has led companies in real estate and construction for over thirty-five years. He now devotes equal time to community service, working in prisons, churches, and with gang-affected youth. He has studied in ashrams, monasteries, and meditation centers in India and Asia, and has been practicing meditation and other yogic disciplines for the past twenty years.